T0255332

APHASIA AND KINDRED DISORDERS OF SPEECH

IN TWO VOLUMES
VOLUME I

APHASIA

AND

KINDRED DISORDERS OF SPEECH

BY

HENRY HEAD, M.D., LL.D. Edin., F.R.S.

CONSULTING PHYSICIAN TO THE LONDON HOSPITAL
HONORARY FELLOW OF TRINITY COLLEGE, CAMBRIDGE

VOLUME I

CAMBRIDGE

AT THE UNIVERSITY PRESS

MCMXXVI

CAMBRIDGE
UNIVERSITY PRESS

32 Avenue of the Americas, New York NY 10013-2473, USA

Cambridge University Press is part of the University of Cambridge.

It furthers the University's mission by disseminating knowledge in the pursuit of
education, learning and research at the highest international levels of excellence.

www.cambridge.org
Information on this title: www.cambridge.org/9781107419018

© Cambridge University Press 1926

This publication is in copyright. Subject to statutory exception
and to the provisions of relevant collective licensing agreements,
no reproduction of any part may take place without the written
permission of Cambridge University Press.

First published 1926
First paperback edition 2014

A catalogue record for this publication is available from the British Library

ISBN 978-1-107-41901-8 Paperback

Cambridge University Press has no responsibility for the persistence or accuracy of
URLs for external or third-party internet websites referred to in this publication,
and does not guarantee that any content on such websites is, or will remain, accurate
or appropriate.

To

*The Memory of the three men who have most influenced
my methods of work and thought*

WALTER HOLBROOK GASKELL, M.D., F.R.S.
Fellow of Trinity Hall, Cambridge

EWALD HERING
Professor of Physiology in the German University
of Prague

JOHN HUGHLINGS JACKSON, M.D., F.R.S.
Physician to the London Hospital and to the
National Hospital for the Paralysed
and Epileptic, Queen Square

PREFACE

THE preface to a book of this kind must always partake somewhat of the nature of an epilogue. The toil of composition is over and the author is anxious to explain how he came to undertake his task. Reasons must be given for the mode in which the facts are marshalled and apology made for the shortcomings of their presentation.

It is nearly forty years since my interest was first aroused in the problem of aphasia. After two years spent in physiological research under the guidance of Professor Hering in Prague I had returned to Cambridge to resume the study of medicine. In November 1886 an elderly woman was admitted to Addenbrooke's Hospital with what I should now call nominal aphasia and right hemianopsia unaccompanied by paralysis of any kind. I spent much time and ingenuity in examining her condition and in reading up the literature on the subject. When she died some seven weeks later from a large recent haemorrhage in the right hemisphere, a smaller well-defined lesion was found to occupy the parts beneath the left supra-marginal and angular gyri; this was evidently the cause of her original symptoms. At the request of the physician in charge, I prepared notes for a clinical lecture on the case, in which every symptom presented by the patient was satisfactorily accounted for by destruction of some centre or internuncial path. At that time the subject was dominated by the theories of Bastian and other diagram makers. Lichtheim's paper had just appeared and exerted a profound influence upon the clinical theories of the day. We believed that every sign and symptom could be deduced from a local lesion in some cortical centre or injury to the paths between them.

But when somewhat later I attended demonstrations on classical examples of aphasia, I lost this robust faith. Moreover I could not make my own observations fit the phenomena which should have been present according to the current theories. It was always necessary to invent some special reason to explain why the patient's condition at the moment did not conform exactly to the proper type.

Later, when working out the consequences of lesions of the peripheral nerves, it became obvious that the changes in function did not correspond to any forms that could be deduced from a priori consideration of the phenomena of normal sensation. The morbid manifestations could not be classed as isolated loss of sensibility to touch, pain, heat or cold, and not infrequently comprised a curious over-activity to certain forms of stimulation, in spite of the fact that the threshold was obviously raised.

As we passed on to investigate the result of functional disintegration at higher levels of the nervous system, this want of correspondence between the actual phenomena observed and the forms of sensation determined by introspection became still more evident. For example, a lesion of the cortex produced results which could only be classed under the heading of defective recognition of certain relations between sensory stimuli and the perceptions to which they gave rise.

I therefore determined to investigate the phenomena of aphasia in the light of these conceptions. But the methods of examination in common use were insufficient for this purpose, and from 1910 onwards I slowly built up a series of tests by repeated trials in suitable instances.

By 1914 my experience with these tests was sufficient to permit their application to the remarkable cases of brain injury produced by the war. But this alone would have been insufficient to lead me to the conceptions I now hold had I not read Hughlings Jackson's long forgotten papers on aphasia. These I subsequently reprinted in *Brain* during the early part of 1915 with an introductory preface. For the first time I began to see light in the confused medley of clinical observations, and with each patient I examined by the new methods, I came to understand more clearly Jackson's attitude to the problems of these disorders of speech.

For, although I was in intimate relation with Dr Hughlings Jackson during the later years of his life, he rarely if ever touched on his views concerning disorders of speech. Many were the talks we had together on evolution and dissolution as manifested in the functions of the nervous system, and he would frequently point out to me the bearing of his theories on my observations concerning disorders of sensibility; but he

seemed to have lost heart with regard to his papers on aphasia, in consequence of the complete neglect into which they had fallen. After his
death, when I read them through in order, they came as a revelation, and
not only explained the observations I was making on patients with war
injuries but also indicated the route of further advance. New methods
and a fresh point of view were fruitful in new results.

My observations demanded consecutive presentation in order to bring
out the new principles upon which they were based. I was anxious to bring
forward my conclusions unhampered by constant reference to the work
of others and have therefore prefaced them with a historical account written
on somewhat unusual lines. More than 125 years have elapsed since the
subject of aphasia first aroused attention, and it was impossible to give
a complete or unbiased history of the views propounded at one time or
another concerning its nature and cause. During this period current
philosophy, physiology and psychology have undergone profound modification, and many of these changes have reacted not only on the theories
but also on the clinical observations made under their influence.

These developments are the subject of my historical sketch. I have
selected certain epochs and men as representing some definite aspect of
thought. I have made no attempt to give a consecutive and coherent
account of the ideas held at any one time concerning such groups of
symptoms as for instance alexia, agraphia and the like. Owing to this
personal method of presenting the historical facts, I have been unable to
notice or give due weight to the admirable contributions of many observers whose conceptions tallied with those held by more prominent
protagonists.

Moreover, since I hold definite views of my own this historical introduction cannot be an unprejudiced account, for it is intended to prepare
the way for fresh facts and new theories, and I could not divert the
narrative to deal adequately with hypotheses which have no direct
bearing on my observations. This must of necessity blind me somewhat
to the work of those with whom I am in fundamental disagreement. I
hope that I have done no man any wrong, and beg those of my fellow-
workers who think they have been neglected or misunderstood to pardon
my want of comprehension.

I have attempted to blaze a track through the jungle, but make no pretence at having reached the end of the journey. I can only hope that some ardent and adventurous spirit may follow in my path and find that my labours have helped him to the solution of the profoundly interesting and difficult problems of disorders of speech.

Finally, it is my pleasant duty to thank those who have helped me in carrying out and presenting this work in the form it has finally assumed.

First of all, I cannot sufficiently express my debt of gratitude to my wife, to whom I have submitted for her unfailing judgment every sentence I have written.

Mr F. C. Bartlett has given me invaluable assistance, especially in the more theoretical portions. His acute and penetrating criticism has saved me from many pit-falls and his sympathy has cheered me through dark and difficult passages.

Further, I must sincerely thank Professor Elliot Smith for the generous way in which he not only placed the resources of the Anatomical Institute of University College at my disposal, but poured out for me his unique knowledge of cerebral topography. In my gratitude I gladly include his assistants, Dr Shellshear, Dr Tudor Jones and the late Dr John Hunter; their enthusiasm helped and guided me in my difficult and laborious task of determining the anatomical site of the cerebral lesion in certain cases of gun-shot injury.

H. H.

52 MONTAGU SQUARE
    LONDON, W. I

August, 1925

CONTENTS OF VOLUME I

CONTENTS

CONTENTS

CONTENTS OF VOLUME II

PART V

LIST OF ILLUSTRATIONS

VOLUME I

VOLUME II

APHASIA
AND KINDRED DISORDERS OF SPEECH

PART I

CHAPTER I

FROM THE SCHOOLMEN TO GALL

THE evolution of our knowledge of cerebral localisation is one of the most astonishing stories in the history of medicine. Throughout the middle ages the brain was supposed to contain three ventricles, each of which was the dwelling-place of one or more aspects of the soul. The anterior chamber received the nerves of taste, smell, sight and hearing, and was the situation of the "Sensus Communis"; in the middle ventricle dwelt the faculty of cogitation and reasoning, whilst the posterior one was the seat of memory[1].

This doctrine appears to have started from Herophilus and, although Galen placed the site of the activities of the mind in the substance of the brain, it persisted until it was rendered untenable by the dissections of Vesalius, in the early part of the sixteenth century. But theories continue to exert a subtle influence on medicine long after they have ceased to be reasonable; in 1798, Soemmering thought the seat of the soul was in the fluid which filled the ventricles, and even as late as 1844, the author of the article on psychology in Wagner's *Handwörterbuch der Physiologie* states that there are facts "which make it very probable that the cerebral ventricles are the organ which stands in the closest relation to consciousness[2]."

With the revival of learning the discussion of the relations between mind and body underwent a fundamental change. A return to the teaching of Aristotle that human reason depends on the senses and imagery made the existence of the mind dependent on bodily activities. This led to the conception that the soul in all its aspects, both higher and lower, was inseparable from the body and incapable of surviving its dissolution.

Accurate anatomical knowledge acquired by dissection destroyed the fantastic dogmas of the Schoolmen about the ventricles, and attempts were made to bring the vital activities of the brain into harmony with the

[1] [124], pp. 179–180, 204. [2] [128], p. 705.

new theories on the functions of other organs. The soul, as the principle of life, was distributed to various parts of the body, and in conjunction with the crude substances it found there was distributed in three forms of "spirits." The liver concocted from the food the "natural spirits," whilst the heart was the centre of the "vital spirits," which rushed through the vessels of the body. In the same way the brain manufactured the "animal spirits," according to Vesalius, out of the blood together with the air which entered through the ethmoid plate and other orifices of the skull. These animal spirits were distributed from the brain through all parts of the nervous system to form the basis of consciousness and voluntary action. He said:

Nerves[1] serve the same purpose to the brain that the great artery does to the heart, and the vena cava to the liver, in as much as they convey to the instruments to which it ought to be sent the spirit prepared by the brain, and hence may be regarded as the busy attendants and messengers of the brain.

He adds:

Meanwhile we will not too anxiously discuss whether the spirit is carried along certain hollow channels of the nerves, as the vital spirit is carried by the arteries, or whether it passes through the solid material of the nerves, as light passes through the air. But in any case it is through the nerves that the influence of the brain is brought to bear on any part, so far as I can certainly follow out the functions of the brain by means of vivisections, with great probability and indeed truth.

But how the brain performs its functions in imagination, in reasoning, in thinking and in memory (or in whatever way, following the dogmas of this or that man, you prefer to classify or name the several actions of the chief soul) I can form no opinion whatever. Nor do I think that anything more will be found out by anatomy or by the methods of those theologians who deny to brute animals all power of reasoning and indeed all the faculties belonging to what we call the chief soul. For as regards the structure of the brain, the monkey, dog, horse, cat, and all other quadrupeds which I have hitherto examined, and indeed all birds, and many kinds of fish, resemble man in almost every particular. Nor do we by dissection come upon any difference which would indicate that the functions of those animals should be treated otherwise than those of man; unless perchance anyone says, and that rightly, that the mass of the brain attains its highest dimensions in man, which we know to be the most perfect animal, and that his brain is found to be bigger than that of three oxen; and then in proportion to the size of the body, first the ape, and next the dog exhibit a large brain, suggesting that animals excel in the size of their brains in proportion as they seem the

---

[1] Translated by Michael Foster [49], p. 255 et seq.

more openly and clearly to be endowed with the faculties of the chief soul. Indeed the more I examine the nature of the heart, the liver, the testes, and the organs secondary to these, the functions performed by which are, there can be no doubt, the same in us as in other animals, and the more I persuade myself that we ought not to draw conclusions concerning the operations of the chief soul, other than those taught by our most holy and true religion, the more I wonder at what I read in the scholastic theologians and the lay philosophers concerning the three ventricles with which they say the brain is supplied.

The revolution in anatomical knowledge produced by the work of Vesalius did not preserve him from enunciating such purely metaphysical doctrines with regard to the functions of the body. These would have been of little historical importance had they not influenced all the theories put forward up to the end of the eighteenth century to account for the relation between the structure and functions of the nervous system. The brain was supposed to secrete thought as the liver forms the bile.

Harvey's discovery that the circulation of the blood obeyed mechanical laws applicable outside the body helped to destroy the idea of a vegetative soul and belief in the existence of vital spirits. Descartes cited it to support his view that all the activities of the body are the mechanical consequence of their structure. Animal life is inanimate and automatic; man alone is endowed with the power of thought and possesses an immaterial soul. The seat of this action of soul upon body is the brain, which from the time of Descartes onwards was universally recognised as the sole organ of mind. For him even the animal spirits which flow along the motor nerves are the result of filtration from the blood; the soul no longer animates the whole body in different forms, but exerts its influence through the pineal gland, chosen for this purpose because of its proximity to the ventricles of the brain[1].

Throughout the eighteenth century the doctrine of the relation between mind and matter became increasingly metaphysical; soul and body were thought to be coexistent but independent factors in the life of man. Knowledge of the structure of the nervous system grew steadily, but up to the end of the eighteenth century the brain was looked upon as a single organ from which flowed vital energy under the influence of the will into all parts of the body. The nerves formed the channels for this distribution, and all of them consequently took their origin in the brain.

Gall was the first to suggest that the apparently uniform mass was made up of organs which subserved the vital, intellectual and moral

---

[1] Even in 1851, Lotze postulated a central seat of the soul in the brain.

faculties of man. We habitually think of him with derision, as a quack who deduced character from the external conformation of the skull, and was directly responsible for phrenology. But it is to this man that we are really indebted for the ideas we now hold of the relation of the constituent parts of the nervous system to one another.

Franz Joseph Gall was born on March 9th, 1758, at Tiefenbronn in Baden. He studied medicine in Strasbourg, and in 1781 settled in Vienna. From 1796 to the end of 1801 he lectured on a new theory of the functions of the brain; but his views were considered so subversive of religion and morals that, on December 24th, 1801, his lectures were interdicted by an autograph letter of the Kaiser. Charles Villers writes to Cuvier: "L'Autriche comme tous les états soumis à un régime militaire et absolu, repousse avec une farouche obstination tout ce qui porte l'impreinte d'une certaine libéralité de pensée." Gall seems to have remained in Vienna for the next three years and then journeyed through Europe with his pupil Spurzheim, lecturing as he went[1]. In 1807 he reached Paris and the following year presented a Memoir to the Institute of France entitled *Introduction au Cours de Physiologie du Cerveau*. This was the first serious attempt made by Gall to put forward the new doctrine in print. In 1798, when his lectures were exciting universal interest in Vienna, he wrote a short account of his views in Wieland's *Der neue Teutsche Mercur*, a monthly popular journal; this consists of a series of dogmatic assertions concerning the localisation of the various human faculties and proclivities in different "organs," or, as we should say, "centres," of the brain. It contains nothing of any permanent value, but is of interest as showing how early the fantastic doctrines of "Craniology" formed an essential part of teaching, which contained so much that was new with regard to the structure and functions of the nervous system.

A fuller account of Gall's views is contained in an open letter of Charles Villers to Cuvier, published at Metz in 1802[2]. This lively description of the new doctrines by one who was greatly impressed by their scientific importance, touches on all the principles subsequently enunciated by Gall in his various publications. The apparently uniform mass of the brain is made up of organs which subserve the manifestations of our vital and moral faculties; these consist of three groups: (1) those which concern purely the exercise of vital force; (2) the inclinations and affections of the soul; and (3) the intellectual qualities of the mind. Each of these groups

---

[1] According to his own account (Preface to vol. i, p. xvi) he left Vienna because his father wrote to him: "Es ist Abend und könnte bald Nacht werden; werde ich dich noch sehen?"   [2] [127].

is localised in a different portion of the brain. The organ of the vital force resides in the brain-stem[1] ("moelle allongée"), which forms the intermediary between the brain and the spine; for butchers kill oxen by thrusting a stylet between the first vertebra and the occiput. The inclinations and affections of the soul belong to the basal ganglia, whilst the intellectual qualities of the mind are situated in various parts of the cerebral hemispheres. Hence the moral and intellectual characteristics can be deduced from measurements of the skull, which is modified in shape by the underlying brain.

Now it is obvious that this doctrine, though logically conceived and developed, consists of two parts of very unequal value to-day. It introduced an entirely new method of approaching the structure and functions of the nervous system, but at the same time formed the basis of what was called "Craniology," or the estimation of character and mental faculties from the shape of the skull. Unfortunately it was this latter aspect of Gall's teaching which excited at the time such widespread interest and subsequently led to its disrepute; but by an odd chance it is this part of the theory that has the more intimate bearing on the history of aphasia.

In the memoir presented in conjunction with Spurzheim to the Institute of France, he devoted his attention solely to general conceptions of the structure and functions of the brain and spinal cord. These have been absorbed so completely into the pool of general knowledge that their importance can only be recognised by studying the current teaching of the time. This has been fairly summarised by Gall himself in the Preface and in the Introduction to vol. I of his complete publication[2].

He insists that when dissecting the brain it should be approached from the spinal cord upwards; the customary method of cutting it into slices from above downwards must be abandoned. For the brain is not the seat of a "sensorium commune," but is the expansion of lower nervous mechanisms which are thus enabled, though independent, to interact upon one another. The spinal cord and brain-stem ("moelle allongée") are not simply downward projections from the brain, but are made up of independent ganglia, from which arise the nerves of the body and head. Amongst other facts in support of this contention, he cites the condition

[1] It must be remembered that the "moelle allongée" is not the medulla oblongata, but the whole of that portion of the central nervous system between the upper end of the spinal cord and the basal ganglia. When the older authorities said that all nerves arose from the brain, they meant the hemispheres and basal ganglia. Thus the "couches optiques" or optic thalmus was so called, because it was supposed to give origin to the optic nerves. [2] [53].

found in certain anencephalic foetuses where a spinal cord exists in spite of the absence of a "brain."

The brain and spinal cord are composed throughout of two substances; one of these, the white matter, consists of nerve fibres and is solely concerned with conduction of the nervous influence; whilst the other, the "pulpy or gelatinous" matter, of a more or less grey colour, forms the cortex of the brain and the ganglia[1].

The nervous system of invertebrates is composed of ganglia united by filaments, and the same organisation is present in the spinal cord of fishes, birds and mammals. Here, however, the ganglia are represented by swellings of grey matter opposite each pair of nerves. These masses, and consequently the size of the spinal cord, are proportional to the nerves which leave it and the brachial and lumbar enlargements correspond to the large outflow for the supply of the upper and lower extremities.

Gall and Spurzheim demonstrated by dissection the crossing of the pyramids, which, though previously suggested, was generally denied by contemporary anatomists. But they went further, pointing out that some such arrangement was necessary to explain the occurrence of paralysis on the opposite half of the body to that of the cerebral lesion. They considered that the cortex of the brain was formed by expansion of the peduncles, and consisted of fibres covered by grey matter; its convolutions were produced by folding and could be unrolled by internal pressure as in hydrocephalus to form a continuous membrane.

Each mechanical system of the "vie animale" is double and is restored to unity by commissures, which subserve the same function, whether they are found in the spinal cord or in the brain; the biggest of these uniting bands is the corpus callosum. Since the central nervous system is composed of many "organs" united from side to side and capable of influencing one another, there can be no common centre for all sensations, thoughts and voluntary actions. Such a conception shows how the brain and spinal cord can have developed out of simpler systems and amongst the conclusions at the end of this memoir occur the following passages:

Nous pouvons dès-à-présent considérer sous un point de vue beaucoup plus relevé, l'ensemble des systèmes nerveux, cette partie de l'organisation animale dont nulle autre n'égale l'importance. Les lois sur leur origine, leur renforcement successif, leur épanouissement, et sur le complément des appareils des fonctions

---

[1] Gall and Spurzheim suggested in this memoir that the grey substance could also be found in the labyrinth of the ear, in part of the mucous membrane of the nose and in the rete malpighi of the skin. But this does not take away from the value of their generalisation concerning the grey and white matter in the central nervous system.

les plus variées, sont en partie découvertes et ramenées à un principe général. Le nerf qui préside au mouvement, au sentiment et aux fonctions des sens, naît et se développe d'après les mêmes lois que l'organe au moyen duquel l'esprit sent, veut et pense.

De quel intérêt et de quelle importance va devenir l'étude du cerveau, maintenant qu'il n'est plus condamné, comme autrefois, à être simplement taillé et en quelque sorte ciselé comme une masse brute et sans but! Ce viscère ne présentera désormais plus de simples débris; l'on y verra partout une disposition pour un but quelconque; partout des moyens d'influence réciproque, malgré la diversité la plus étonnante des fonctions. Toutes ces anciennes formes et ces connexions mécaniques se transforment aujourd'hui en une collection merveilleuse d'appareils matériels pour les facultés de l'âme. De même que l'action des différens viscères, et la sensation des différens sens se trouvent subordonnées à un appareil nerveux particulier, de même aussi chaque instinct, chaque faculté intellectuelle, se trouvent subordonnés dans l'homme et dans tous les animaux, à une partie quelconque de la substance nerveuse du cerveau.

This remarkable memoir was handed over to a committee consisting of Tenon, Sabatier, Portal and Pinel with Cuvier as "rapporteur"; the result was the sort of half-hearted judgment that might have been expected from men of such established reputation and public eminence. They allowed that the description of the grey and white matter was novel, and agreed that Gall and Spurzheim had overthrown the theory that all nerves descended from the "brain" (i.e. the hemispheres and basal ganglia). But they failed to appreciate the revolutionary significance of this new conception of the nervous system and damned it with faint praise, suggesting that what truth it contained was already familiar, whilst the rest was of doubtful value.

Gall and Spurzheim responded by publishing in full their original memoir with comments on the report of the committee[1]. A year later (1810) appeared the first volume of the *Anatomie et Physiologie du Système Nerveux en général et du Cerveau en particulier*. Here they insist[2] that man and the animals, whatever their respective faculties, are links in a chain of living beings. The human nervous system does not differ fundamentally in structure from that of the beasts; its functions are identical in quality but more highly developed. How is it possible, they ask, to look on the brain as the seat of the faculties of the soul, if it is nothing but a secretory or excretory organ or is solely destined to secrete the principle of voluntary movement? It is impossible to explain the successive development, isolated activity and fractional diminution of the different

---

[1] [52].   [2] [53], Preface p. x.

intellectual faculties by postulating a central point, where all the nerves unite, the unique and exclusive organ of the soul.

The brain, cerebellum and spinal cord, together with the sympathetic nervous system, are composed of grey and white matter. The white substance wherever it occurs consists of fibres; it must not be compared with the medullary substance or grey matter from which all nerves take their origin[1].

All special systems of the brain and other parts of the nervous apparatus are reinforced and made perfect gradually. For this purpose the fibres of the brain are brought together and enclosed in ganglionic masses just as other neural systems unite to form sometimes plexuses and sometimes ganglia.

Each particular system of the brain terminates by an expansion of fibres disposed in layers ("en couches") in the same way as other neural endings expand in fibres at their peripheral extremity; these are brought into connection with their neighbours by communicating branches.

Every such special cerebral apparatus is double, like those of the spinal cord and of the senses. All these double portions, whether they belong to the cerebrum, cerebellum, the same organs or vertebral column, are reunited by commissural mechanisms.

Those parts of the brain which are the prolongation or reinforcement of the pyramidal bundles are in connection by crossing with the nervous system of the spinal column, and it is for this reason that a cerebral lesion causes paralysis on the opposite side of the body.

Sometimes one and sometimes another of the integral portions ("parties intégrantes") of the same system, whether in the brain or elsewhere, are developed to a different degree in individuals of the same species. Any one of these mechanisms or even a part of it may be attacked alone by disease, just as any single organ of the body can suffer without the others being affected.

The second volume, issued in 1812, has little direct bearing on the history of cerebral localisation as we understand it to-day. Gall insists that the instincts, aptitudes, sentiments and faculties are not situated in the viscera, nervous plexuses and ganglia of the chest and abdomen (sympathetic nervous system) and that they are not determined by the temperament or general constitution of the body. They are associated solely with the active life of the nervous system. The "vie animale" can be divided into two classes; firstly, the faculty of sensation, voluntary movement and the sensory functions; secondly, the moral and intellectual

[1] [53], vol. I, p. 317, et seq.

faculties, inclinations and feelings. The brain is the exclusive seat of the second group; moreover, these moral and intellectual dispositions are innate, contrary to the teaching of Locke.

Volume III did not appear till 1818. By this time Gall had parted from Spurzheim, who meanwhile had written a book on what he called *Phrenology* greatly to Gall's annoyance. In the fourth volume[1] Gall reveals the course of reasoning which led him to pitch on the anterior portion of the brain as the situation of the faculty of speech. He again tells the story of how he was sent in his ninth year to an uncle who was a *curé* in the Black Forest. Here he was educated with another boy of his own age who excelled him in learning his lessons. The two youths passed on to school at Baden, and Gall discovered that, when it was a question of learning by heart, he was beaten by those who were greatly inferior to him in written composition. Two of his new schoolfellows surpassed even his first companion in the ease with which they learnt by heart, and because they had large and prominent eyes ("yeux à fleur de tête") they received the nickname of "Ox eyes." Three years later at Bruchsal and again at the University of Strasbourg he continued to notice that those who learnt easily by heart had the same sort of eyes. He began to associate this conformation with a good verbal memory, and so arrived at the conclusion that this faculty was situated in that part of the brain which lay behind the orbits. From such fantastic beginnings sprang the idea that the memory for words was situated in the frontal lobes.

This was confirmed in his mind by subsequent cases of injury to these parts of the brain. Gall mentions an officer who received a sword thrust just above the eye, and another young man injured in the same situation by the point of a fencing foil; both had lost the "memory for words" and could not recall the names of relatives or friends. But the following remarkable case[2], which forms the first complete description of aphasia due to a wound of the brain, seems to have escaped the notice of medical historians.

M. Edouard de Rampan was sent to Gall by Baron Larrey, Napoleon's famous surgeon. He was 26 years of age and had received a wound from a foil, the point of which broke on the padded front of his fencing jacket. It entered the cheek in the middle of the left "canine region" close to the ala nasi and passed obliquely from below upwards and a little from without inwards. The instrument penetrated for a depth of about three inches and a half across the left nasal fossa and traversed the perforated plate of the ethmoid close to the insertion of the falx cerebri. It appears

[1] [53], vol. IV, p. 68.   [2] [53], vol. IV, p. 76, et seq.

to have penetrated in a vertical direction and a little obliquely from before backwards to a depth of five to six lines (half an inch) into the inner and posterior portion of the left "anterior lobe" of the brain. The patient suffered from considerable haemorrhage at the moment of the wound and a large number of sequestra came from the nose and mouth. At the same time all the sense organs were paralysed but recovered their functions little by little. The following changes alone remained, when the patient was seen by Gall.

The sight of the left eye, which was lost for a month, had recovered, but the patient saw double. Smell and taste were also abolished at first; the former returned completely, whilst taste remained defective on the left half of the tongue. The tongue was "dragged over to the right in opposition to the hemiplegia, which occupied the right side, the mouth being drawn to the left." Hearing, at first lost in the ear on the side of the wound, gradually returned and nothing abnormal remained but a humming sensation. The voice, which was also lost, was restored except for a slight stammer. At first the injury produced hemiplegia of the whole of the right side of the body; but Gall found paralysis for walking only, sensibility remaining intact.

Memory for names was completely destroyed and they could be re-called with great difficulty only, whilst the memory of images and all that was susceptible of demonstration remained intact. The mental aberration which existed in the organs of the intellect during the earlier days had passed away entirely; but all that bore on his "amour propre," his military success, etc., threw him into a state of alienation and profound melancholy, whilst conversation bearing on his family, relatives and friends restored his faculties. The patient recalled perfectly the person, face and characteristics of M. le Baron Larrey; he recognised him without difficulty. In the words of the patient he "sees him before his eyes"; and yet he could not remember the Baron's name and called him "M. Chose."

Gall describes another patient[1] where the loss of speech was due to a vascular lesion. In consequence of an attack of apoplexy a soldier found it impossible to express in spoken language his feelings and ideas. His face bore no signs of a deranged intellect. His mind ("esprit") found the answer to questions addressed to him and he carried out all he was told to do; shown an arm-chair and asked if he knew what it was he answered by seating himself in it. He could not articulate on the spot a word pro-nounced for him to repeat; but a few moments later the word escaped from his lips as if involuntarily. In his embarrassment he pointed to the

---

[1] [53], vol. IV, p. 83.

lower part of his forehead; he showed impatience and indicated by gestures that his impotence of speech came from there. It was not his tongue which was embarrassed; for he moved it with great agility and could pronounce quite well a large number of isolated words. His memory was not at fault, for he signified his anger at being unable to express himself concerning many things which he wished to communicate. It was the faculty of speech alone which was abolished. This soldier was also unable to read or to write.

Had Gall laid more stress on such cases, the history of aphasia would have been considerably advanced; but, although many instances came before him, he appears to have looked upon them as confirmatory of a localisation of faculties determined on other grounds[1]. For him normal speech was due to the perfect exercise of certain aspects of memory, each of which was situated in some particular part of the anterior lobes of the brain. He distinguished verbal memory, including the "sense of words and names," grammatical memory with "talent for language and philosophy," and the "sense of relation of numbers." Man was also endowed with a sense of "locality," of "colours" and of "tonic harmony and music." The "organs" responsible for these "intellectual faculties" are situated in those convolutions of the brain which abut on the orbit and immediately adjacent parts of the skull. That is to say the faculty of normal speech depends upon the activity of the convolutions situated on the inferior aspect of the frontal lobes. This localisation was reached by fantastic deductions from portraits or casts of the skull of persons preeminent or deficient in certain mental characteristics.

This insistence on the distinction between the various intellectual and moral faculties as the basis of the activities of the mind, led Gall to a complete misunderstanding of the nature of speech. He rightly took up the position that we do not think in words or signs; but on the other hand he made all such symbols depend immediately on one or more of the faculties he had described. Destul-Tracy[2] had suggested that every sign is the expression of the answer to a complete calculation or analysis; it fixes and states this result in such a way that a language is in reality a collection of determined formulae, which in turn facilitate and simplify subsequent calculations or analyses. Gall, on the other hand, appears to have looked upon speech as the direct mechanical expression of the concepts, inclinations, feelings and talents of man, each of which he localised in a particular part of the brain. He cites his pathological cases to show

---

[1] [53], vol. IV, p. 79.
[2] *Projet d'éléments d'idéologie*, chaps. XVI and XVII. Quoted in [53], vol. IV, p. 93.

that "full knowledge of things" is compatible with inability to discover or pronounce their names.

In 1813, Gall contributed the article "Cerveau" to the *Dictionnaire des Sciences Médicales*[1]. This forms an excellent summary of his anatomical views and all reference to "Craniology" is postponed to be dealt with under "Crane." All the material points in his general conception of the nervous system are clearly and succinctly stated and it is possible, with the help of this article, to obtain a bird's eye view of Gall's real contribution to knowledge without labouring through his complete work.

The four volumes of the *Anatomie et Physiologie du Système nerveux*, accompanied by its superb atlas of a hundred plates, proved too costly for general circulation; and in 1825 Gall published an octavo work in six volumes. It was without plates and did not contain the anatomical considerations which occupied the first volume of the earlier publication. This in all probability accounts for the failure of the medical world to recognise Gall's true scientific position; his reputation became permanently attached to the fortunes of what others had named the "Science of Phrenology" and by the middle of the nineteenth century he had sunk to the position of a discredited charlatan.

He remained in Paris, delivering annual lectures, until his death from progressive disease of the cerebral vessels, on August 22nd, 1828. His skull according to his wishes was added to his collection, subsequently deposited in the Museum of the Jardin des Plantes.

[1] [51], vol. IV, pp. 447–479.

CHAPTER II

BOUILLAUD TO BROCA

THE doctrines of Gall exerted considerable influence and attained widespread popularity. Societies were formed in all the great capitals of Europe for the study of Phrenology, and the subject assumed the pseudo-scientific position of "Psychical Research" to-day. On the other hand, many physicians rejected the phrenological elements in Gall's teaching, although they accepted the principle of localisation of function. They insisted that the brain did not "act as a whole," but was composed of centres each of which could be affected independently of the others.

Of the younger men who adopted these views, the most important for the history of aphasia was Bouillaud, who was born in 1796 and did not die till 1881. He rose rapidly to a brilliant position as a teacher of medicine, and, at the time when Broca described his first case of aphasia, was Doyen of the Faculty, Membre de l'Institut and the powerful head of the Charité. In 1825 he published a paper entitled "Recherches cliniques propres à démontrer que la perte de la parole correspond à la lésion des lobules antérieurs du cerveau et à confirmer l'opinion de M. Gall, sur la siège de l'organe du langage articulé[1]." After expressing surprise that according to Flourens the brain exerts no immediate and direct influence on the phenomena of muscular movement, he sets out to show that the tongue and correlated organs can be paralysed for the act of speech, although there is no loss of power in other parts of the body. Moreover, the tongue may still be capable of all its ordinary movements, although speech is gravely affected[2]. He cites cases, some of which are original, whilst others are culled from publications of the time, and sums up as follows[3]:

The brain of man plays an essential rôle in the mechanism of a large number of movements; it governs all those which are under the empire of the intelligence and the will. In the brain there are several special organs, each one of which has certain definite movements depending upon it. In particular, the movements of the organs of speech are regulated by a special cerebral centre, distinct and independent. This is situated in the anterior lobes of the brain. Loss of speech depends sometimes on lack of memory for words, sometimes on want of the muscular

[1] [12].   [2] [12], p. 29.   [3] [12], p. 44.

movements of which speech is composed; or what is probably the same thing, sometimes on a lesion of the grey, and at others of the white matter of the anterior lobes. Loss of speech does not necessitate want of movements of the tongue considered as an organ of prehension, mastication, deglutition of food; nor does it necessitate loss of taste. Many nerves have their origin in the brain itself, or rather communicate with it by anastomotic fibres; for example, the nerves animating the muscles, which combine in the production of speech, arise from the anterior lobes or at any rate possess the necessary communications with them.

In the same year (1825) he published the *Traité clinique et physiologique de l'Encéphalite*[1], selecting from Magendie the motto "La pathologie est la physiologie de l'homme malade." Given the symptoms it is the business of the physician to discover the site of the malady; for it is evident that, if the functions are known, their disturbance will indicate some change in the organ which brings them into being.

With this aim in view he narrates a series of cases of cerebral disease, attempting to show that the symptoms differ according to the site of the lesion. He devotes his attention to disorders of motion, of sensation and of the intellectual functions, particularly speech; but it is in the deductions he draws from various cases of motor paralysis that he is most original and approximates most closely to modern conceptions. He contends[2]:

The plurality of the cerebral centres devoted to motion is proved by the existence of partial paralyses, corresponding to a local lesion of the brain; for it is evident that if the brain were not composed of many centres, motor or conductors of muscular movement, it would be impossible to conceive how the lesion of one of those parts could bring in its train paralysis of a given portion of the body, without in any way affecting the movements of all the other parts.

Commenting on one of his cases, followed by an autopsy, he suggests that isolated paralysis of the arm is associated with a lesion of the posterior aspect of the middle part of the opposite cerebral hemisphere. "Should this turn out to be a constant phenomenon, we must conclude," he says, "that this limb receives from this point in the brain the principle of voluntary movement."

He lays down clearly the difference between higher or voluntary, and lower or automatic acts[3].

The brain as the organ of the intelligence and centre of the will, is the nervous force which holds in dependence intellectual movements, that is to say, those the animal executes by virtue of intellectual acts; consequently, a lesion of this organ will paralyse more or less completely the movements of this order and

[1] [13].   [2] [13], p. 279.   [3] [13], p. 280.

leave intact those of a different order. Hence the paralysis of voluntary movement, of which we have reported so many examples; and here clinical observation is not in contradiction to physiological experience, because on the one hand animals from whom the cerebral lobes have been removed are incapable of all movement directed by intellectual combinations, and on the other hand, patients incapable of all voluntary movement in consequence of an affection of the brain, can in spite of this execute diverse automatic and instinctive movements; for example, they can withdraw a limb that is pinched, a movement that cannot be evoked simply by the will.

Let us not forget that the muscular system is obedient to many different nervous powers. For example, the nervous power which presides over the movements of the internal muscles, such as the heart, the intestinal muscles, etc.; that which rules over the respiratory muscles and all those designated under the name of conservative or instinctive movements; that which governs voluntary movements, reflective, intellectual, all these are essentially different and their respective site has been rigorously determined by modern physiologists.

These principles he applied to elucidate the loss of speech produced by a cerebral lesion[1]. He writes:

It is evident that the movements of the organs of speech must have a special centre in the brain, because speech can be completely lost in individuals who present no other signs of paralysis, whilst on the contrary other patients have the free use of speech coincident with paralysis of the limbs. But it is not sufficient to know that there exists in the brain a particular centre destined to produce and to coordinate the marvellous movements by which man communicates his thoughts and feelings, but it is above all important to determine the exact situation of this coordinating centre. From the observations (cases) I have collected, and from the large number I have read in the literature, I believe I am justified in advancing the view that the principal lawgiver of speech is to be found in the anterior lobes of the brain. Let us admit for an instant that this portion of the brain is the site of the nervous principle which presides over the movements of speech; following this hypothesis, it would be necessary that, in those cases where the anterior lobes of the brain were altered, speech should be more or less deranged, and this should be true of the inverse condition also. It would follow moreover, that speech should remain, when the affection occupies other parts of the brain than the lobules indicated.

It might be asked how it is that the tongue continues to execute a great number of movements, even in those cases where the anterior portion of the brain is profoundly disorganised, if it is true that this part presides over the production of speech[2]. This objection, which I foresaw, is more specious than real. In effect

<hr>

[1] [13], p. 158.   [2] [13], p. 169.

the tongue is an extremely complicated organ, which fulfils many different and distinct functions; in consequence it is possible to conceive that one of these functions may be abolished without of necessity disturbing the others; this conclusion reached by logic is confirmed by experience. Since certain movements of the tongue such as those of prehension, mastication, deglutition, etc., persist, although those necessary for the articulation of sounds are abolished by a lesion of the anterior lobes of the brain, it follows that the tongue has in the nervecentre several sources of distinct action.

Later in his treatise[1] he says:

It is important to distinguish the two causes which may be followed by loss of speech, each one in its own manner; one by destroying the organ for the memory of words, the other by alteration of the nervous principle which presides over the movements of speech.

If we are asked why animals do not speak we should not reply with many naturalists that they have no suitable external organs, but we should add that this phenomenon arose from a more potent cause, to wit the absence of the internal organ, the cerebral centre, which dictates, so to say, and coordinates the complicated movements by means of which man expresses the operations of his understanding.

He points out that from the beginning man possesses all the movements of his larynx, tongue and cheeks; but is obliged to acquire speech by education, because the actions necessary for speech belong to the intellectual life, whilst those of the external organs are purely instinctive. Even the loss of memory for words may be partial, and he cites several cases, including a splendid instance of jargoning, to prove this point[2].

In order to explain these facts, so bizarre in appearance, it is necessary to admit that the cerebral organ responsible for articulated language is itself composed of several distinct parts, each one of which can be altered independently. It is necessary also to admit, however strange this opinion may seem, that this organ is composed of several different portions, each of which presides over the formation and the memory of one of the words, such as the substantive, adjective, verb, etc., which taken together compose speech.

These views met with much opposition; and nearly fifteen years later Bouillaud, now a popular professor of medicine, dealt with his most important critics in a lecture delivered before the Académie de Médecine, on October 29th, 1839[3]. He began by a precise statement of his position, pointing out that Gall had considered the "sense of words" from an intellectual aspect, whilst he proposed to study the localisation of the faculty of speech from the mechanical point of view. "I wish," he said[4],

---

[1] [13], p. 285.   [2] [13], p. 289.   [3] [14].   [4] [14], p. 284.

"to apply to the brain, considered as agent or principle of coordinated movements, that system of plurality which Gall invented for the same organ in as far as it is the instrument of intellectual and moral phenomena." Speech or articulated language constitutes a complex act, which demands for its perfect execution three diverse factors: (1st) instruments of articulation, such as the tongue and lips, representing the agent or "executive and articulatory power"; (2nd) an internal or cerebral organ, which may be called the "law-giver, the creator and coordinator of speech"; (3rd) the means of communication between the seat of the executive and legislative power. He reaffirmed his contention that the centre in the brain, which presides over the faculty of speech, is situated in the anterior lobes, and criticised the cases advanced to the contrary.

This paper was followed by a lengthy discussion, which led to no conclusive result. For on the one hand his opponents were obsessed by the bogey of phrenology, whilst Bouillaud failed to explain why speech was sometimes gravely affected although the lesion was not situated in the frontal lobes. No one suspected that the left half of the brain might differ functionally from the right. Marc Dax of Sommières had, it is true, already made the suggestion that loss of speech depended on a lesion of the left hemisphere, but this fact remained entirely unknown in Paris until 1865[1].

Bouillaud was an important and assiduous member of the Académie de Médecine, ready to intervene in any discussion on cerebral localisation. When therefore a paper was presented by Belhomme in January, 1848, on "The localisation of speech, or rather of the memory of words, in the anterior lobes of the brain," Bouillaud was stimulated to open another full-dress debate on the subject[2]. Some few fresh cases were cited, but he met his old opponents on the same ground and with the same weapons. Rochoux boasted that he had opposed craniology ever since 1814 and continued to disbelieve in cerebral localisation. Discussion grew warm and Bouillaud offered five hundred francs to anyone who would bring him an example of a severe lesion of the anterior lobes of the brain unaccompanied by disturbance of speech[3].

It is customary to speak of Broca's discovery as if it came like a clap of thunder from a clear sky; this was by no means the case. In 1861, the air was again full of the localisation of cerebral functions, and this question was liable to crop up with any excuse, in scientific discussions. Thus, in February, 1861, before the recently formed Société d'Anthropologie,

---

[1] [34].   [2] [15], pp. 699–719, 778–816.   [3] [15] p. 813.

Gratiolet[1] exhibited a Totonac[2] skull, and gave his views on the signifi-cance of the volume of the brain. This started a discussion which was continued through the sittings of the Society until the end of June and rapidly became divided into two parts. Firstly, what is the relative value of form or volume in determining the cultural level of the brain; and secondly, does the brain function as a whole, or is it composed of many organs or centres acting more or less independently?

The treatment of this second question by the various speakers in the debate is of fundamental importance, if we wish to understand the history of aphasia. After Gratiolet had made his communication, Auburtin[3], the pupil and son-in-law of Bouillaud, insisted that the total volume of the brain did not give an exact measurement of intelligence; but, if instead of considering the organ as a whole its different parts were examined, it was possible to arrive at some precise data. "We know for example," he said, "that the highest functions of the brain stand in relation to the develop-ment of the anterior lobes." He pointed out that an apoplexy produced different results according to whether it occupied the cerebellum, corpus striatum, optic thalamus, or the anterior lobes of the brain.

Broca[4], who was secretary of the Society, joined in the debate, but on this occasion spoke solely on the value of the weight of the brain as a measure of the intelligence. It was a remark made by Gratiolet towards the end of this meeting which had such an important bearing on the subsequent form assumed by the discussion. He said[5], "In a general manner I agree with M. Flourens that the intelligence is one, that the brain is one, that it acts above all as a whole; but this does not exclude the idea that certain faculties of the mind stand in special relation, although not exclusively, with certain cerebral regions."

So much interest was excited in this question that Broca reopened the discussion on March 21st[6] with a long address devoted firstly, to the importance of the volume of the brain, and secondly, to whether it acted as a whole or as a group of coordinated organs. He paid a high tribute to the anatomical work of Gall and to the great principle of cerebral localisa-tion "which has been, one may say, the point of departure for all the discoveries of our century on the physiology of the brain." He warned his auditors against confounding the principles of Gall with the applica-tions that had been made of them; "I, for my part," he said, "believe in the principle of localisation," and he found support by appealing to the facts of embryology and anatomy.

[1] [41], p. 66.   [2] A primitive race descended from the Maya of Yucatan.
[3] [41], p. 71.   [4] [41], p. 75.   [5] [41], p. 78.   [6] [41], p. 139.

The sitting of April 4th was opened by Auburtin[1], who insisted on the importance of the facts of pathology as opposed to those of physiological experiment, and cited several cases from Lallemand and from Bouillaud's *Traité de l'Encéphalite*; he dwelt particularly on the association of speech with the frontal lobes. So strong was his belief that he offered to recant his faith in this doctrine, if anyone would show him a single definite case of loss of speech, such as he had described, in which there had been no lesion of the anterior lobes of the brain. The source of his inspiration was obvious, and it might have been Bouillaud who was speaking.

These statements impressed Broca so deeply that he asked Auburtin to see with him a patient suffering from loss of speech, who had just been admitted to the surgical wards of Bicêtre (April 11). In spite of the right hemiplegia and other complications, it was agreed to accept this patient as a test case; for Auburtin allowed that the clinical condition corresponded to that in which a lesion of the anterior lobes might be anticipated.

Death occurred on April 17th, and Broca demonstrated the brain[2], in support of the views of Bouillaud and Auburtin, at a meeting of the Société d'Anthropologie held next day. But so little effect was produced on the opponents of localisation, that this case was not mentioned throughout the whole of the subsequent discussion. Even Broca[3], when he intervened again towards its close, after a brief allusion to the specimen, confirmed his arguments to general principles and confessed "although I inclined towards the opinion of M. Auburtin, I had not intended to take sides in the debate. I do not pronounce either for or against particular localisations; I seek only to establish a general principle by considering the cerebral convolutions, not one by one, but in groups or if you will by regions."

Broca was a superb anatomist and in August, 1861, he gave a complete account of this first case, and of the structural changes discovered in the brain, before the Société anatomique de Paris[4]. Here he first spoke of the disorder of speech as "Aphemia," laying down clearly what he understood by this term. He pointed out that the faculty of articulated language was a totally different thing from the "general faculty of language." This is the power of establishing a constant relation between an idea and a sign, whether it be a sound, a gesture, a figure, or an outline; if it were destroyed all language would become impossible. But this general function may remain intact, the auditory apparatus be normal, all

[1] [41], p. 209.   [2] [41], p. 235.   [3] [41], p. 320.   [4] [19], p. 347 et seq.

muscles, not excepting those responsible for the voice, lips and tongue may act perfectly, and yet a cerebral lesion can abolish articulated speech.

The two aspects of the question have never been so clearly formulated as in the first communication by Broca, which is worthy of the closest study. For he recognised that the phenomena in which he was interested were due to disorder of the "special faculty of articulated language" and not to an affection of speech as a whole; it was an intellectual disturbance on the executive side. On the other hand he hoped by precise anatomical observations to discover the exact site of the cerebral "organ" or centre which governed this function.

The patient was a man named Leborgne who, though subject to epileptiform attacks since his youth, had been able to exercise his trade up to the age of thirty, as a last-maker. He then lost the use of his speech and was subsequently admitted in 1840 to the Hospital of Bicêtre. Broca could not discover whether the loss of speech occurred suddenly or slowly nor whether it was accompanied by any other symptoms. For three or four months he was unable to speak at all, but did not differ from a normal man in any way, except in the loss of articulated language. He went about the Hospital, where he was known by the name of "Tan." He understood all that was said to him and his hearing was perfect; but whatever question he was asked he always answered, "Tan, tan," accompanied by the most varied gestures, through which he succeeded in expressing most of his ideas. When the questioner failed to understand his mimicry, he became angry and added to his vocabulary an oath. "Tan" passed for an egoist, vindictive, malicious, and his comrades detested him, even accusing him of being a thief. These defects may have been due in great part to the cerebral lesion; but they were not sufficiently pronounced to appear pathological, and at no time was any suggestion made that he should be transferred to the insane department of the Hospital. On the contrary he was always considered to be completely responsible for his acts.

Ten years later (1850) the right arm became weaker and was finally completely paralysed. "Tan" continued to walk without difficulty; but gradually the loss of power invaded the right lower extremity and, after dragging it for some time, he was compelled to remain permanently in bed. About four years elapsed from the time when power began to be lost in the arm until the moment when he was no longer able to stand.

For some years he remained bed-ridden, and but little information could be collected with regard to this period; but his sight became more feeble during the last two years. On April 11th, 1861, however, he was found to be suffering from wide-spread diffuse cellulitis of the right lower extremity, and was therefore transferred to the surgical ward, where he came under the care of Broca.

Examination of this man who could neither speak nor write was beset with difficulties. But Broca was able to determine the following condition. All power was lost in the right arm and leg; on the left half of the body every movement could be carried out feebly. There was no squint. The face moved equally; but in the act of whistling the left cheek appeared to be a little more swollen than the right, which seemed to show that the muscles of this side were somewhat weakened[1]. The tongue moved perfectly in every direction and did not deviate on protrusion. There was some difficulty in deglutition due to commencing paralysis of the pharynx. The tone of the voice was natural and the muscles of the larynx did not appear to be affected. General sensibility was everywhere preserved, but the right half of the body was less sensitive than the left. Micturition and defaecation were normal.

Hearing retained its acuity; "Tan" heard perfectly the sound of a watch, but his vision was weakened. When he wished to look at the time, he was obliged to take the watch himself with his left hand and to place it in a particular position about 20 cm. from the right eye, which appeared to see better than the left. The state of his intelligence could not be exactly determined. It is certain that "Tan" understood almost all that was said to him; but since he was unable to express his ideas or his desires except by movements of the left hand, he could not make himself understood as well as he understood others. Numerical answers were those which he carried out the best, by opening or closing his fingers. Asked how many days he had been ill, he answered sometimes "five days" and sometimes "six days." How many years he had been at Bicêtre? He opened his hand four times in succession and then raised one finger; this made twenty-one years, an answer which was perfectly correct. Next day on repeating the same question the same reply was obtained. Broca says:

But when I wanted to return the third time, "Tan" understood that I was making him do an exercise; he became angry and articulated the oath, which I have only heard from his mouth on a single occasion. I gave him my watch two days in succession. The second hand did not go; he was not in consequence able to distinguish the three hands excepting by their form and length;

[1] Broca adds in explanation the incorrect statement, "Il est inutile de rappeler que les paralysies de cause cérébrale sont croisées pour le tronc et les membres, et directes pour la face."

nevertheless after having examined the watch for some moments, he was able on each occasion to indicate the time exactly. It is incontestable that this man was intelligent, that he could reflect, and that he had preserved in a certain measure, the memory of past things. He could even understand somewhat complicated ideas; thus, when I asked him in what order his paralyses followed one another, he made a little horizontal gesture with the index of the left hand, as much as to say, I understand; then he showed successively his tongue, his right arm and his right leg. This was perfectly exact in as far as he attributed the loss of his speech to paralysis of the tongue, which was a natural mistake. All the same, certain questions, which a man of ordinary intelligence would have found means to answer by gestures even of the left hand, remained without reply. At other times it was not possible to catch the meaning of certain responses, and this appeared to make him very impatient. Occasionally the answer was clear but false; thus, although he was childless, he pretended that he had a family. The intelligence of this man was undoubtedly diminished, either in consequence of the cerebral lesion or owing to the effect of the fever from which he suffered. But he evidently possessed much more intelligence than was necessary for speech.

This patient died on April 17th at 11 o'clock in the morning and the autopsy was made after an interval of twenty-four hours. The body presented no signs of putrefaction, but there was diffuse cellulitis of the whole right lower extremity. The skull was somewhat thicker than normal and the diploë was replaced by compact tissue; the internal surface of the cranial vault presented a somewhat worm-eaten appearance. The external aspect of the dura mater was red and vascular; it was thickened and covered on its inner surface with a pseudo-membranous layer, infiltrated with serous fluid. The dura mater and the false membrane together had a medium thickness of 5 mm. (minimum 3 mm., maximum 8 mm.) On removing the dura the pia mater was seen to be much injected, at certain points thickened and in places opaque, infiltrated with yellowish plastic material, which had the colour of pus but was solid, and when examined under the microscope did not contain "purulent globules." On the lateral aspect of the left hemisphere, at the level of the fissure of Sylvius, the pia mater was raised by a collection of transparent serous fluid which lay in a large and deep depression of the cerebral substance. When this liquid was evacuated by puncture, the pia mater sank profoundly, and there resulted an elongated cavity with a capacity equivalent in volume to that of a hen's egg, corresponding to the fissure of Sylvius. This lesion extended back to, but was entirely in front of, the fissure of Rolando, and the parietal lobe was relatively healthy, although no part of the hemisphere was in an entirely normal condition. Broca continues:

On incising and turning back the pia mater at the level of the cavity which I have described, it is at once seen that this corresponds not to a depression, but to a loss of substance in the mass of the brain; the liquid which filled it was poured out consecutively to fill the void as it was formed, as happens with chronic softening of the superficial layers of the brain or of the cerebellum. The state of the convolutions which limit the cavity shows that they are the seat of chronic softening, whose march is sufficiently slow to permit of the molecules of the brain, dissociated one by one, being absorbed and replaced by the serous exudate. A considerable portion of the left hemisphere had been destroyed gradually in this manner, but the softening extends well beyond the limits of the cavity; this is not in any way circumscribed and cannot be compared to a cyst. Its walls, almost everywhere irregular and broken, are constituted by the substance of the brain itself which is extremely softened at this level, and the innermost layer in direct contact with the serous exudate was on the way to slow and gradual dissolution when the patient died. The inferior wall only is smooth and of a sufficiently firm consistence. It is clear that the original focus of softening existed in that place where the loss of substance is found to-day, that the morbid condition extended little by little by continuity of tissue, and that the point where it began must have been situated, not in the organs actually softening, but amongst those which are more or less completely destroyed.

Broca sums up the extent of the loss of substance as follows:

The small inferior marginal convolution (first temporal); the small convolutions of the lobe of the insula together with the subjacent parts of the corpus striatum; finally, in the frontal lobe, the inferior portion of the transverse convolution (ascending frontal) and the posterior half of the two large convolutions, designated by the name of the second and third frontal. Of the four convolutions which form the frontal lobe, the first and most internal, has preserved its continuity; but it is not normal for it is softened and atrophied.

All the parts which surrounded this cavity were distinctly affected. Even the second temporal convolution was softened on its surface, and those portions of the frontal lobes, which bounded the lesion, were almost diffluent. Moreover, it was possible to make out without incising the brain that the whole of the corpus striatum was softened, although the optic thalamus retained its normal colour, volume, and consistence. The remaining portions of the hemispheres were superficially wasted, but had preserved their shape and continuity.

In November, 1861, Broca demonstrated the brain from another patient[1], Lelong by name, who had been transferred to the surgical side

---

[1] [20].

of Bicêtre for a fracture of the neck of the femur. He was a man of eighty-four years of age, admitted eight years before for senile debility.

In April, 1860, when descending the stairs he suddenly collapsed and was found to be unconscious. On his recovery he was not paralysed, but had lost the power of speech. He could pronounce certain words only, and these were articulated with difficulty. His intelligence was not apparently affected; he understood all that was said to him, and his small vocabulary, accompanied by expressive mimicry, was comprehensible to those who lived with him habitually.

So he remained till October 27th, 1861, when he fell, breaking the neck of his left femur; this led to his transfer to Broca's care. There was no loss of power except in the fractured limb. Sensation was unaffected; sight and hearing were good. The tongue was not paralysed and did not deviate on protrusion.

When questioned, he replied by signs accompanied by one or two syllables articulated quickly and with effort. These were the French words "oui," "non," "tois" (trois), and "toujours"; when asked his name he said "Lelo." Each of the first three words correspond to a definite idea; to express approval or affirmation he said "oui," whilst "non" was used in the opposite sense. The word "tois" expressed all numbers or numerical ideas. On every occasion, when these three words failed to express his meaning, Lelong employed "toujours." Asked if he knew how to write, he answered, "Oui"; questioned as to his ability to do so, he said, "Non," and, when told to try, failed completely.

He always accompanied the use of the word "tois" by signs on his fingers; for he knew that his speech was faulty, and so corrected his error by gestures. Asked, "How many years have you been at Bicêtre?" he replied, "Tois," and raised eight fingers. "Have you any children?" "Oui"; "How many?" "Tois," lifting four fingers. "How many boys?" "Tois," lifting two fingers; "How many girls?" he again lifted two fingers. All these answers were exact. "Can you tell the time?" "Oui," "What is it?" "Tois," and he lifted ten fingers; it was in fact ten o'clock. When asked, "How old are you?" he did not lift his ten fingers eight times, and then add four, to make it eighty-four, as was expected; but he said "Tois," first raising eight fingers and then four. As soon as he saw he was understood, he said, "Oui."

His gestures were most expressive; asked what work he did before entering the hospital, he made the movements of taking a spade into his hands, driving it into the earth and turning a spadeful of soil. "You were a navvy?" "Oui," he answered with an affirmative movement of the head.

This patient died on November 8th, 1861, and the autopsy revealed the following condition. All the sutures were ossified, and the walls of the skull were a little thickened, but not harder than usual. The dura mater was not thickened, and appeared to be unaffected. There was a considerable quantity of serous fluid in the cavity of the arachnoid. The pia mater was neither thickened nor congested. The whole brain with its membranes weighed 1136 grammes, far below the average, and scarcely equal to the minimum weight of that of an adult male of normal mentality. This was due not only to general senile atrophy but to distinct wasting of the left hemisphere.

When the brain was placed on the table, it was evident that a superficial lesion occupied the left frontal lobe immediately below the anterior extremity of the fissure of Sylvius. At this level the surface of the hemisphere was sunken and through the transparent pia mater could be seen a collection of serous fluid, occupying an area almost equal to that of a franc. The third frontal convolution was completely cut in half and had suffered a loss of substance extending over about 15 mm. This excavation was continuous on the one side with the fissure of Sylvius, at the level of the insula. In the other direction it encroached on the second frontal convolution, which was profoundly eaten away, though the innermost portion remained for a thickness of 2 mm.; this minute tongue alone maintained the continuity of the convolution. The first and also the ascending frontal convolution were perfectly normal. Broca concludes, "In this patient, therefore, the aphemia was the result of a profound, but accurately circumscribed lesion of the posterior third of the second and third frontal convolutions." Its origin was probably apoplectic, for it must be remembered that the patient lost his speech suddenly, and haematin crystals were discovered on microscopical examination at the site of the lesion.

These communications produced the greatest excitement in the medical world of Paris. They were specially selected for comment by the Secretary of the Société anatomique, in his Annual Report for the year 1861. Bouillaud and his son-in-law, Auburtin, greeted Broca as a convert to their doctrines. Localisation of speech became a political question; the older Conservative school, haunted by the bogey of phrenology, clung to the conception that the brain "acted as a whole"; whilst the younger Liberals and Republicans passionately favoured the view that different functions were exercised by the various portions of the cerebral hemispheres. During the next few years every medical authority took one side or other in the discussion.

Numerous cases were collected in favour of Broca's doctrine, but it was not long before autopsies were reported which told against the localisation of a centre for speech in the third frontal convolution. Of these, the most striking was the post-mortem examination carried out in the presence of Broca on one of Charcot's patients[1]. This woman suffered from right hemiplegia, with inability to utter more than two or three words and was a characteristic example of loss of speech in Broca's sense of the term; but the third frontal convolution was not materially affected, and the lesion occupied the neighbourhood of the posterior portion of the fissure of Sylvius. It had destroyed the first and part of the second temporal convolutions, a great part of the insula, the whole of the extra-ventricular and the posterior half of the intra-ventricular nucleus of the corpus striatum. We now recognise that such a condition was amply sufficient to account for the phenomena observed during life; but Broca was staggered by this observation and wondered whether the faculty of language was confined to the third frontal convolution. Might it not extend backwards to the supra-marginal area? If such were the case, a lesion in this part of the brain might also produce an aphemia, although the frontal lobe itself was completely intact. He pointed out that among the twenty cases collected by himself and his friends, all showed some pathological change in the left half of the brain, and in nineteen of them it had been situated in the third frontal convolution. In view, however, of so serious an exception, it was necessary to await further facts before expressing a definite opinion concerning the exact position of the cortical centres connected with articulated speech. Here, we see how close Broca came to a correct anatomical opinion; he was too scientific and too modest to adopt the dogmatic tone of Auburtin, to whom Charcot administered a well-deserved castigation[2].

In 1868, the British Association for the Advancement of Science held its Annual Meeting at Norwich; Broca opened the discussion on the Physiology of Speech and was followed by Hughlings Jackson. No record of this discussion is to be found in the *Proceedings of the British Association*, but Broca's paper was published in the *Tribune Médicale*[3]. In his

[1] [32].

[2] On July 20th, 1864, Broca was present at another autopsy on one of Charcot's patients [11], Anselin by name, who had formed the subject of one of Trousseau's lectures on aphasia ([126], p. 587). The patient had suffered from right hemiplegia and gross defects of speech of embolic origin associated with mitral regurgitation and stenosis. There were several lesions scattered about the cortex, none of which affected the third frontal convolution; but there was softening of the anterior and superior portion of the intraventricular nucleus of the left corpus striatum.   [3] [27].

comments on the post-mortem at the Salpêtrière, he had hovered on the verge of a correct anatomical localisation, and in his contribution to the discussion at Norwich, he came near to defining the different forms that might be assumed by affections of speech. He rejects first of all those due to gross intellectual changes, and those produced by some defect of function of the organs of articulation. He then divides disorders of speech, due to a central lesion, into two main groups, "aphémie" and "amnésie verbale" and lays down clearly the difference between them. The aphemic patient has a profoundly reduced vocabulary and may be speechless except for some monosyllables, oaths or words that do not seem to belong to any language. His ideas are intact, as shown by gestures, and he can understand what is said to him, and recognise words and phrases which he cannot pronounce or even repeat. On the other hand, the amnesic patient no longer recognises the conventional associations established between ideas and words. He can pronounce them, but they do not seem to have any bearing on the ideas he wishes to express; he is able to show by gestures that he has not lost all kinds of memory; it is the special memory, not only of spoken but of written words, that he has lost.

So far Broca's statements are admirably clear and consonant with fact. When, however, he tried to determine the site of the lesion responsible for such conditions, he became confused and indefinite; he saw clearly that the larger number of cases did not correspond to these two clean-cut divisions. In practice both states can exist together and this greatly hampers the determination of the causative lesion. He utters a wise warning on the necessity for drawing conclusions from selected cases only, and insists that it is aphemia alone which is caused by a lesion of the third frontal convolution. Had he been able to combine his previous anatomical suggestions with this hypothesis concerning the nature of the functions that are disturbed, he would have approached the position held by most neurologists to-day.

Meanwhile cerebral localisation, as exemplified by disorders of speech, formed the subject of innumerable communications. In 1864, Trousseau[1], at the height of his fame as a teacher of medicine, gave a series of lectures at the Hôtel Dieu on loss of speech. He objected to the word "aphemia" and coined in its place "aphasia" because a Greek physician of his acquaintance appears to have persuaded him that "aphemia" signified "infamous" and had nothing to do with want of speech. He therefore replaced it by a term of his own invention, which unfortunately gained

[1] [125].

uniform acceptance and enabled him to impress his personality upon the question of the moment. His lectures were brilliant, and he proceeded to divide aphasia into three varieties, which bore no relation to any fundamental principles, but were supposed to correspond to "clinical entities." Such fictitious classification of disease is one of the familiar methods adopted by popular teachers for stamping their image on the history of medicine. He added nothing that deserves to be remembered. Broca's letter of protest is a model of respectful irony and he justly complained that Trousseau had "brought back into pathology, the very confusion I thought to dissipate [1]."

Broca's conception that the left half of the brain was endowed with functions which differed from those of the right, was hotly contested by the older school of clinicians. Marc Dax [2] of Sommières had, it is true, nearly thirty years before, brought forward this hypothesis at a meeting in Montpellier; but the suggestion passed unnoticed until his son presented a Memoir on this subject to the Académie de Médecine in 1864 [3]. He seems to have been entirely ignorant of Broca's work, and the sort of material he offered in proof was not up to the anatomical knowledge of the day. This Memoir was handed over to a committee consisting of Bouillaud, Béclard and Lélut, the last of whom prided himself upon having opposed cerebral localisation for forty years. He took the remarkable course of not calling together his colleagues, but presented a report scarcely occupying two pages of print, in which he said that he had taken up his position once and for all and he was not going to alter his attitude towards cerebral localisation for anybody. Bouillaud was not the sort of man to accept such conduct lightly, and he called for a formal debate on the matter which lasted over many meetings [4]. Two of these he occupied in expounding his conception of cerebral localisation, and accepted Broca's work as confirming these doctrines. Many clinicians, including Trousseau, took part in the debate, which elicited no new facts; but the medical papers were filled with reports and communications on cerebral localisation of disorders of speech. The *Gazette Hebdomadaire* summed up the state of the question in two excellent articles, which assumed that speech consists of a physiological and intellectual aspect. The former comprises language in the form of mimicry, writing and articulated speech; the latter is a special function concerned with the memory of words. Internal speech was assumed to be a purely intellectual phenomenon.

[1] [25].   [2] In 1836 [34].   [3] [35].   [4] [42].

Had research proceeded along these lines, clinicians would have approached almost the position subsequently assumed by Marie. There was a wide tendency, clearly formulated by Broca in his Norwich address, to believe that disorders of speech produced by cerebral lesions consisted of an intellectual and an executive side; many of the less prejudiced observers felt that the third frontal convolution was not the only situation where a lesion could produce disorders of speech. But the younger men were concerned mainly in the doctrine of anatomical localisation, which seemed to have received such strong support from the work of Broca and his followers. They were not interested in a detailed examination of the forms assumed by the loss of function; their attention was concentrated on the remarkable fact that a local lesion of the brain could produce destruction of the power of speech. Those who had come to Paris in the sixties to study medicine returned to all corners of the civilised world bearing with them this doctrine; they gloried in demonstrating to their fellow-countrymen, on the post-mortem table, that some peculiar and little understood affection of speech was the result of a definite cerebral lesion, and thus they paved the way for the physiological discoveries of the 'seventies.

CHAPTER III

HUGHLINGS JACKSON[1]

INTEREST in the association of cerebral lesions with disorders of speech rapidly spread to England, and in 1864, Hughlings Jackson made his first contribution to this subject. He was at that time twenty-nine years of age, and had been recently appointed to the Staff of the London Hospital. Here he delivered his famous clinical lecture on "Loss of Speech, etc." based on a profound study of the disorders of function which accompany right hemiplegia, and follow epileptiform convulsions. He was one of the most remarkable pioneers in this field of research. Between 1864 and 1893, he published a series of papers on this subject, and throughout the whole of this period he would enunciate his views to anyone who visited the wards under his care. But even amongst the younger men his aphoristic dicta fell upon deaf ears. Until Arnold Pick dedicated *Die agrammatischen Sprachstörungen* to "Hughlings Jackson, the deepest thinker in neuropathology of the past century," no one attempted to understand his contribution to the subject. Moutier mentions his name along with those of other English-men who held more popular views, not knowing how closely in some respects Hughlings Jackson's conceptions agreed with those of Pierre Marie. Von Monakow mentions four only of Hughlings Jackson's papers amongst over 3000 which form the references at the end of his volume on *Die Lokalisation im Grosshirn*, and there is nothing in the text to show that at that time he understood Jackson's point of view or recognised how completely it diverged from the popular conceptions.

Four reasons may be offered for this extraordinary neglect of Jackson's work. Dr Hughlings Jackson was a man of such profound personal modesty that he laid little value on the publication of his views, although firmly convinced of their utility in explaining the phenomena of disease. Thus, most of his papers are to be found in Journals which are not accessible to foreigners, and many cannot be consulted even by English workers except in the great medical libraries.

Secondly, the style in which they are written makes them peculiarly difficult to read. He was so anxious not to overstate his case that almost every page is peppered with explanatory phrases or footnotes, so that

[1] Throughout this chapter all the references are to the reprint of Jackson's papers on Aphasia in *Brain*, 1915 [81].

the generalisation can scarcely be distinguished from its qualifications. English students, accustomed to the fluent facility of his contemporaries, turned away from the bristling difficulties of Hughlings Jackson's papers.

Thirdly, Jackson derived all his psychological knowledge from Herbert Spencer, and adopted his phraseology almost completely. This has tended to alienate psychologists, blinding them to the truths underlying this somewhat uncouth nomenclature.

Finally, the nature of the ideas he propounded was foreign to the current views of the day. He was always accustomed to say that "it generally takes a truth twenty-five years to become known in medicine," a dictum certainly founded on his personal experience. Each generation of house physicians and clinical clerks at the National Hospital passed out impressed by the beauty of his character and his simple-hearted sincerity. Some carried away with them one or more of his broad generalisations to bear fruit in their subsequent work. Thus, for instance, his doctrine that "destructive lesions never cause positive effects, but induce a negative condition which permits positive symptoms to appear," has become one of the hall-marks of English neurology.

But no one assimilated his views on defects of speech and applied them to a series of actual examples of this condition. We failed to appreciate how much closer these conceptions would have led us to the phenomena of aphasia than the glib generalities founded on the anatomical facts of cortical localisation.

Although the study of the phenomena of aphasia is one method of elucidating the mechanism of speech, it is by no means the only one. In the last forty years philologists, psychologists, and students of philosophy have steadily progressed away from the conceptions expressed by neurologists, even in their most recent monographs and text-books. Neurology has become frozen stiffly in the grip of pseudo-metaphorical classifications which neither explain the conditions nor correspond to the clinical facts. The dangers of such false classification were recognised by Jackson in 1878. "We must not," he said, "classify on a mixed method of anatomy, physiology and psychology, any more than we should classify plants on a mixed, general, and empirical method as exogens, kitchen herbs, graminaceae and shrubs." Thus, by an irony of fortune the advance of knowledge, in other than neurological fields, has resulted in attainment of a position in many ways corresponding closely with that held by Jackson more than forty years ago.

Throughout the whole of his work on affections of speech Hughlings Jackson insisted on the necessity of studying and classifying the phenomena before any attempt was made to correlate them with morphological changes. Speech is a function of mental activity; and however much that mental activity may ultimately be linked up with the integrity of some portion of the brain-substance, the problem is primarily a psychological one.

We shall, to start with, consider our subject empirically and afterwards scientifically; we first arbitrarily divide and arrange for convenience of obtaining the main facts which particular cases supply, and then try to classify the facts in order to show their true relations one to another, and consider them on the psychical side as defects of mind and on the physical side as defects of the nervous system[1].

Every worker on the affections of speech has claimed to deal with the "facts" of each case; but no one except Jackson recognised that all the phenomena are primarily psychical and only in the second place susceptible of physiological or anatomical explanation. Even most modern accounts attempt to deal with the clinical facts as if they could be deduced from the physiological activity of morphological centres. A visual centre or an auditory centre demands a visual or auditory aspect of affections of speech, and attempts are made to classify the psychical phenomena as a direct expression of the activity of such centres. Still greater chaos was introduced by the theory that affections of speech were due to destruction of morphological "visual psychic" or "auditory psychic" centres. Here we are, indeed, in the middle of that confused classification against which Jackson uttered a solemn warning in 1878.

As far back as 1868, when Jackson took part in the discussion on Broca's paper at the Norwich meeting of the British Association, he recognised the law that a destructive lesion can never be responsible for positive symptoms; pure destruction produces negative effects, and any positive symptoms are the consequences of the released activity of lower centres. This general law of nervous activity he applied rigidly to the phenomena of affections of speech.

To say that the disease "caused" these (abnormal) utterances, a positive condition, is absurd, for the disease is destruction of nervous arrangements, and that could not cause a man to do something; it has enough to answer for in leaving him unable to speak. The utterances are effected during activity of nervous arrangements which have escaped injury. This remark may seem a truism here, but in more complicated cases it is very common to hear of positive symptoms being ascribed to negative lesions, to loss of function of nervous elements. It is common, at any rate, for disease to be thought of vaguely as something "dis-

---

[1] [81], p. 112.

ordering the functions of the brain." ... It is an error to ascribe such positive symptoms as the recurring utterances of speechless men, the erroneous words uttered by those who have defect of speech . . . etc., to loss or to defect of function. These positive mental symptoms arise during activity of lower centres or lower nervous arrangements which have escaped injury[1].

Every case of affection of speech exhibits, therefore, two sides—the negative and the positive; on the one hand, the patient may not be able to speak, to write or to read, and expression by signs may be impaired. This is the negative aspect, whilst his power of writing his signature, and of swearing, or uttering other emotional expressions, form the positive symptoms, and are the expression of lower mental activities.

Some critics have imagined that Jackson's ideas were built up on a priori reasoning; but anyone who will attempt to examine a case of aphasia according to his conceptions will find himself led to the discovery of phenomena which will elude any other theoretical method. He will discover that in many cases it is impossible to say that a man can or cannot speak; for he can utter a phrase or a word which he cannot repeat to order. He can write his name and address, but not that of his mother with whom he lives. He may understand all ordinary commands to fetch this or that object, but, told to close his eyes, opens his mouth. He may not be able to draw a square or a triangle to order, but draws them without difficulty spontaneously. The "golden rule" upon which Dr Jackson insisted—"Put down what the patient *does* get at and avoid all such terms as amnesia, etc.," had it been habitually followed, would have saved neurologists from many years of wandering in the wilderness.

Jackson's attitude was strictly phenomenal. He never deduced his observations from his hypothesis, but any hypothesis he enunciated sprang, as it were, ready-made from some clinical fact. He never experimented or arranged a series of observations to elucidate a definite point. He stood like an observer on a bridge formulating the extent of the flood from matter carried down by the stream. The acuteness and rapidity of the conclusions he drew from some minute indication made his slower-witted companions believe that he had produced the hypothesis from his inner consciousness; whereas, in truth, the view he enunciated was the direct outcome of some phenomenon accurately observed and carried to a strictly logical conclusion.

He did not choose those cases which exhibited the most perfect conditions for experimental observation; he would watch a patient in the

[1] [81], pp. 154–155.

throes of delirium tremens as he tossed in the padded room, or listen to the laughter of a man with pseudo-bulbar paralysis, or the recurrent utterance of some partly demented aphasic, and from such observation would spring the luminous exposition of a principle. We did not see how much closer he was to the clinical facts than those who talked glibly of "centres" for psychical processes.

He never failed to recognise that the phenomena of aphasia did not stand alone; they illustrated the same principles and were governed by the same laws as other functions of the nervous system. Above all he insisted on the importance of remembering that dissolution occurred first in the most highly organised products of neural or mental activity, leaving the more lowly at liberty to express themselves freely in the resulting symptoms.

The consideration of such facts will help us to classify the phenomena of cases of aphasia on a deeper basis than that of language. To use an expression somewhat loose in this connection, there is loss of certain voluntary actions in some cases of aphasia with conservation of the more automatic—a dissolution affecting more than language processes, and affecting language processes not so much as language processes but as they are some of the voluntary actions. We have to consider speech on this wider basis in order that we may be better able to see how speech is part of mind, and to get rid of the feeling that there is an abrupt and constant separation into mind and speech[1].

§1. CLASSIFICATION OF AFFECTIONS OF SPEECH

Dr Jackson's first clinical lecture in the *London Hospital Reports* for 1864 was devoted to the classification of defects of speech. He laid stress on the importance of separating articulatory difficulties due to paresis of tongue, lips, or palate from true affections of speech. He pointed out that patients with speechlessness due to such paralysis could write, but had difficulty in swallowing, whilst aphasics, who could neither speak nor write freely, could swallow perfectly.

Somewhat later he described cases of speech defect where the patient could not protrude the tongue on being commanded to do so, but could use it perfectly in all such automatic movements as licking his lips[2].

In 1868 the British Association for the Advancement of Science held its annual meeting at Norwich, and M. Broca opened a discussion on aphasia; he was followed by Dr Jackson. Unfortunately no full account of this paper is extant, for the official record gives the names only of the

[1] [81], p. 168.　　　[2] [81], pp. 37, 48, 104.

speakers; but a synopsis appeared in the *Medical Times and Gazette* from which we can obtain some knowledge of the views expressed by Dr Jackson[1]. He said:

Healthy language could be divided into two distinct forms which may be separated by disease:

(1) Intellectual, i.e. the power to convey propositions.

(2) Emotional, i.e. the ability to exhibit stress of feeling.

Intellectual language suffers throughout not only in its most striking manifestations such as words, but also in writing and sign-making. It is the power of intellectual expression by "movements" of any kind which is impaired, those most special, as of speech, suffering most; those of simple sign-making least or not at all.

Emotional language is conserved throughout not only in its most striking manifestations by variations in voice, but in smiles, etc., and in its most simple manifestation by gesticulation.

Here he strikes the note which sets the key of all his subsequent work. Speech, apart from its articulatory aspect, is double, consisting of intellectual and emotional language, and it is the former that is usually disturbed in consequence of cerebral disease. What, then, is the special nature of these defects of intellectual language? Jackson pointed out that patients with affections of speech fell into two groups:

Class 1. Severe cases in which the patient is speechless or nearly so, or in which speech is very much damaged. In the worst of these cases the patient can only utter some one unvarying word or two words of some jargon[2].

Class 2. Cases in which there are plentiful movements, but wrong movements, or plenty of words but mistakes in words.

In this class the phenomena show that speech suffers in proportion to the mental complexity of the task the patient is asked to perform. He is not wordless, and knows what he wants to say; but he uses wrong words, has difficulty in consecutive exposition both by word of mouth and writing, and his speech may be reduced to jargon. The extent to which all these defects are manifested at any moment depends on the nature of the mental processes necessary to the successful carrying out of the task.

Then he asks, "What is the degree of intelligence these patients have?" and expressly guards himself against any implication that language and thought exist separately. "The question," he says, "is

[1] [81], p. 59.

[2] Throughout the whole of Dr Jackson's subsequent papers the term "speechless patient" refers definitely to this class of aphasic. This definition of his use of "speechless" occurs again in the first paper he wrote for *Brain*. ([81], p. 116.)

not 'How is general mind damaged?' but 'What aspect of mind is damaged?'"

(*a*) Sign-making is least affected, sometimes seeming to escape altogether.

(*b*) Writing suffers more or less in nearly every case of defect of speech from disease of the hemisphere, but varies as much as the defect of speech itself does. "Indeed writing, and we may add reading, is the same defect in another form. For in each we have to reproduce motor symbols of the words. Written or printed symbols are 'symbols of symbols.'" The patient who cannot write can usually copy and can often sign his own name when he cannot write anything else. Moreover, he may find no difficulty in copying exactly the contents of a printed document in fluent handwriting although he is quite unable to write any of these words spontaneously or to dictation.

(*c*) Do they know what is said to them? In Class 1, where the patient is speechless except for some recurrent utterance or jargon, they usually do understand; but in Class 2, where they have free but disorderly utterance, they often do not quickly understand words said to them.

(*d*) Can they repeat words said to them? In Class 1 they cannot, whilst in Class 2 they can with or without blunders.

(*e*) They cannot read but they can often understand what is read to them.

He then passes on to show that the general law underlying these disturbances of speech is that voluntary power is diminished with retention of the power to carry out the same movement in a more automatic manner. This is illustrated by the example of the speechless man who was unable to protrude his tongue when told to do so, although he could perform this movement perfectly to lick a crumb from his lips.

These "speechless" patients are not "wordless," for they can swear and even ejaculate appropriately on occasion; a man usually speechless may even at times get out an actual proposition. But the words of a "speechless" patient are not at his disposal for voluntary use; they exist for comprehension and can also be called upon under emotional stress but, like the movement of the tongue, they cannot be reached by the will.

This aspect of the phenomena in speechless patients had been elaborated by Jackson in a previous paper[1]. He says:

In some cases of defect of speech the patient seems to have lost much of his power to do anything he is told to do even with those muscles that are not paralysed.

---

[1] [81], p. 48 et seq.

Thus a patient will be unable to put out his tongue when we ask him, although he will use it well in semi-involuntary actions, e.g. eating and swallowing. He will not make the particular grimace he is told to do, even when we make one for him to imitate. There is power in his muscles and in the centres for the coordination of muscular groups, but he, the whole man or the "will," cannot set them agoing. Such a patient may do a thing well at one time but not at another. In a few cases the patients do not do things so simple as moving the hand (i.e. the non-paralysed hand) when they are told...

Although the difference in the execution of voluntary and involuntary movements is very striking in some cases of loss of speech, the degree of loss of power to utter words must not be taken as a certain index of this difference. ... Anyone who has tried to use the ophthalmoscope in many cases where speech is lost or defective, will find how great the difference is in different cases. ... A few months ago a patient came under my care who could only say "pooh! pooh!" and an examination of his eyes was almost impracticable. He made efforts, but he never did what I told him, whether it was to look in a particular way or to keep his eyes still. Instead of opening them, he opened his mouth or screwed his face, or shut his eyes and could not be got to look in any particular direction, although he seemed to be on the alert to act and was all the time doing something with his muscles. ... Now it may be said that patients do not know what we wish them to do. But (one) patient, when told to look at my finger, seemed to know what was wanted, for when I was about to give up in despair he took hold of my little finger, as I guessed deprecatingly, and as much as to say he knew what was wanted but could not do it. ... It will be observed that a speechless patient who cannot put out his tongue when told will sometimes actually put his fingers into his mouth as if to help to get it out; and yet not infrequently when we are tired of urging him he will lick his lips with it. Now, as a rule, the worst of these patients can generally smile, and all such involuntary processes go on well enough. I say generally, for a physician who has seen many cases of defective speech will be obliged to use the word "generally."

Here we have a clear recognition of the variability of response in all such cases of affection of speech. This variability and uncertainty of obtaining the same result throughout a series of observations is one of the characteristics of defective cortical activity and is responsible for much of the difficulty in recording results of a clinical examination in cases of aphasia.

Not only do the results of any series of similar observations vary enormously, so that at one moment the patient seems to possess a faculty of which he is devoid at the next, but all use of such words as "agraphia," "alexia," "amnesia verbalis," and the like is rendered impossible and highly dangerous to the truth of the record by the selective nature of the loss in any one group of tests.

How, for instance, are we to characterise in one word the condition of the man who can write his name, that of his house, the number and the street, the county and kingdom correctly, and yet cannot do the same for his mother with whom he lives? Is he suffering from agraphia or not? What name is to be applied to the state of a man who cannot read a word of a letter he has received when asked to do so, but who carries out the instructions it contains accurately with regard to time and place? Is he a case of alexia or not? In a similar way the use of the phrase amnesia verbalis lands us in numerous difficulties. Supposing that after the patient has failed to name several common objects he says, when shown the ink, "That's what I should call a china pot to hold ink"— has he amnesia or not? On Jackson's view the significance of such an answer is clear; the disturbance of voluntary speech destroys the power of making the more selective answer "ink" but permits a more descriptive response. What, again, is the condition of a man who cannot draw a "square" when asked to do so, but, asked to draw a "block of wood," at once draws a perfect square?

§2. SUPERIOR AND INFERIOR SPEECH

The idea that speech is a mental process which can be split by disease into emotional and intellectual expression was developed by Jackson into the differentiation of superior and inferior speech.

Figuratively speaking, emotion uses propositions in a largely interjectional manner, that is to say, reduces them to or towards inferior speech. Emotion, as it were, appropriates and subordinates an intellectual utterance[1].

The words uttered by an otherwise speechless patient can be divided into "recurring utterances" and "occasional utterances."

Recurring utterances may be:

(1) Jargon such as "yabby," "me, me committimy, pittymy, loss, deah." They have no propositional value whatever.

(2) Sometimes the utterance is a word such as "man" "awful"— this is not a word to the patient; for, although a single word may have a propositional value to a healthy person, these words have none for the patient. The speechless man's "one" comes out at any time and not appropriately as when a normal person is asked, "How many oranges will you have?" and answers, "One."

[1] [81], p. 163.

(3) The recurrent utterance may be a phrase such as "Come on," "Oh, my God!" These phrases, which have a propositional structure, have in the mouths of speechless patients no propositional value. They are at best interjectional.

(4) It is common for the patient to retain as his sole utterance "yes" or "no," or both these words. To speak is to propositionise, and "yes" and "no" are "proposition-words." But they are not always used for assent and dissent, and in so far they are not propositions and are therefore liable to be retained by the speechless patient. He may utter "yes" and "no" without any sort of application, or even the one when he means the other. But although the actual word used may be incorrect, the tone in which it is uttered and the smile or gesture which accompanies it may correctly express the patient's meaning.

In some cases, however, of loss of speech, there may be a use of "yes" and "no" higher than a mere emotional service; the patient can reply with them. But even in such cases they may not reach the level of normal speech. The patient cannot utter the word in all the ways healthy people can. He may be able to reply "no" to a question requiring dissent, although he cannot say the word when he is told and when he tries to do so.

Occasionally he can not only use "yes" and "no" correctly, but can even repeat them. Here, then, we have propositional speech and voluntary utterance, although otherwise these powers have been destroyed.

Hughlings Jackson then deals with the occasional utterances which may occur in the speech of the aphasic patient. These may be:

(1) Utterances which are not speech, such as swearing and ejaculation. The patient may say, "Oh dear," or, "Bless my life," but cannot repeat them voluntarily. In some people oaths have become very deeply automatic, almost as much so as smiles and frowns; they are, so to speak, "detonating commas."

(2) Occasional utterances may be true, though inferior, speech. A speechless patient said, "Whoa, whoa," when standing by his horse, another could say, "Goodbye," when a friend was leaving the room, and yet neither patient could repeat the word he had used appropriately when asked to do so.

(3) He records still higher degrees of utterance by speechless patients —a woman suddenly asked, "How is Alice getting on?" A man who was asked where his tools were, answered, "Master's." Both of these were of highly propositional value, especially the latter; in neither case, however, could they be repeated or recalled voluntarily. They rose to expression under the influence of great emotional stress.

Passing on to a higher level of utterance he points out that many patients who can say a word such as "Battersea" cannot say either "batter" or "sea." The whole word rises in speech on account of its appropriateness, whilst the two halves are in reality two fresh words in no way required by the circumstances.

Perseveration or "barrel-organism" he refers to automatic repetition analogous to the automatic acts which occur in other states, when the activity of the higher levels of consciousness is reduced, and quotes a case of Dr Buzzard's of high-grade automatic acts following fracture of the base of the skull.

§3. SPEAKING AND THINKING

It is precisely in his handling of the problems of speaking and thinking that Jackson lies furthest from the ideas of the neurologist and anticipates in a remarkable manner the present views of students of language. "Of course," he says[1], "we do not either speak or think in words or signs only, but in words or signs referring to one another in a particular manner.... Indeed, words in sentences lose their individual meaning, if single words can be strictly said to have any meaning, and the whole sentence becomes a unit, not a word heap." We must not forget that in 1866, when this view was put forward, scientists were dominated by the idea that we "think in words." No one had considered that words might disappear in the unity of a sentence, still less that behind the sentence might be a general verbal proposition.

Jackson stated that disease might separate these processes, which lie on the way from thinking to speaking, and that the phenomena of aphasia were analytical examples of the mechanism of normal speech. Moreover, he laid stress on the importance of recognising that there is no such thing as the "faculty" of language and "the use of the word 'memory' in the sense of its being a distinct faculty is likely to lead to confusion." There is no faculty of memory apart from the things remembered. It is necessary to bear these points clearly in mind if we wish to comprehend his attitude towards affections of speech. Their interest for him lay in their value as illustrations of general neurological laws and of the mechanism of normal speech.

It is not enough to say that speech consists of words. It consists of words referring to one another in a particular manner; and, without a proper inter-relation of its parts, a verbal utterance would be a mere succession of names

---

[1] [81], p. 56.

embodying no proposition. A proposition—e.g. gold is yellow—consists of two names, each of which, by conventional contrivance of position, etc., . . . modifies the meaning of the other. All the names in a random succession of words may, it is true, one after the other, excite perception in us, but not perceptions in any relation to one another deserving of the name of thought. The several perceptions so revived do not make a unit. We are told nothing by a mere sequence of names, although our organisation is stirred by each of them. Now a proposition is not—that is to say, in its effect on us—a mere sequence.

When we apprehend a proposition, a relation between two things is given us—is for the moment, indeed, forced upon us by the conventional tricks which put the two names in the respective relations of subject and predicate. We receive in a two-fold manner, not the words only, but the order of the words also[1].

Single words are meaningless, and so is any unrelated succession of words. The unit of speech is a proposition. A single word is, or is in effect, a proposition, if other words in relation are implied. . . . It is from the use of a word that we gather its propositional value. The words "yes" and "no" are propositions, but only when used for assent and dissent; they are used by healthy people interjectionally as well as propositionally. A speechless patient may retain the "no," and yet have only the interjectional or emotional, not the propositional use of it; he utters it in various tones as signs of feeling only. He may have a propositional use of it, but yet a use of it short of that healthy people have, being able to reply "no" but not to say "no" when told. . . . On the other hand, elaborate oaths, in spite of their propositional structure, are not propositions, for they have not, either in the mind of the utterer or in that of the person to whom they are uttered, any meaning at all; they may be called "dead propositions."[2] . . .

Loss of speech is, therefore, the loss of power to propositionise. It is not only loss of power to propositionise aloud (to talk) but to propositionise either internally or externally, and it may exist when the patient remains able to utter some few words. We do not mean by using the popular word "power," that the speechless man has lost any "faculty" of speech or propositionising; he has lost those words which serve in speech, the nervous arrangements for them being destroyed. There is no "faculty" or "power" of speech apart from words revived or revivable in propositions, any more than there is a "faculty" of coordination of movements apart from movements represented in particular ways. We must here say, too, that besides the use of words in speech there is a service of words which is not speech; hence we do not use the expression that the speechless man has lost words, but that he has lost those words which serve in speech. In brief, speechlessness does not mean entire wordlessness[3].

[1] [81], p. 66.　　　[2] [81], pp. 113–114.　　　[3] [81], p. 114.

On the psychical side (we) must look on the condition as one of loss of words used in speech. The expression "loss of memory for words" is too indefinite.... We must, indeed, bear most vividly in mind that the patient has words remaining; it will not do to think of this positive condition under the vague expression that "he retains a memory of words." If we do use such redundant expressions, we must be thorough in our application of them, and say two things: (1) that the speechless patient has lost the memory of the words serving in speech; and (2) that he has not lost the memory of words serving in other ways. In healthy people every word is in duplicate. The experiment which disease brutally makes on man seems to me to demonstrate this; it takes one set of words away and leaves the other set[1].

The words removed are those employed in the formation of propositions; those which remain to the speechless patient are the same words used non-propositionally or in the lowliest form of proposition. Less extensive damage of speech disorders the use of words in such a way, that, the higher or more abstract the proposition, the more likely is the patient to fail, not only in the emission of a correct verbal equivalent, but in the recognition within himself of the full value of the proposition.

§4. INTERNAL AND EXTERNAL SPEECH

One of the greatest obstacles to mutual understanding amongst students of speech has been the diverse use of the expression "internal speech." "Internal speech," "langage intérieur" and "innere Sprache" have not even been used consistently in any one language. But if we combine all the various uses to which these expressions have been put by different writers, we shall find that they have been made to comprehend at least three different processes. They have been used for unspoken speech, as for instance when we move our lips but utter no sound whilst writing; they have been used for the verbal formulation which precedes utterance, and even for those general processes of thought which result in propositions spoken or unspoken.

Fortunately Jackson leaves no doubt in which sense he uses the expression "internal speech" and throughout his writing he remains steadfast to his original definition.

After demonstrating that speech is not simply the utterance of words but is essentially the formation of propositions, he points out that there is no difference in this respect between external and internal speech. He says[2]:

[1] [81], p. 149.   [2] [81], p. 182.

I do not mean that propositionising occurs only when we speak to tell others what we think, but that it occurs when, so to say, we are telling ourselves what we think. Whether "gold is yellow" is said aloud or whether it is thought that gold is yellow, there is propositionising, a relation of images to one another in a particular way.

Jackson thought of internal speech as identical in form and nature with uttered speech except that it was not passed over the vocal organs. He therefore sought for some means of investigating disturbances of internal speech, and believed that writing was invariably defective whenever internal speech was disturbed; writing is the key to the condition of internal speech.

The speechless patient not only cannot speak aloud, he cannot propositionise internally. This is shown by the fact that he cannot write. He may copy accurately, and can copy print in written characters, but cannot express himself in writing. He can say nothing to himself, and therefore has nothing to write. For its character as speech, it matters nothing whether the proposition be said to oneself or spoken aloud.

So, then, the speechless patient has lost speech, not only in the popular sense that he cannot speak aloud, but in the fullest sense; he cannot propositionise in any fashion. If this be really so, we must not say that speech is external thought, for there is no essential difference betwixt internal and external speech. We speak not only to tell other people what we think, but to tell ourselves what we think. Speech is a part of thought, a part in which we may or may not exteriorise. Again, it is not well to say that thought is internal speech, for the man who is speechless (the man who has no internal speech) can think. How well or ill he can think we will discuss later. ... There are two ways in which words serve in thought; speech is but one way, and this, whether it be internal or external, is, physiologically, a function of the left cerebral hemisphere.

Those who do not limit the definition of speech as we have done, would suppose that if a man had lost speech altogether (internal as well as external) there could be nothing further to say about words in his case; for it is sometimes assumed that words serve only in speech. But the cases of persons who have lost speech show that speechlessness does not imply wordlessness; for if I say to a man who cannot speak at all, "gold is yellow" (or anything not difficult or novel to him) he readily understands it[1].

Internal speech and internal reproduction of words are not therefore synonymous. There is a voluntary internal reproduction of words in new and propositional forms which occurs when we write, and there is an automatic internal reproduction

---

[1] [81], p. 82 et seq.

of words in old and acquired forms, or in forms given us when we receive and understand words in propositions spoken to us[1].

Thus, the speechless man can think because he has in automatic forms all the words he ever had; he will be lame in his thinking because, not being able to revive words, he will not be able to register new and complex experiences of things.

To receive a proposition and to form one are plainly two different things. It is true that in each case our own nervous centres for words are concerned; but when we receive a proposition the process is entirely automatic, and unless we are deaf, or what is for the time equivalent, absorbed, we cannot help receiving it. When anyone says to me "gold is yellow," I am, so to speak, his victim, and the words he utters rouse similar ones in me; there is no effort on my part, the revival occurs in spite of me if my ears are healthy. Moreover, the speaker makes me a double gift; he not only revives words in my brain, but he revives them in a particular order—he revives a proposition. But if I have to say "gold is yellow," I have to revive the words, and I have to put them in propositional order. The speechless man can receive propositions, but he cannot form them, cannot speak[2].

Internal and external speech differ in degree only. Such a difference is insignificant in comparison with that betwixt the prior unconscious or subconscious and automatic reproduction of words and the sequent conscious and voluntary reproduction of words; the latter alone is speech either internal or external[3].

Thus both external and internal speech are processes which do not differ from one another in principle; they differ solely in that the one leads to articulatory verbalisation, the other to no utterance except in writing.

But behind these varieties of formulated speech lie more "subjective," more automatic, processes which precede the revival of words. In the next section we shall try to set out Jackson's views of the nature of these processes and the extent to which they are disturbed in the speech of the aphasic.

§5. THE "PROPOSITION" ANTECEDENT TO INTERNAL AND EXTERNAL SPEECH

So far Jackson's nomenclature can lead to no serious misunderstanding. Internal and external speech or their equivalents in other languages have been used with such diverse meanings by various authorities that his clear definition of the use to which he puts these terms cannot lead

---

[1] [81], p. 78.   [2] [81], p. 84.   [3] [81], p. 124.

to confusion. But, when he deals with the processes behind internal speech, his use of the words "subject" and "object" is liable to lead the reader to reject his views incontinently. If, however, an attempt is made to discover the principles underlying such phrases as "subject and object proposition," the observer will find an idea which enables him to understand the phenomena of aphasia and to invent tests which bring out the limits and nature of the loss of speech in any particular case. He says:

In all voluntary operations there is preconception. The operation is nascently done before it is actually done; there is a "dream" of an operation as formerly doing before the operation; there is a dual action. Before I put out my arm voluntarily I must have a "dream" of the hand as already put out. So, too, before I can think of now putting it out I must have a like "dream," for the difference betwixt thinking of now doing and actually doing is, like the difference between internal and external speech, only one of degree[1].

Jackson saw clearly that the process of forming a proposition to be expressed by internal or external speech was a double one. First the mind must be aroused in propositional form and then the words must be fitted to the proposition. The fitting of words to the proposition is internal or external speech, according as it finds utterance to oneself or to the outside world; the process which precedes this is what he called the "subject-proposition."

If we coin the term verbalising to include the whole process of which speech is only the end or second half, we may say that there are in it two propositions: the subject-proposition followed by the object-proposition.... The subject-proposition symbolises the internal relation of two images, internal in the sense that each of them is related to all other images already organised in us and thus it symbolises states of *us*. The object-proposition symbolises relation of these two images as for things in the environment, each of which images is related to all other images then organising from the environment; thus it stands for states of the environment. The two propositions together symbolise an internal relation of images in relation to an external relation of images[2].

At first sight this attempt to divide the formation of a proposition into two stages may appear fanciful hair-splitting. But not only is its truth obvious, but the necessity of some such discrimination will appear to anyone familiar with two languages. A proposition may be built up in the mind and be registered in memory to be uttered indifferently in either language. Whichever language is ultimately the vehicle for its

[1] [81], p. 168.　　　　　　[2] [81], pp. 151–152.

emission there is no feeling of translation, no bias against the proposition making its appearance in one rather than in the other language. Once uttered, however, in one particular language its use in the other is accompanied by a feeling of translation, a bias which not infrequently destroys its freedom of use.

Not only does introspection show the necessity of some such hypothesis, but the phenomena of aphasia cannot be understood without it. For although the process standing directly behind internal and external speech is distinctly affected in the majority of cases of aphasia, it may be less affected than internal and external speech because it is not so definitely verbalised. It is more automatic and aroused by the incoming stream of impressions. Moreover, it serves more closely in the processes of thought than internal and external speech. He says[1]:

For the perception (or recognition or thinking) of things, at least in simple relations, speech is not necessary, for such thought remains to the speechless man. Words are required for thinking, for most of our thinking at least, but the speechless man is not wordless; there is an automatic and unconscious or subconscious service of words.

It is not, of course, said that speech is not required for thinking on novel and complex subjects, for ordering images in new and complex relations, and thus the process of perception in the speechless, but not wordless, man may be defective in the sense of being inferior from lack of co-operation of speech; it is not in itself a fault, it is left unaided.

In many persons the processes of thought are accompanied in part at any rate by internal, and in some, especially the less educated, by external speech. But internal and external speech are not necessary to perfect logical thought, whilst the process called by Jackson "subject-proposition" forms an essential portion of the act of thinking.

Behind this "subject-proposition" stands that mental process included by Jackson under the name of "image" or "symbol"; this forms the subject of the next section and completes his views on speaking and thinking.

§ 6. "IMPERCEPTION" AND THE CONDITION OF THE "IMAGES" IN A SPEECHLESS PATIENT

No aspect of this work exhibits Jackson's peculiar insight more clearly than his treatment of the mental processes which stand behind the birth

---

[1] [81], p. 123.

of a propositional statement. For at a time when everyone assumed that
the destruction of auditory and visual word images was a sufficient
explanation of the phenomena of aphasia, he saw that in the speechless
man these images might be intact.

He divided cases of speech defect of central origin into two groups:
those where images were intact and those in which they were defective.
To the latter he gave the name "imperception" and pointed out that
this state corresponded on the afferent side to aphasia in the word
series. Many years before the invention of the term "agnosia" Jackson
clearly described this condition under the term "imperception" and
illustrated his description with clinical instances.

In many cases met with in practice, aphasia and imperception are
combined; but the great merit of Jackson's observations is the clearness
with which he saw the necessity of separating these two factors in any
particular example. At that time everyone believed that the destruction
of "images" was a simple explanation of aphasia. Jackson showed that
there were affections of speech in which "images" might be defective,
but, on the other hand, they were certainly not abolished in a large
number of cases of aphasia. He says[1]:

We must then briefly consider the patient's condition in regard to the images
symbolised by words. For although we artificially separate speech and perception,
words and images co-operate intimately in most mentation. Moreover, there
is a morbid condition in the image series (imperception), which corresponds
to aphasia in the word series. The two should be studied in relation.

The speechless patient's perception ... (propositions of images) is unaffected,
at any rate as regards simple matters. To give examples: he will point to any
object he knew before his illness which we name; he recognises drawings of all
objects which he knew before his illness. He continues able to play cards or
dominoes; he recognises handwriting, although he cannot read the words written;
he knows poetry from prose, by the different endings of the lines on the right
side of the page. One of my patients found out the continuation of a series
of papers in a magazine volume and had the right page ready for her husband
when he returned from his work; yet she, since her illness, could not read a word
herself, nor point to a letter, nor could she point to a figure on the clock. There
is better and simpler evidence than that just adduced that the image series is
unaffected; the foregoing is intended to show that the inability to read is not due
to loss of perception nor to non-recognition of letters, as particular marks or
drawings, but to loss of speech. Written or printed words cease to be symbols

---

[1] [81], p. 121 et seq.

of words used in speech for the simple reason that those words no longer exist to be symbolised; the written or printed words are left as symbols of nothing, as mere drawings. The simplest example showing the image series to be undamaged is that the patient finds his way about; this requires preconception, that is "propositions of images" of streets, etc. Moreover the patient can, if he retains the propositional use of "yes" and "no" or if he has the equivalent pantomimic symbols, intelligently assent or dissent to simple statements as that "racehorses are the swiftest horses" showing that he retains organised nervous arrangements for the images of the things "swiftness" and "horse"; this has already been implied when it was asserted that he understands what we say to him, a process requiring not some of his words only, but also some of his "images" of things of which the words are but symbols. ...

These facts as to the retention of images are important as regards the writing of speechless patients. The printed or written letters and words are images, but they differ from the images of objects, in being artificial and arbitrary, in being acquired later; they are acquired after speech and have their meaning only through speech; written words are symbols of symbols of images. The aphasic patient cannot express himself in writing because he cannot speak; but the nervous arrangements for those arbitrary images which are named letters are intact, and thus he can reproduce them as mere drawings, as he can other images, although with more difficulty, they, besides lacking their accustomed stimulus, being less organised. He can copy writing and can copy print into writing. When he copies print into writing, obviously he derives the images of letters from his own mind. He does not write in the sense of expressing himself, because there are no words reproduced in speech to express. That series of artificial images which make up the signature of one's name has become almost as fully organised as many ordinary images; hence in many cases the speechless man who can write nothing else without copy can sign his own name[1].

Jackson recognised that in the speechless person we possessed a means of analysis of the processes behind the formation of speech. Images, whether direct or symbolic, together with those unconscious mental processes on which they may depend, remain intact in the speechless patient. He cannot speak, he cannot write, he cannot read, not because he has lost "images" or "memories" of words, but because he cannot propositionise. He has lost the use of words in speech.

Those cases where images are affected suffer from a distinct and definite defect which he calls "imperception." Speechlessness may exist without imperception, and it is from such cases only that we can obtain a clear analysis of the processes which make up speech.

[1] [81], p. 123.

§7. THE MIND OF THE APHASIC

Jackson's method of treating the phenomena of loss of speech entirely from the psychical aspect, robs the question as to the condition of intelligence in the aphasic patient of half its significance. In his Norwich address he laid down that the question was not "How is general mind damaged?" but "What aspect of mind is damaged?" He then proceeded to indicate one by one the changes we have considered in previous sections of this chapter.

But when a man has lost the power of propositionising and cannot speak or write, when both internal and external speech have been destroyed and the process which stands between them and his perceptions is also disturbed, it is obvious, as Jackson points out, that he will be "lame in thinking." The reception of complex and novel propositions demands internal speech for that formulation which must precede their committal to memory. Thus the existence of "inferior speech" is associated with distinctly "inferior comprehension."

Suppose, however, "imperception" is added to the defect of speech, the formation of images, arbitrary symbols and those unconscious processes which precede their development will be disturbed. The "general intelligence" will then appear to suffer greatly; for the mind will be struck, not only on its emissory, but also on its receptive side.

Thus Jackson saw that the question was not one of loss of "general intelligence," but the disturbance of certain activities of the mind associated with those lesions of the brain which could affect speech.

§8. SPEECH AND CEREBRAL LOCALISATION

It is not to be wondered at that a man who held these views on aphasia and analysed the phenomena exhibited by the speechless patient in this manner remained incomprehensible to his contemporaries and even to the younger generation. The air was thick with schematic representations of centres of all kinds; there were "auditory," "visual,"and "motor-word centres," "centres" for writing and naming, and even for ideation. He says:

It is well to insist again that speech and words are psychical terms; words have of course anatomical substrata or bases as all other psychical states have. We must as carefully distinguish betwixt words and their physical bases, as we do betwixt colour and its physical basis; a psychical state is always accompanied by a physical state, but, nevertheless, the two things have distinct natures. Hence we must not say that the "memory of words" is a function of any part of the nervous system, for function is a physiological term[1].

A method which is founded on classifications which are partly anatomical and physiological, and partly psychological, confuses the real issues. These mixed classifications lead to the use of such expressions as that an idea of a word produces articulatory movement; whereas a psychical state, an "idea of a word" (or simply "a word") cannot produce an articulatory movement, a physical state[2].

The anatomical substratum of a word is a nervous process of a highly special movement of the articulatory series. That we may have an "idea" of a word it suffices that the nervous process for it energises; it is not necessary that it energises so strongly that currents reach the articulatory muscles. How it is that from any degree of energising of any kind or arrangement of any sort of matter we have "ideas" is not a point we are here concerned with[3].

The notion that movements or cerebral nervous arrangements for them serve in mentation is grotesque. The statement is that a word, a psychical thing, is concomitant with discharges of certain cerebral arrangements representing one or more articulatory movements—and that words serve in mentation[4].

From his first paper in 1864 throughout the whole series he emphasises the psychical nature of the phenomena of loss of speech. These changes in mental activity are associated with material destruction of the cerebrum, but it is fallacious to attempt to localise the various activities into which speech may be analysed by introspection, or by disease, in various portions of the cortex. He says[5]:

Whilst I believe that the hinder part of the left frontal convolution is the part most often damaged, I do not localise speech in any such small part of the brain. To locate the damage which destroys speech and to localise speech are two different things. The damage is in my experience always in the region of the corpus striatum.

He also pointed out that the nearer the disease lay to the corpus striatum the more likely is defect of articulation to be the striking feature of the case; whilst the further off the disease lies from this part, the more likely will the main characteristic be mistakes in words.

In his Norwich address in 1868 he pointed out that affections of speech of cerebral origin could be divided into two classes:—Class 1 in which the patient is speechless, or nearly so, or in which speech is very much damaged; Class 2 in which there are plentiful words but mistakes in words. In the first class the disease tends to lie in the neighbourhood

---

[1] [81], p. 114.   [2] [81], p. 108.   [3] [81], p. 85.

[4] [81], p. 177.   [5] [81], p. 81.

of the corpus striatum, whilst in the second class it reaches further back or deeper in the brain.

Even in 1866 he indicated the fundamental error in Broca's localisation of the "faculty of speech" and the "memory of words." In an extract from the *Bulletin de la Société anatomique* for July 1863[1], Broca says, "Pour expliquer comment un aphémique comprend le langage parlé, sans pouvoir cependant répéter les mots qu'il vient d'entendre, on pourrait dire qu'il a perdu, non la mémoire des mots, mais la mémoire des moyens de co-ordination que l'on emploie pour articuler les mots." Jackson takes up this definition[2], and points out that the use of the word memory in the sense of its being a distinct faculty is likely to lead to confusion. The speechless man understands because words remain to him in as far as they are excited from without; he cannot speak because he has lost the service of words in propositions. The words he retains in non-propositional forms may be perfectly articulated. To say that he has lost "la mémoire des moyens de co-ordination que l'on emploie pour articuler les mots" when he can still articulate some words, is most misleading. Moreover Broca entirely missed the significance of the fact that the speechless man cannot write.

Jackson believed that the automatic service of words was associated with activity of the right hemisphere. In right-handed people the left hemisphere was the leading one and subserved the use of words in propositional forms; it also had its lower use in the automatic service of words. The lower, more automatic activities were centred in both hemispheres; but the left alone possessed the power, sequent to its neural action, of exciting words in propositional forms.

I think the facts of cases of loss of speech from damage to but one—the left—half, show conclusively that as regards the use of words the brain is double in function. But the very same cases show that the two hemispheres are not mere duplicates in this function. Both halves are alike in so far as each contains processes for words. They are unlike in that the left alone is for the use of words in speech[3].

Summary

In spite of its occasional obscurity, Jackson's work is of peculiar importance to the neurologist of to-day, both as a practical guide to an understanding of the clinical phenomena of aphasia and, theoretically, because of his conception of the processes which underlie the production of speech. I have attempted to present his views as a coherent whole,

---

[1] [21], p. 399. [2] [81], p. 55. [3] [81], p. 81.

and for every statement to be found in my account of his work a reference has been given to one or more of his papers. But in consequence of the fortuitous manner in which many of his views were presented, there is much repetition, and some of his most valuable conceptions appear amongst a good deal that is no longer of importance to us.

It will be well, therefore, to sum up the points in which Jackson's observations and views can help us to-day. In this summary I shall begin with those points of more practical importance in revealing the clinical phenomena of aphasia, and shall end with those of more theoretical significance.

(1) In 1868 Hughlings Jackson pointed out that patients with aphasia could be divided into two main groups. In Class 1 the patient was almost speechless, or, at any rate, speech was gravely damaged; but in the worst of these cases he can utter some one or two unvarying words or jargon. Class 2 comprises those who have "plentiful words," but habitually use them wrongly.

(2) The loss of power to carry out an order depends on the complexity of the task. The more abstract the conception the more likely is the patient to fail in executing it, although he may succeed when it is put before him in a simpler and more descriptive form. Thus the patient who could not find the word "kitten" called it a "little fur-child," and one who could not draw a square when asked to do so, drew a perfect square when told to draw a "block of wood." It is more important when asking an aphasic patient to carry out some order, to present it to him if possible in several forms, noting accurately his response in each case; because a man cannot write the alphabet we must not assume he cannot write a letter.

(3) The higher and voluntary aspects of speech tend to suffer more than the lower or automatic. The least voluntary speech is that which is emitted under the effect of emotion, such as exclamations, oaths, and words, such as "good-bye," rising to utterance under the impulse of a moment. In many cases "yes" and "no" can be used appropriately as propositions, and even words or phrases of true propositional value may spring to the lips of the aphasic patient. But in such cases he is usually unable to repeat at will the phrase he has just used under an appropriate impulse. The "speechless man is not wordless," and the apparent inconsequence of observations on persons with aphasia, is to a great extent removed by an analysis of the conceptual value of the words and phrases which are actually uttered.

(4) Writing is affected, not as a separate "faculty," but as a part of the failure to propositionise in words. There is no such condition as pure

"agraphia." A man who cannot write spontaneously may be able to copy printed matter in perfect handwriting. The "faculty" of relating handwriting to print is intact; he cannot write voluntarily because he has lost the use of written words in propositions. Hence he can usually write his name and address, because in most of us this has reached with time more nearly the level of an automatic act.

(5) Patients with such affections of speech may not be able to read aloud or to themselves when asked to do so; but they can understand what is read to them and may even obey written commands although unable to reproduce them in words. This is not due to some loss of function called "alexia," but to an inability to reproduce a proposition which, on the other hand, they may be capable of receiving accurately.

(6) "Imperception" (agnosia) is on the receptive side what aphasia is in the "word series." In many cases the two conditions are combined; but they may exist separately, and where aphasia is present without "Imperception," images remain intact. Thus the patient may be able to point to colours and objects when they are named; he continues able to play cards or dominoes, he recognises handwriting, although he cannot read the words written; he knows poetry from prose by the different endings of the lines on the right of the page.

Thus affections of speech are caused (a) on the emissive side by inability to form or to express a proposition in words, (b) on the receptive side by failure of those mental processes which underlie perceptual recognition.

(7) External and internal speech are identical, except that the one leads to the utterance of articulated words, whilst the condition of internal speech can be discovered by writing only.

(8) Behind external and internal speech stands the proposition which, when verbalised, can be expressed in speech or writing.

This proposition is necessary for clear and logical thought, but not for all thinking. When this aspect of speech is affected the patient cannot retain a sequence of abstract propositions because he is unable to formulate them at will to himself. He can think, but he is "lame in thinking."

(9) If, however, "Imperception" (agnosia) is added to such defect of speech the patient will not only suffer from "Inferior Speech" but will show signs of "Inferior Comprehension."

(10) In the majority of cases of affections of speech mental images are unaffected. This extremely important contribution to the theory of aphasia has been entirely neglected by neurologists. For almost every hypothesis propounded in the last forty years presupposes some defect in "auditory" or "visual word images."

CHAPTER IV

THE DIAGRAM MAKERS

§1. THE ENGLISH SCHOOL

JACKSON'S earlier papers excited universal interest amongst that band of young Englishmen who were attracted to the novel study of the structure and functions of the nervous system. In 1862, he had been appointed to the National Hospital for the Paralysed and Epileptic, which had been recently founded, and came under the influence of Brown Séquard, then practising in London. Here, those who worked in the wards became familiar with the most recent advances in French medicine, not only from the teaching of this renowned physiologist and clinician, but in daily intercourse with his relative and famulus, Victor Bazire, the translator of Trousseau's lectures, then in charge of the electro-therapeutic department.

At first, Jackson's insight and clinical industry caused his name to be cited by all the writers on aphasia, alongside that of Broca; but gradually they began to complain that he was obscure. They failed to comprehend why he denied the existence of a centre for the faculty of speech, and why he contended that the loss of function consisted in failure to formulate a proposition. For after all no one could deny the categorical existence of speech, reading and writing; and if anatomical localisation were a fact, these various human aptitudes must be disturbed more or less independently by lesions of specific centres and their commissural fibres.

In 1869, Bastian published his famous paper, which had so profound an influence on the subsequent development of the question[1]. His whole work was founded on the axiom that "we think in words," and that "these words are revived as sound impressions in the auditory perceptive centres of the cerebral hemispheres." He believed "that words become nascent in consciousness primarily and perhaps principally as revived auditory impressions[2]." Based upon this conception he divided the higher forms of the disorders of speech into two main groups, amnesia and aphasia proper[3]. In the former condition the thinking power of the individual is impaired almost in direct proportion to the loss which he experiences in his power of expression. There is a distinct defect in the memory for words, not only for use in articulate speech, but also in silent thought. True aphasia, on the other hand, is a condition in which silent

---

[1] [3]; see also [4].   [2] [5], p. 619.   [3] [3], pp. 214–216.

thought is possible; the words are revived as sound impressions in the auditory perceptive centres. But, when this thought has to be spoken articulately, impulses arising from these revived impressions must be transmitted to the more immediate motor centres for speech. In the same way, when the individual attempts to write, the revived sound-perceptions call up visual impressions, which are transmitted to the motor centres for the hand.

In *amnesia*[1] there is an inability to recall words, i.e. they cannot properly be revived in the auditory perceptive centres, and there is an almost proportional impairment of the thinking power. Now it would appear that this condition must be due either to some abnormal state of the auditory perceptive centre itself, where words have to be revived, or else to some defect in those portions of the cortical grey substance, which have to do with the exercise of that marvellous power of voluntary recall of past impressions to consciousness, which occurs in the processes of recollection. In this condition we obviously have to do principally with defects of the cortical grey matter of the hemispheres, rather than with defects of afferent or efferent fibres connecting this with lower nerve centres. But in *aphasia*, as we have seen, the individual is able to think and understand what is said to him, though he cannot express himself either by speaking or writing. Now, we can well imagine that this will be precisely the condition of a person in whom those efferent fibres are damaged (and functionally inert) along which the motor stimuli are wont to pass that primarily incite those combined muscular contractions necessary, for speech on the one hand, and for writing on the other. There being no notable injury to the cortical or convolutional grey matter, the individual can carry on processes of thought as before, and the afferent fibres not being damaged, he can understand what is said to him. But he cannot translate his thought into articulate speech or into written language because the first part of the path along which the motor stimulus would have to pass, in order to incite the necessary combined muscular movements, is broken up or damaged. A lesion of both these sets of fibres in any part of their course between the cortical grey matter and the corpus striatum, or in this body itself, would therefore produce such a result. Just so, a lesion of either one of these sets singly, would produce the corresponding simple condition of which aphasia is compounded.

He then proceeds to explain that if the fibres emerging from the auditory centre were injured in any part of their course, the individual would be able to think and to write, but not to speak. If, on the other hand, the damage destroys efferent fibres from the visual centre alone, the patient would be able to speak, but could not express himself in writing.

[1] [3], p. 478.

Ogle[1] had already described agraphia, and had laid down that the loss of power to write might belong either to the amnesic, or to what he called the "atactic group" of disorders of speech. In the former, the patient writes a confused series of letters which have no apparent connection with the words intended, whilst, in the latter case, all attempts to write result in a mere succession of up and down strokes bearing no resemblance to letters. This view was woven by Bastian into the texture of his theory that all high-grade disorders of speech are due either to the destruction of the auditory and visual centres, or to some affection of the fibres transmitting impressions between them and the lower motor mechanism for the tongue and lips, or for the hand in writing.

Here we see the origin of the conception that disorders of speech can be classified as affections of independent centres, or of the paths between them. It inevitably led to the production of a diagram[2]. As each case arose, it was lopped and trimmed to correspond with a lesion of some cortical centre or hypothetical path. Bastian early developed the idea that the so-called motor centres of the cortex were in reality sensory in function; they were occupied with the appreciation of the data of "muscular sense" and were therefore what he called "kinaesthetic." Thus, his well-known diagram showed not only an auditory and a visual word centre, but also one for the tongue and one for the hand, which he spoke of respectively as "glosso-" and "cheiro-kinaesthetic[3]."

By the time his book was issued, he and his followers had come to believe so firmly in this form of a priori explanation, that in any case of speech defect they thought it was possible to foretell the situation of the lesion with perfect assurance. Four pages are therefore devoted to a list of the clinical manifestations and the site and the nature of the lesion which produces them.

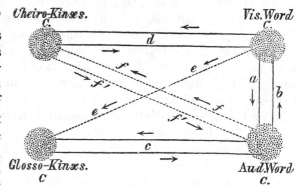

Fig. 1. A diagram illustrating the relations of the different word centres and the mode in which they are connected by commissures. The connections represented by dotted lines indicate possible but less habitual routes for the passage of stimuli. From Bastian [8], p. 106.

For eighteen years, at University College Hospital, Bastian had demonstrated to generations of students a man who had been seized with

---

[1] [112],   [2] The first diagram seems to have been that of Baginski [2].
[3] [6], p. 937 and [8], p. 106.

loss of speech in December, 1877[1]. On each occasion the famous diagram
was drawn and we were told what commissural fibres were affected, and
why the visual centre must be intact, although that for hearing was in a
state of lowered vitality. But, alas, the post-mortem examination revealed
unexpectedly profound changes. The whole of the area supplied by the
middle cerebral artery, with the exception of that of its first cortical
branch, showed the grossest destruction. The angular and supra-marginal
convolutions had disappeared together with the superior temporal, excepting only its anterior third; the superior and inferior occipital convolutions were intact, but the atrophy had extended into the middle
occipital convolution; the trunk of the middle cerebral and all its branches
were blocked. Much of the posterior segment of the internal capsule
together with the greater part of the thalamus had disappeared; anteriorly the atrophy had extended into the white substance up to the
corpus striatum which was also much diminished in size. No wonder
Bastian admitted that "the difficulties in reconciling the persistent and
often-verified clinical condition with the post-mortem record are extreme." He did not recognise that what he called the "clinical condition" was nothing more than a translation of the phenomena into
a priori conceptions, which had no existence in reality.

    Moreover, all this school of observers believed that they could interpret
the clinical manifestations directly in terms of anatomical paths and
centres; each one added one or more cases to those that had already
become classical. Thus, Bastian's first paper contained two original
observations only. It was an era of robust faith and nobody[2] suggested
that the clinical data might be insufficient for such precise localisation;
still less could they believe that the conclusions reported by men of
eminent good faith might be grossly inaccurate. In reading these admirably written papers, we are astonished at the serene dogmatism with
which the writers assume a knowledge of the working of the mind and
its dependence on hypothetical groups of cells and fibres.

    But we must not forget that Bastian was the first person to describe
"word-deafness" and "word-blindness"; in 1869, he wrote as follows[3]:

Most aphasic patients can understand perfectly what is said to them, and can
follow and feel interested when they hear others read aloud. In these cases we may
presume that the afferent fibres connecting the auditory centres of the medulla
with the auditory perceptive centres of the cerebral hemispheres and also these
latter centres themselves are intact, so that the spoken sounds revive their accustomed

---

[1] [7]; see also [8], p. 254 et seq.
[2] The sole dissenting voice was Maudsley [102].
[3] [3], p. 482.

impressions in the hemispheres, these being perceived as words, symbolic of things or ideas, which being duly appreciated by the individual as they are conjured up, suggest to him the thoughts which they are intended to convey. In certain of the severe cases of aphasia however, as in that recorded by Dr Bazire and in Dr Gairdner's case, it is distinctly stated that the patient either did not gather at all, or with difficulty and imperfectly, the import of words when he was spoken to, although he could be made to understand with the utmost readiness by means of signs and gestures. Must we not suppose that in such a condition either the communication of the afferent fibres with the auditory perceptive centres is cut off, or that this centre itself, in which the sounds of words are habitually discriminated and associated with the things to which they refer, is more or less injured? In either of these cases, though the sound is not appreciated as a word having its definite meaning, we must not expect that there would be deafness; the sound would be still heard as a mere sound, only it does not call up that superadded intellectual discrimination, by the ingrafting of which upon it, it can alone be made to serve as a symbol of thought. Hence the individual does not adequately comprehend when spoken to, though he may be quite capable of receiving and appreciating fully the import of sounds and gestures, which make their impression upon his visual perceptive centres. ... And[1], where the individual cannot read, I am inclined to think that this must be owing either to some lesion of the afferent fibres to the visual perceptive centre, of the visual perceptive centre itself, or of the communications between the cells of this centre and those of the auditory perceptive centre. If lesions existed in either of the first two situations, the visual impression could not receive its intellectual elaboration, and consequently it could not call up its associated sound (word) in the auditory centres, and hence no meaning would be conveyed by the hieroglyphic marks of the printed or written pages. They would be to the person mere meaningless strokes, just as we have assumed that if similar defects existed in the auditory perceptive centres, or in the afferent fibres with which they were connected, the individual could not appreciate the meaning of spoken words; these would be to him mere sounds.

Broadbent accepted this view of the auditory and visual centres, insisting however on the dual aspect of word formation; words are not only articulate sounds, but also serve as symbols of an idea. In spite of his admiration for Jackson's teaching, he was constitutionally inclined to a mechanical view of disorders of speech. He held[2] that "if the nervous system is the instrument of language and of thought, then the objective aspect of the operations concerned in what are subjectively mental processes will be changes in cells and fibres, and we shall understand the physiology of intellectual operations only so far as we can represent them in terms of cells and fibres."

[1] [3], p. 484.   [2] [16], pp. 145–146.

He restated the close functional relation of the act of articulate speech with "that part of the upper edge of the fissure of Sylvius, which forms the posterior end of the third frontal convolution of the left hemisphere[1]," and asserted that he had never met with a single example of the opposite kind. This portion of the cortex is not the seat of a faculty of language, "but simply a part of the nervous or cell and fibre mechanism, by means of which speech is accomplished, which mechanism may be damaged elsewhere above or below this particular node[2]." He insisted that to look for a lesion in precisely the same part of the hemisphere in amnesia and aphasia could only lead to confusion. The formation of motor word or sound-groups and their intellectual elaboration are two entirely different and independent processes. The latter is the result of the convergence of impressions from the various perceptive centres upon an intermediate cell-area in the super-added convolutions, where they are combined and elaborated into an idea of which the word is a symbol.

In 1879, Broadbent[3] reported a beautiful case of "jargoning" aphasia and accompanied his comments by a diagram. This contains an auditory centre and one for executive speech, united by a commissure. But the most remarkable feature is that "naming" and "propositioning" are separated from one another and to each is assigned a centre at a higher level in the hierarchy than that for hearing or for speech. He was led to this conclusion from the fact that his patient could formulate ideas but could not express them or name objects correctly.

As the result of his beautiful dissections, Broadbent[4] had already arrived at the conclusion that "the convolutions which are not in immediate relation with crus, central ganglia or corpus callosum by means of fibres are those of the island of Reil, those on the under-surface of the temporo-sphenoidal lobe and of the orbital lobule, those on the flat inner aspect of the hemisphere, and those along the middle of the convex surface of the hemisphere from the occipital extremity as far forwards as the first ascending parietal gyrus."

Now these convolutions, he argues, are the latest in order of development, and "on this ground alone might be supposed to be concerned in the more strictly mental faculties, which are the latest in their manifestation.... It would, moreover, seem to accord with the general plan of construction of the nervous system and with what we know of the mental operations, that these convolutions which are withdrawn, so to speak, from direct relation with the outer world, should be the seat of the more purely intellectual operations, receiving the raw material of thought

[1] [16], p. 172.   [2] [16], p. 174.   [3] [17].   [4] [16], p. 178.

from the convolutions on which sensory impressions impinge, and employing for the transmission outwards of the volitional product those convolutions which are in communication with the motor ganglia and tract."

Thus, he mapped out by indirect means those portions of the cortex which must contain the perceptive centres for hearing and vision. But it was Ferrier's[1] experimental researches that led the English school to place the auditory centre in the first temporal convolution, whilst that for vision was located in the supra-marginal and angular gyri. To Broca's area

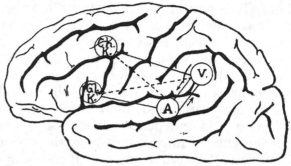

Fig. 2. Diagram showing the approximate sites of the four word centres and their commissures. From Bastian [8], p. 19.

was assigned the glosso-kinaesthetic centre, whilst that for writing was placed in the posterior portion of the second frontal convolution.

§2. THE GERMAN SCHOOL

Flourens taught that all parts of the cerebral hemispheres were equally endowed with those functions proper to them. Vision, hearing, memory and voluntary action disappear step by step with ablation of the cortex and, although no sense-organ is thereby totally deprived of sensibility, all specific perceptions are destroyed. Perceptions and the will depend on the integrity of the cerebrum exactly as coordination of voluntary movements is the result of cerebellar activity. As a corollary to this conception he held that any part of the hemispheres could carry on, to a greater or less extent, the general functions exercised by the whole; conversely, when the surface of the brain was gradually sliced away, all of them were more or less affected.

This doctrine had a profound effect on physiology and continental medicine for nearly fifty years; and in spite of Jackson's demonstration of the nature of those convulsive seizures which bear his name, the cerebral hemispheres were held to be an inexcitable mass of nervous tissue with uniformly distributed functions.

In 1870, Fritsch and Hitzig succeeded in producing isolated movements of various muscle groups by electrical stimulation of certain spots

[1] [46], p. 445.

on the surface of the brain. Excision of these areas was followed by disorders of motion in the same parts of the body and they concluded that some, and probably all, psychical functions depend for their material existence on the activity of certain circumscribed centres in the cerebral hemispheres. From the very first they insisted that these were not strictly "motor," but were concerned with the mental aspect of the muscular act.

Ferrier[1], instigated by Hughlings Jackson, entered the experimental field in 1873 and profoundly influenced the English school; he localised the site of Bastian's auditory centre in the temporal lobe, but unfortunately placed that for vision in the region of the angular gyrus. Munk followed in 1877, and determined the true position of the visual centre in the occipital lobes, adding the conception of "mind-blindness" ("Seelenblindheit").

Meanwhile Goltz asserted, as the result of his experiments, that the same disturbance of motion, sensation and vision followed extirpation of any part of the hemispheres; the more extensive the destruction the graver was the loss of function, and he believed that his observations were incompatible with the theory of specific cortical centres. Thus every school of clinicians could draw experimental support from the statements of one or other of these observers.

Germany had just emerged victorious from her war with France and the awakened national consciousness influenced even so remote a subject as cerebral physiology. In 1874, Wernicke[2] published his pamphlet entitled *Der aphasische Symptomencomplex* based entirely on the work of his fellow-countrymen. The names of Ogle and Jackson are cited, but in such a way that it is evident he had not read their papers; Bastian he consistently ignores.

Wernicke's theory of the nature of aphasia was the direct outcome of Meynert's researches on the projection systems of the cortex. This observer was able to show by tracing afferent tracts, particularly the visual fibres, to their expansion on the hemispheres, that the posterior part of the brain was "sensory" in function[3]. Conversely, by following centrifugal paths, the anterior portion appeared to be obviously "motor." But, since the cerebrum is essentially the organ of consciousness, these "motor" centres must be occupied with conceptions of movement, whilst the "sensory" areas are the seat of memory images of sense

[1] [45], and [46].   [2] [129].
[3] In order to understand how the temporal lobe is included in the "posterior" part of the brain, vide Wernicke's diagram ([129] p. 19).

impressions. The actual cells of the cortex are neither motor nor sensory, but have one fundamental property, the power of receiving impressions; their diverse functions depend upon the nature of the apparatus with which they are connected by projection fibres, either centripetal or centrifugal. The vital process within them is in nature identical.

Following up this reasoning Wernicke placed the auditory centre, the seat of sound memories, in the first temporal convolution and the conceptual basis of articulated speech in Broca's area. He then proceeded to construct a diagram with commissures and incoming and outgoing paths, deducing from it the phenomena which should follow interruption at each point in this mechanical system. Every part of this hypothetical representation he endowed with profound and definite functional significance. A lesion of the first temporal convolution, by destroying the auditory centre, must abolish "sound-images" ("Klangbilder") and so lead to want of understanding of spoken words. At the same time the patient cannot name objects and shows aphasic defects in speaking because he cannot appreciate and correct his faulty utterances. This form of "sensory" aphasia can be recognised by the flow of words and lack of auditory recognition. It is accompanied by agraphia, but the educated patient can understand print though he cannot read aloud.

Destruction of the third frontal convolution, the seat of images of movement for articulated speech, leads to "Broca's aphasia." The patient is more or less dumb, but can understand all that is said to him both orally and in print. Should the commissure between these two centres be interrupted, he can understand everything in whatever manner it may be presented to him; but his choice of words is restricted, he cannot read aloud and usually is unable to write.

Ten cases are cited in support of these deductions; of these the first was a good example of auditory imperception that ended in recovery. There is nothing to indicate the situation of the lesion and yet Wernicke considers he is justified in "assuming a focal lesion in the first temporo-sphenoidal convolution[1]." Of the remaining examples it can only be said that the clinical records are inadequate, or the details of the post-mortem findings unconvincing.

In his text-book[2], published in 1881, Wernicke makes no attempt to justify his theory by an appeal to observation. The diagram with its two centres and commissural paths appears again and the clinical forms of disordered speech are deduced from it as from a figure in Euclid[3]. These are now four in number: (1) Motor aphasia, equivalent to the aphemia

[1] [129], p. 46.   [2] [130].   [3] [130], p. 205.

of Broca, due to destruction of the third frontal convolution. The patient can utter at most a few words only, but can understand all forms of speech. (2) Conduction aphasia, due to interruption of the paths between the two centres. In this form there is no lack of words but they are misapplied; understanding is perfect. (3) Sensory aphasia[1], produced by destruction of the auditory centre in the first temporal convolution. The number of words is unlimited and words are wrongly used, but the most important symptom is complete inability to comprehend oral speech. (4) Total aphasia; here both expression and comprehension of speech are destroyed in consequence of a lesion comprising both centres.

Wernicke was completely satisfied with his attempts to deduce the clinical manifestations from hypothetical lesions; every unprejudiced person will be convinced, he says, how firmly the facts support the theory. In 1903, he published "A case of isolated agraphia[2]"; no better example could be chosen of the manner in which the writers of this period were compelled to lop and twist their cases to fit the procrustean bed of their hypothetical conceptions. Such a title can only mean that in this patient every other act of language could be perfectly performed, except that of writing. But the recorded symptoms show that the patient had much difficulty with spontaneous speech and in comprehending what she read. She was unable to understand some spoken words, nor could she carry out perfectly oral commands. She is said to have shown almost complete inability to write, and it was with great difficulty that she could be brought to make the attempt. She was unable to draw to command, although she could copy drawings and writing. She failed to say the days of the week or the months in their proper order and had forgotten the alphabet and the Lord's Prayer. Wernicke failed to recognise the wide-spread nature of the affection owing to the fixed preconceptions with which it was approached; in the solemn discussion that follows the report we can only wonder at his clinical obtuseness and want of scientific insight.

It is a pleasure to turn from this work to the monograph of Kussmaul, published in 1877 as part of *Ziemssen's Handbuch*[3]. He regards speech as primarily an organised reflex. We become conscious of some thought and are urged by our feelings to express it; we then choose suitable words and say them to ourselves. Finally, we let loose the reflex apparatus, which gives the words an outward form. All verbal expression follows three stages, preparation, internal diction and articulation.

[1] ([130], p. 206.) He will have nothing to do with word-deafness ("Worttaubheit") suggested by Kussmaul ([83], p. 174).   [2] [131].   [3] [83].

The further development of Kussmaul's exposition shows the influence of a remarkable paper read in 1870 by Finkelnburg[1] before a provincial medical society. Asked to compile a report on the fashionable subject of aphasia, he began by pointing out that these disorders of speech were part of a wider disturbance, which he called lack of symbolic representation. He brought forward five cases to show that the conventional manifestations of amnesia and aphasia were accompanied by other morbid conditions, not directly associated with word-formation. All the disorders of function he united under the term "Asymboly[2]"; this consists of inability to express concepts by means of acquired signs, together with want of comprehension of their significance. In fine, it is a more or less profound disturbance of the power to receive or impart knowledge in as far as this depends on sensory symbols. This morbid condition is essentially both motor and sensory and an organic lesion must disturb both aspects of function.

Kussmaul[3] accepts this view and points out that it is incompatible with the existence of a special centre for speech; "we turn away with a smile from all those naïve attempts to seek a 'seat of speech' in this or that cerebral convolution." The cerebral organ is composed of a large number of ganglionic mechanisms widely separated from one another, but connected by numerous tracts and fulfilling certain intellectual, sensory and motor functions; no part of this apparatus subserves speech only. Local lesions of the brain must therefore be associated with some partial damage to this complex group of symbolic activities. We must abandon the old view which regards memory as a special storehouse in the brain where images and ideas lie together arranged in separate compartments[4].

He insists that visual and auditory images may remain unaffected although their symbolic significance can no longer be recognised. Conversely "word-blindness" and "word-deafness" are disorders essentially independent of defects of speech. Unwittingly he adopted exactly Jackson's view of imperception and he gives Bastian full credit for first describing these morbid states.

Unfortunately he was seduced into constructing a diagram[5]; but his views were not susceptible of schematic formulation and the figure was of such complexity that it failed to make a general appeal. It lacked that definite localisation of centres and paths demanded by the popular taste; but Kussmaul's monograph can be read with profit to-day for its shrewd insight into the problems of disorders of speech.

¹ [48].   ² [48], p. 461.   ³ [83], pp. 33, 127.   ⁴ [83], p. 36.   ⁵ [83], p. 182.

On the other hand Lichtheim's paper, which was greeted with enthusiasm and issued simultaneously in German and English, reads like a parody of the tendencies of the time[1]. It was definite and precise; his famous diagram was easily reproduced and every form of aphasia could be anticipated by postulating destruction of one of its centres or commissural paths. Even a dominant centre for consciousness was not forgotten. Seven forms of disordered speech were built up categorically from this figure. But, when the actual records of cases were examined, lamentable deficiencies were discovered; sometimes the clinical manifestations ran counter to those expected. "In a large number of instances, however, the probability is that they do really belong to one of two forms. But one readily obtains examples in which this is not the case; they seem to differ in one point or another from these morbid types. Do they constitute a serious objection to my theory? I do not think so; most of them can be shown to be reducible to the schema[2]."

Here we have the high-water mark of this school of thought. It enabled teachers of medicine to assume an easy dogmatism at the bedside and candidates for examination rejoiced in so perfect a clue to all their difficulties. But serious students could not fit these conceptions of aphasia to the clinical phenomena; incredulous of such scholastic interpretations, they lost interest in a problem of so little practical importance.

Most of the observers mentioned in this chapter failed to contribute anything of permanent value to the solution of the problems of aphasia, because they were dominated by a philosophical fallacy of their day, which can still count its victims amongst writers on the subject. They imagined that all vital processes could be explained by some simple formula. With the help of a few carefully selected assumptions, they deduced the mechanism of speech and embodied it in a schematic form. For every mental act there was a neural element, either identical with it or in exact correspondence. From diagrams, based on a priori principles, they deduced in turn the defects of function which must follow destruction of each "centre" or internuncial path. They never doubted the validity of their postulates, based as they were on the rules of human reason.

They failed to appreciate that the logical formulae of the intellect do not correspond absolutely to physical events and that the universe does not exist as an exercise for the human mind. To them an explanation that appealed directly to reason must of necessity correspond to the

---

[1] [86], and [87].   [2] [86] p. 464.

facts of observation; the form assumed by the manifestations of organic disease could be therefore confidently anticipated from study of a well considered diagram. They believed that a simple explanation must conform more closely to reality than one so complex that it defies the ordinary means of human expression. Lip service was paid to the theory of evolution; but they could not conceive that the intellect of man was not a paramount and all sufficing instrument for resolving the riddle of the universe.

These observers used analysis as their instrument. So far they were right; but most of them fell into the subtle error of assuming that the elements reached by analysis could be treated as independent entities, which had entered into combination. They thought they had got hold of the sole and ultimate factors in mind and life, and all that happens must be capable of statement in these terms. They did not doubt the completeness of the analysis or its finality.

Hence all psychological problems were stated in terms of sensory processes or laws of association. When difficulty was found in applying these conceptions to action, "kinaesthesis" and "motor" presentations were invented to fill the logical gap.

Most of the English school, accustomed to the positive philosophy of the day, started axiomatically with the idea that we think in words. When the Germans entered the field they found it thickly strewn with theoretical assumptions, both positive and negative. Diagrams were multiplied until the subject of aphasia became the despair of the clinician, especially if he had been trained in the vigorous physiological atmosphere of the 'eighties. The time was ripe for a ruthless destruction of false gods and a return to systematic empirical observation of the crude manifestations of disease.

CHAPTER V

MARIE THE ICONOCLAST

IN 1906 Pierre Marie startled the medical world with three papers in the *Semaine Médicale* on "Revision of the Question of Aphasia[1]." The first of these bore the aggressive title, "The third frontal convolution does not play any special rôle in the function of language." In his second communication he fell foul of the popular conceptions of sub-cortical aphasia, whilst the third was a fascinating historical essay on Broca and his times; this contained an account of a re-examination of the hemispheres of Broca's two first patients, still preserved in the Musée Dupuytren.

Marie attacked the orthodox doctrines of aphasia from two aspects: he denied the validity of the clinical observations on which the symptomatology of the various forms had been erected, and refused to acknowledge the current views concerning their cerebral localisation.

Now before it is possible to determine the anatomical basis of a disorder of function, it is obviously necessary to make certain of its nature and clinical manifestations. Observers had complacently accepted the whole paraphernalia of belief in the fundamental importance for the genesis of aphasia of motor, visual and auditory word-images. Sub-cortical destruction was supposed to produce a distinctive group of manifestations, whilst lesions of the cortex, by interfering with motor or sensory centres, were associated with demonstrably different disorders of speech. These and many other analogous beliefs were founded on a priori considerations and the actual manifestations were twisted into more or less conformity with these preconceptions. Marie's criticism passed like a harrow over a weed-choked field and I shall therefore begin with an exposition of his views on the nature of aphasia in general, before considering his treatment of anatomical localisation.

He insisted that every true aphasic shows some want of comprehension of spoken words. The patient, it is true, may carry out a simple command to close his eyes or to put out his tongue; but, if the difficulty of the task is increased, he will ultimately fail to execute it correctly. This insistence on the necessity for graduating the tests employed was an advance of the first importance.

[1] [97], [98] and [99].

Secondly, in every case of aphasia intellectual capacity is diminished as a whole. The patient is in no sense demented, but he shows an inability to carry out many operations which are not an integral part of speech. He cannot solve simple problems in arithmetic, or is unable to imitate actions performed silently in his presence. Marie gives as an instance of such loss of intellectual aptitude a professional cook with slight aphasia who failed to produce a dish of fried eggs.

Wernicke's or "sensory" aphasia consists essentially of such loss of intellectual capacity. This is not a disturbance of mental power as a whole, but a defect of all those intellectual operations which are concerned with the use of language in its widest sense. The patient has difficulty in understanding what is said to him, in reading, in writing and in executing many other simple acts spontaneously or to command. But he can talk; speech, it is true, may be hampered by his defective processes of thought, yet he can find words in which to express himself, however haltingly.

The "aphasia of Broca" is this condition plus what Marie called "anarthria." In this composite form all the symptoms of a true aphasia just described may be present to a greater or less degree, but in addition the patient cannot talk. He is dumb, or utters a few ejaculatory words only; in addition, he cannot read or write with ease.

The most adventurous part of Marie's theory was his use of the term "anarthria." This defect of function does not consist solely of articulatory troubles, or of a disturbance of the motor power in the tongue or lips; it comprises loss of control of all those complex mechanical aptitudes which are employed in the exteriorisation of language. Anarthria has, however, no direct affinity with aphasic manifestations. It can exist alone, and if so internal speech is intact; the patient can understand what is said to him, can read, can write and his intellectual capacity is in no way diminished. Such a condition, corresponding to the "subcortical motor aphasia" of other observers, can be evoked by a lesion of either hemisphere.

Thus, according to Marie, there is only one true or primary aphasia, that of Wernicke, characterised by some loss of intellectual aptitude. When to this is added "anarthria," we have the syndrome known as "Broca's aphasia." But "anarthria" can exist alone and has nothing to do with the phenomena of aphasia, for the intellect remains completely intact.

Such views necessitated a complete revision of the prevailing ideas concerning cerebral localisation of speech. Marie developed his two lines of attack on the current doctrine simultaneously, but it is more convenient to arrange his arguments in their natural sequence rather than to follow the order in which they were published. He traced the historical development of the view that the third frontal convolution was the centre for speech and showed on what flimsy grounds it was based. He re-examined and described the hemispheres of Broca's two first patients, preserved in the Musée Dupuytren. The lesion in Leborgne[1] far exceeded the limits of the third frontal; it destroyed the lower half of the Rolandic convolutions, the greater part of the first temporal and, to a considerable extent, the supra-marginal gyrus. That is to say, the loss of tissue included not only the third frontal, but also Wernicke's zone. This was exactly the lesion predicated by Marie for the composite syndrome known as "Broca's aphasia." The second brain revealed no definite local lesion, but was probably an example of the changes which accompany senile atrophy[2]. The base of the second frontal convolution was considerably diminished in size and on the surface there was one of those collections of serous fluid so common in the wasted brains of the aged.

This examination of the original specimens destroyed the historical basis of the doctrine that aphasia was of necessity associated with a lesion of the third frontal convolution. For in the first case the destruction was far more extensive and in the second there was little evidence that the loss of tissue affected this area to any preponderating degree.

Marie did not attempt to attack the question of cerebral localisation of function at the root. Although he denied the validity of the current conceptions of "sensory word-centres," he allowed that what he called true aphasia was caused by lesions in the region of Wernicke's zone. If, in spite of defective power to employ language, the patient could still articulate, the destruction of tissue would probably be found somewhere in the neighbourhood of the supra-marginal, angular and posterior portion of the upper temporal gyri. There are, however, no separate centres for the visual or auditory aspect of words and no areas of the cortex where a localised lesion produces pure alexia or agraphia. Whenever Wernicke's zone is destroyed, the loss of capacity extends over a wide range of intellectual functions. The patient can talk, but shows more or less inability to understand spoken words, to read, to write, to solve problems in arithmetic and to perform other actions not usually associated by clinicians with the use of language.

On the other hand, pure anarthria, consisting of loss of speech

---

[1] [99], p. 565.

[2] This statement was denied by Dejerine ([43], pp. 1005–1006) who described a lesion of both the second and third frontal convolutions.

uncomplicated by any diminution in intellectual capacity, is the result of sub-cortical lesions in what Marie called the "lenticular zone" either of the right or the left hemisphere. This extensive area includes the insula, claustrum, external and internal capsule, the nucleus caudatus and lentiformis.

The "Aphasia of Broca," a combination of true aphasia with anarthria, depends on destruction both of this lenticular zone and of Wernicke's area of the cortex or the sub-cortical paths passing to and from it in various directions.

Dejerine, as the representative of the current views, at once took up the challenge and responded with two papers, "L'aphasie sensorielle et l'aphasie motrice[1]." He failed to appreciate the radical nature of Marie's destructive criticism and concentrated his attention on the more anatomical aspects of the question. He began by stating that motor and sensory aphasia are universally admitted, together with the existence of a zone of language containing motor and sensory images of words. To-day, he asserted, there is no dispute about the motor aphasia of Broca and the sensory aphasia of Wernicke. Since everybody is agreed on these points, researches on aphasia aim at the study of certain special disorders of language, with motor or sensory symptoms, designated sub-cortical or "pure" aphasia, in which internal speech remains intact; these comprise pure motor aphasia, pure word-deafness and pure word-blindness.

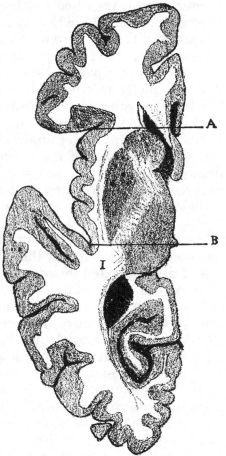

Fig. 3. To show the "quadrilateral" of Pierre Marie in horizontal section. It comprises the structures between the lines *A* in front and *B* behind. From Moutier [104], p. 145.

All psychologists, neurologists and alienists admit the existence of language images and the defects of intelligence universally recognised in all aphasias of cortical origin are due to the suppression or loss of such

[1] [36].

images. On the other hand, sub-cortical lesions produce forms of pure aphasia in which intelligence remains completely intact.

After these vast assumptions, he turned to the anatomical questions raised by Marie's views on the cerebral localisation of the various forms of defective speech, subjecting the use of the term "anarthria" and the limits of the "lenticular zone" to severe criticism. He failed, however, to recognise that, apart from any questions of localisation, Marie denied the validity of the current ideas concerning motor and sensory aphasia, language images, word-blindness, word-deafness and the conception that there were separable centres in different parts of the cortex for the use of words.

In 1908 appeared Moutier's monograph[1], in which he gave an interesting history of our knowledge of aphasia, followed by an authoritative statement of the nature and symptoms of disorders of speech from the point of view of his master Pierre Marie. The second part of the book is prefaced by a scheme for examining patients, which is singularly complete and far in advance of any set of systematic tests in common use. Moutier also described a number of examples of aphasia where a careful post-mortem examination was carried out in the laboratory of Bicêtre. But in most of them the loss of power to use language was so gross that they threw little light on the different forms of disordered function, and the organic destruction was too extensive and profound to demonstrate the finer points in dispute with regard to cerebral localisation. Most of the cases are frankly acknowledged to conform to a mixed type of combined aphasia and anarthria, due to a correspondingly diffuse lesion usually situated in sub-cortical areas of the left hemisphere.

By this time the difference of opinion in Paris had become so acute, that three sittings of the Société de Neurologie (June 11, July 9, and July 23, 1908)[2] were devoted to a discussion of the nature and causes of aphasia. Although a strenuous attempt was made to keep the clinical and pathological aspects of the question apart, this was impossible in practice. Anatomical data perpetually intruded on the consideration of the various forms actually assumed by these disorders of speech, and the discussion on the locality of the cerebral lesions was frequently interrupted by the description of signs and symptoms.

The debate opened with the following question, "Are motor and sensory aphasia clinically different from one another, or is motor aphasia simply sensory aphasia accompanied by anarthria?" This was followed by a discussion on the significance of Marie's use of "anarthria" and

---

[1] [110].　　　　　　　　　[2] [43].

the justification for the separation of pure motor aphasia from that form with agraphia and alexia. Can we say that motor aphasia exists as a primary manifestation, or is it the residue of a complete aphasia where partial recovery has occurred? Finally, what is to be understood by "total aphasia" and how often do we actually encounter "total aphasia," "sensory aphasia," "motor aphasia of Broca" and "pure motor aphasia"?

As might have been expected, a debate on these lines led to much repetition by the two protagonists of the arguments they had brought forward on previous occasions. Marie held strictly to the views he had originally expounded. There is one true aphasia only, that known by the name of Wernicke and called by the opposing school "sensory." A cerebral lesion can also produce a disturbance of the higher aspects of articulation, which has nothing to do with aphasia and must be classed as an "anarthria." Broca's aphasia, on the other hand, is a complex syndrome due to the coexistence of these two morbid conditions.

Dejerine defined his position as follows[1]: The aphasia of Broca is a motor aphasia and is accompanied by lack of words, marked defects in writing and some alexia, though this is not excessive. Any trouble that may exist on the sensory side is very slight compared with that found in "sensory aphasia," which is characterised by "word-blindness" and "word-deafness." "Total aphasia" is a combination of the motor and sensory forms. He laid great stress on the fact that a patient with motor aphasia can transcribe print into cursive script, whilst the sensory aphasic is unable to do so, copying servilely letter by letter. He attacked the use of the word anarthria, which should, he contended, be kept for definite troubles of articulation, such as occur in pseudo-bulbar paralysis.

Ballet pointed out the essential difference between want of power to evoke words and a true anarthria or articulatory defect, suggesting that motor aphasia was in reality an apraxia. Marie[2] replied that the anarthric patient had no difficulty in evoking a word, but solely in pronouncing it, and agreed to substitute the term "aphemia," provided the meeting would acknowledge that anarthria was not associated with any disturbance of internal speech.

Meanwhile Souques[3] argued that it was futile to divide aphasia into motor and sensory, for all true aphasics showed want of comprehension of spoken or written words together with more or less agraphia; the difference is one of intensity and not of quality. On the other hand, anarthria is an independent morbid condition, which may supervene on these manifestations in consequence of a subsequent cerebral lesion and

---

[1] [43], p. 614.   [2] [43], p. 628.   [3] [43], p. 615.

so produce what is known as "total aphasia." André Thomas agreed that motor and sensory aphasia merged into one another, but contended that the differences between them could be discovered by studying the more extreme forms.

Dupré[1] struck the first frankly psychological note in the discussion. He insisted that motor aphasia was not a trouble in articulating words, but a difficulty in discovering the correct verbal expression. All aphasia, whether motor or sensory, is a psychical defect of the use of language; anarthria, on the other hand, is a motor syndrome and a disorder of speech. In a case of aphasia the motor images of the word are recalled with difficulty; its kinaesthetic representation becomes impossible owing to interference with associations and other habitual modes of recall.

Before considering the debate which followed on anatomical localisation, it will be well to summarise shortly the results of the latter half of the third sitting devoted more strictly to the nature of these disorders of function. In reply to the question, "Are these disturbances of intelligence both in motor and sensory aphasia, and if so what form do they take?" Marie[2] re-stated his views on the evident diminution of intellectual capacity in all true aphasia, whether of the Wernicke or Broca type. All such changes are absent in cases classed by him as "anarthria." This loss of intellectual capacity is in no sense a dementia or affection of the mind as a whole and requires for its discovery careful and direct examination. It is a specialised defect concerned not only with the use of language, but also with other forms of knowledge acquired didactically. Marie therefore proposed the term "intellectual" instead of "sensory" to describe the loss of function in Wernicke's aphasia.

Ballet replied that, when an aphasia was said to be "sensory," the disturbance was always presumed to be psychical, and Dupré[3] pointed out that the disorder of function consisted essentially in a want of collaboration of sensory and psychical elements. The word "sensory" serves to designate the highest activity of the elaborated image possessing a symbolic value. On the material side, this view does not prevent the acceptance of special sensory centres, which are situated in the neighbourhood of the receptive foci for the visual or auditory elements involved; this total area forms the "zone of language." Aphasia does not result from destruction of a stock of images deposited in different localities of the brain, but is due to changes in the mechanism by which the elements constituting these images are evoked and associated with one another.

[1] [43], p. 630.   [2] [43], p. 1031 et seq.   [3] [43], p. 1033.

Marie[1] expressed his readiness to accept "language images," if they were supposed to represent the psychological aspect of acts of language, but he denied that they could be "localised" in different anatomical centres. Dejerine[2] asked if internal speech was possible without such images and re-asserted his belief in the existence of two varieties of word-blindness, one of which, associated with agraphia, was a true "sensory" aphasia with a centre in the angular gyrus; the other was a "pure" word-blindness accompanied by right hemianopsia and no other defects of any kind. This was produced by a lesion destroying the fibres passing to the visual centre.

Souques[3] pointed out that we know nothing of these verbal images beyond the fact that, when we read, write or talk to ourselves silently, we hear the words of our internal speech. The so-called "images" are not sensory, but essentially intellectual phenomena. The "word-deaf" hears the words, but does not understand them; the "word-blind" sees them and cannot comprehend their meaning. It is consequently impossible to localise these "images" in the cells of different areas of the brain; for, in reality, they exist only at the moment of recall and are simply memories, that is, manifestations of intellectual activity.

The second meeting and the first half of the final one were devoted to an attempt to settle the lesions responsible for the various forms of aphasia. But, as no satisfactory and unanimous clinical definition had been reached during the earlier phase of the debate, the greater part of the time devoted to anatomy was spent in discussing the limits of Marie's "lenticular zone" and its justification. He repeated his view that destruction within this "quadrilateral" caused a pure anarthria; on the other hand, a lesion of the posterior part of the "language area" or the fibres which supply it causes a true aphasia, that is, an intellectual change.

Nothing could have been more unfortunate than his original statement that the third frontal convolution played no part in the production of aphasia. This pronouncement, so startling and subversive to those who held the classical conceptions, was in reality of secondary importance in view of his main doctrine. For, if he could have established that there is but one form of aphasia due to destruction of Wernicke's zone and that the defects of speech due to lesions elsewhere are anarthric, the smaller question of the functions of the third frontal convolution and its relation to his lenticular area would have been swallowed up in the larger hypothesis. As it was, he laid himself open to a brilliant attack by Mme Dejerine[4], who gave a learned and convincing demonstration on

¹ [43], p. 1038.   ² [43], p. 1044.   ³ [43], p. 1039.   ⁴ [43], pp. 977–990.

the anatomy of this region of the brain and the constitution of the
"quadrilateral" area. She pointed out that any lesion of its upper,
anterior and external parts must cut fibres from the third frontal convolution. Motor aphasia, she concluded, was dependent on destruction,
cortical or sub-cortical, of fibres issuing from the front portion of the
zone of language; sensory aphasia, on the other hand, was due to a lesion
in Wernicke's area. Dejerine added that this could be split up still
further; the centre for visual word-images was situated in the angular
gyrus, whilst that for word-hearing occupied the posterior part of the
first and second temporal convolutions.

Marie fought hard for simplification and made a bold attempt to sweep
away the vast concretion, which obscured the nature of these disorders
of speech. He saw that the clinical manifestations were psychical defects
and attributed them to "intellectual" changes. This led to profound
misunderstanding and he was obliged to insist repeatedly that aphasics
suffered from a specialised loss of intellectual capacity and not from a
dementia, although the abnormal responses covered a wider ground than
is usually attributed to misuse of language.

As a corollary he ejected from aphasia all examples of pure anarthria,
true verbal apraxia and other cases where articulation was at fault. This
was a useful distinction. But he refused to acknowledge the existence of
"motor" aphasia, asserting that the clinical manifestations so described
were either a form of anarthria or a combined syndrome, consisting of
this defect of speech with the addition of true aphasia. Thereby he undoubtedly fell a victim to his desire for theoretical simplification.

When examining a case of aphasia, we must investigate systematically
the patient's power to speak, to understand what is said to him, to read
and to write. No one of these acts is solely and exclusively affected in
any one instance; the disturbance of these "intellectual" functions is
distributed more or less over the whole group. This tendency to massive
rather than to specialised defects is, according to Marie, characteristic
of true aphasia.

Before it is possible to "localise" the site of the anatomical destruction,
it is necessary to classify the various forms of aphasia in psychical terms
and not in those of some lower or more elementary function, such as
motion, vision, or hearing. Nobody suggested any such categories and
the greater part of the discussion became a verbal battle. Had the dis-
putants been familiar with the work of Hughlings Jackson, they would
have recognised that, from the point of view of the question at issue, all
such expressions as "motor aphasia," "Broca's aphasia," "total aphasia,"

"word-blindness" and "word-deafness" did not correspond exactly to any fundamental groups of clinical phenomena. Since no satisfactory agreement was reached on this head, the debate on the anatomical site of the various lesions responsible for aphasia ended inconclusively. Marie held to his original opinion that destruction of Wernicke's zone was alone capable of producing true aphasic manifestations, whilst Dejerine adhered to the conception that motor, visual and auditory defects were evoked respectively by lesions of the frontal, angular and supra-marginal gyri.

CHAPTER VI

CHAOS

§1. HENSCHEN AND ANATOMICAL LOCALISATION OF FUNCTION

MARIE'S simultaneous attack, both on the nature and causes of aphasia, rudely disturbed traditional belief in the classical doctrines. His views aroused violent and often unreasoning opposition; but, especially after the publication of Moutier's monograph, many observers accepted his destructive criticisms, although they rejected the full consequences of his theory.

The whole problem of disorders of speech was thrown into the melting pot and each worker was free to take up an individual position. This state of chaos was emphasised by the fact that the leaders in this field of research held views which were mutually incompatible. Some, like Henschen, assumed the strictest parallelism between anatomical structure and the use of language. On the other hand, von Monakow, applying his doctrine of diaschisis to defects of speech, showed that aphasia and amnesia, like apraxia and agnosia, were temporary disorders of function, which tended to diminish greatly if the lesion remained stationary. Moreover, an acute exacerbation of the disease might produce manifestations far exceeding in severity and extent any loss of function that could be attributed directly to the injured portion of the brain. This makes it impossible to establish a strict and detailed relation between the site of the anatomical lesion and the specific forms assumed by the defects of speech. The incursion of Liepmann into this field and his attempt to classify disorders of speech as forms of apraxia and agnosia also shook the foundations of traditional belief and offered a new and at first sight plausible explanation of the phenomena.

Further, as the result of more careful investigation, auditory and visual imperception in man turned out to be less simple than "mind-deafness" and "mind-blindness" as described from experiments in animals. Closer examination of the pathological records also showed that there was little or no evidence to justify belief in the existence of pure "word-deafness" or "word-blindness," apart from true imperception. For isolated words do not form the units of thought or even of speech.

Gradually a tendency grew to regard disorders of speech from their mental aspect. Stress was increasingly laid on the psychological factors in the use of language and to a limited extent this method was applied to the phenomena of aphasia. But it was not until the war produced unique examples of local wounds of the brain accompanied by definite defects of speech that this line of research was utilised fully in clinical cases.

I found it impossible to give a consecutive account of these mutually incompatible ideas and have therefore selected one aspect of the subject for consideration in each section of the present chapter, attempting as far as possible to correlate the observations of the different workers in the same field. By this means alone is it possible to give any account of the cross-currents of thought to which the problems of aphasia have been subjected since Marie first put forward his subversive ideas.

Henschen was the first to show that limited lesions of the area striata produced distinct local defects of the visual field. This portion of the cortex, which has a special structure, lies within and around both lips of the calcarine fissure and extends to the pole of the occipital lobe. Destruction of the upper part of this area on the one side produces a defect of vision in the lower quadrant of the opposite half of the field and vice versa. This undoubted fact, which has been amply confirmed by the study of gun-shot injuries during the war[1], led Henschen to conclude that each retina is represented point by point on the surface of the cortex in the calcarine region and that this forms the primary centre for sight. Here visual impulses are received, transformed and redistributed to other portions of the cortex, to participate in responses of ever-increasing complexity.

For many years Henschen strove to discover the analogous receptive centre for hearing, which had been loosely assumed to lie somewhere in the upper part of the temporal lobe. By the investigation of pathological cases, where the lesions could be strictly localised, he determined that the primary centre was situated in the gyrus transversus (Heschl's convolution) and not in either the first or second temporal.

Impressions, whether of sight or hearing, are received within these specialised sensory areas and transmitted respectively to other parts of the occipital or temporal lobes, which contain centres for the elaboration of higher psychical processes. Here, by new transformations, more complicated reactions are built up to form elementary factors in the production of thought. Such a theory demands the existence of many different centres not only of diverse function, but of separate locality, where these new and various combinations can take place.

[1] [78].

Granting these postulates, it is obvious that even such high-grade acts as reading and writing, which depend primarily on vision and hearing, can be analysed into a series of stages; these differ not only in functional complexity, but in the cortical locality where they are worked up mechanically. Thus, by examining an extensive series of cases where the autopsy revealed a well localised lesion, it should be possible to discover the anatomical site of the centres engaged in manufacturing the highest psychical products out of these primary sense elements.

Henschen therefore undertook the colossal task of abstracting the records of every case of aphasia, sensory or motor, together with their subsidiary forms, which contained a sufficiently detailed description of the post-mortem appearance[1]. Each group of anatomical lesions was then presented in tabular form together with the recorded symptoms and an attempt was made to discover some correlation between them. He started with the anatomical facts and deduced from them the specific functional disorders for which they were responsible.

"Sensory" disorders of speech are considered under the headings of temporal, angular and occipital aphasia, according as the lesion was situated within one of these portions of the hemisphere. Henschen concludes that within the left temporal lobe there are two sharply defined centres, one of which in the gyrus transversus (Heschl) is associated with general hearing, whilst the other is responsible for the auditory comprehension of words. He insists on the importance of recognising that these two centres are anatomically and functionally separable. A bilateral lesion of the gyrus transversus produces inability to appreciate the meaning of sounds, whilst destruction of the posterior and middle portion of the first temporal convolution on the left side is commonly followed by "word-deafness." This he defines as inability to understand spoken words with perfect comprehension of the significance of sounds and for this condition he proposes as far as possible to substitute the term "speech-deafness."

A lesion of this "word-hearing" centre produces a special form of disordered speech; the patient cannot recall the expressions he requires and uses wrong or misformed words. He cannot repeat or understand what is said to him, although he may be able to read to himself or to write. But since most temporal lesions are diffuse, the optic radiations are liable to suffer and the pure clinical picture is then disturbed by complications such as "word-blindness" and "agraphia."

---

[1] [73 a, b and c.]

Destruction of tissue confined to the cortex of the angular gyrus is followed by "word-blindness." This defect, which consists essentially of inability to read words, may assume various forms and arise in several different ways. Thus, for instance, the patient may be unable to appreciate the significance and use of an object shown to him; he is in fact "mind-blind" and suffers from visual agnosia. Or the want of understanding may be confined to words and letters; such pure "word-blindness" is peculiarly associated with lesions of the angular gyrus, which forms the essential "reading-centre." Occasionally this variety of alexia is complicated by right hemianopsia, due to destruction of the fibres of the optic radiators which lie just below the surface in this region.

Lesions of the occipital lobe produce a more complex series of disorders, all of which depend fundamentally on disturbance of visual impulses. The patient may be "mind-blind" or incapable of understanding what he sees, although sight is otherwise intact; his want of comprehension may be confined to words and letters, or he can suffer from pure "agraphia." All these morbid conditions are found independently of one another and Henschen therefore assumed the existence of at least three separate centres in the occipital lobe, apart from the primary visual centre in the neighbourhood of the calcarine fissure. In addition he felt compelled to postulate one for the visual appreciation of figures and still another for reading and translating into action musical notes.

Clinically, articulated speech, repetition and the comprehension of spoken words are not materially disturbed by occipital lesions. But the power of understanding what is read and of writing spontaneously or to dictation is more or less diminished. In every instance where it was looked for, copying was grossly affected, whether the "agraphia" was otherwise partial or complete.

In addition to these varieties of "sensory" aphasia, Henschen came to the conclusion that the so-called "trans-cortical" form, due to a lesion situated between the principal groups of centres, "seems to stand on an assured basis." It is characterised by "word-deafness" associated with intact power of repetition; that is to say, the patient is capable of hearing the words although he does not understand them.

Before passing to the much debated question of the effects produced by lesions of the frontal lobe and the deeper parts in the neighbourhood of the Sylvian fissure it is necessary, he says, to adopt a clear and definite nomenclature. Many authors employ the terms aphasia, aphemia, anarthria and dysarthria without describing exactly the nature of the defects of articulated speech. Verbal expression is a complex manifestation demanding, according to Henschen: (1) an impulse from the auditory or visual speech centre; (2) its transmission to the motor centre; (3) from this a motor impulse passes by way of motor paths to the bulbar nuclei; (4) these in turn innervate the peripheral mechanism of speech.

After long and elaborate analysis he comes to the conclusion that the first and second frontal convolutions play no serious part in the mechanism of articulated speech. On the other hand, the foot of the third frontal forms a psychical centre for these movements. It acts as a kinaesthetic station of a high order, where impulses from the sensory speech areas are regulated and combined before they pass on in the cortico-bulbar tracts. Thus, a lesion of the cortex in the third frontal region produces a want of power of coordinating letters and syllables to form words; the patient knows what he wants to say, but cannot find the suitable forms of verbal expression. He has forgotten the movements of speech; to this high-grade motor loss of function, Henschen prefers to apply the term "aphemia."

On the other hand, under the terms "anarthria" and "dysarthria," he includes solely that condition in which words well known to the speaker cannot be perfectly enunciated or phonated; speech fails because of defective vocalisation and not from lack of vocal memory. This is not an aphasia and, although at times it may be so severe as to result in mutism, is not associated with lesions of the third frontal convolution.

These two forms of defective speech are profoundly different in origin and can be distinguished pathologically and clinically. A lesion confined to the lower portion of the third frontal produces aphemia; but, if it also affects the adjacent parts of the precentral gyrus, this is accompanied by dysarthria, for the operculum Rolandi is known to be the centre for the organs of speech such as the lips and tongue.

Are "word-deafness" or "word-blindness" always associated with true aphemia; that is to say, does the patient of necessity fail to comprehend what is said to him or what he reads to himself? This is one of the most vexed questions in the symptomatology of motor aphasia. Henschen concludes that a lesion of the frontal lobe, even when extensive, does not lead to "word-deafness" unless the temporal lobe or its connecting fibres are destroyed. Although the patient may be almost mute, he can understand what is said to him and execute oral commands, provided the destruction of tissue is confined to the frontal lobe. On the other hand, as far as "word-blindness" is concerned, some true aphemias of frontal origin may be accompanied by "alexia" and yet the power of writing is usually retained.

This led him to a comprehensive study of the pathological conditions which are attended with "agraphia." On the sensory side, inability to write may be produced by a lesion either of the occipital or angular region, which causes some variety of "word-blindness," by a lesion of the temporal lobe associated with "word-deafness," or by destruction of the conducting paths between the various centres. In addition, a parietal lesion may cause apraxia and so be responsible for profound changes in writing. But apart from all these factors, Henschen came to the conclusion that there was definite anatomical evidence for the exist-ence of a "writing centre" in the second frontal convolution, which could be separated from the motor speech centre in the base of the third frontal. He rejected the view of Dejerine, enunciated long before by Jackson, that a disturbance of writing was mainly an expression of disorders of internal speech.

Henschen was fully aware of the steps by which an aphasia of frontal or even more complex origin either increases in severity or recovers. Mutism may gradually pass away until nothing remains but a scarcely perceptible aphemia, or a slight "motor" defect may deepen into in-ability to utter a word. The intervening stages, either in an upward or downward direction, follow a definite law and are almost exactly the converse of one another.

He holds as an axiom that this restitution of speech, when it occurs, is often due to the activity of the opposite hemisphere[1]. Normally in right-handed persons the right half of the brain is a vast uncultivated field, which plays a subservient or secondary part in the mechanism of speech. Impressions received by the sensory surfaces are worked up by centres of the left hemisphere into factors, which underlie the highest forms of logical thinking. These are transferred to the opposite side, to be stored up as unconscious memories in this special seat of latent and automatic psychical activities. Under normal conditions centres in the right hemi-sphere are responsible at most for affective or interjectional speech; but as the result of suitable education and training they may play a material part in the re-acquisition of power to employ language.

In spite of the enormous labour and care expended on this analysis of cases of aphasia and kindred disorders of speech in the light of the ana-tomical lesions discovered by post-mortem examination, Henschen's method suffers inevitably from several grave defects. He repeatedly complains of the insufficient nature of the clinical data. Sometimes the most important details were entirely omitted. This can arise from the

[1] [73 c.], p. 294 and [73 b.], p. 113.

fact that a considerable number of patients who become the subjects of an autopsy are not suitable for the finer methods of clinical examination. Or it may be that, although the condition on admission to the hospital was carefully recorded, the patient remained subsequently for months or years without sufficient further investigation to determine whether his state at death corresponded to that set out in the earlier records. A still more tantalising fault is the employment by the observer of comprehensive terms, such as "paraphasia," "word-blindness," "agraphia," and others of a like kind, without indication of the exact form assumed by the disorder.

But frequently the fullest and most detailed reports cannot be summarised in tabular form[1]. The patient may have been able to carry out simple orders, but not those which were more complex; he could read with understanding, provided the word did not contain a command to act, or he was able to write his name but not his address. Can such a case be tabulated as one of "word-deafness," "alexia" or "agraphia"? Comprehension of spoken words, reading and writing were possible under certain conditions, but not if the task was rendered more difficult or made to assume a less familiar form.

Another serious hindrance to this method of anatomical analysis arises from the transitory nature of the phenomena[2]. Even with severe and permanent destruction of tissue the first grave symptoms may in great part pass away; the patient recovers his power to speak, to understand what is said to him, to read, or to write at any rate to a considerable extent. For some time before death the report states that no trace of aphasia could be discovered.

Moreover, capacity to execute the various tests may vary from time to time; it is a common observation in the best observed cases that on a certain day tasks could be executed with ease, which were otherwise quite impossible. Familiar surroundings, friendly people, sympathetic handling and the mode of examination have a profound effect on the results obtained, a fact which has been widely neglected.

In spite of these difficulties in fitting the clinical manifestations into the rubric of anatomical terms, Henschen propounds the most extreme views of cerebral localisation. He not only upholds the classical separa-

---

[1] Consider, for instance, the case reported by Henschen himself with limited destruction in the third frontal region (No. 18, vol. V [73 a.], pp. 21, 22) and his comments upon it (vol. VII [73 c.], p. 302).

[2] "The tables can never give an exact expression of the changing symptoms of aphasia." (Preface to [73 c.].)

tion of the varieties of aphasia into "word-blindness," "word-deafness" and the motor forms, but constructs a diagram[1] showing centres for speaking in the third frontal, for writing in the second frontal and for reading in the angular gyrus. He starts from the idea that there are different speech centres, more or less independent of one another[2], and states that "every cell or cell-complex is endowed by education with a special capacity to receive, to store up, and then to compare visual, auditory and tactile images or perceptions with new impressions." When we learn to read or acquire the use of a language, "engrams" are written in appropriate brain-cells "as the form of a seal is impressed upon wax." Functional or organic disturbances of these "word-cells" are followed by "word-deafness," "word-blindness," or some abnormal form of constructive speech.

Such extreme mechanical conceptions have been adopted by few observers, although Mingazzini[3] and his school have strongly supported Henschen's anatomical views. But however much we may differ from the conclusions drawn from this vast pathological material, it is of fundamental importance to know the situation of the various lesions which can disturb the use of language and we can frequently gather, even from the insufficient clinical records, the main features assumed by the disorder of speech.

Round and round like a stage army moves the procession; the clinical appearances are identical, but each fresh group of observers views them with new eyes and with different preconceptions. It is often possible to recognise through the hazy reports and diverse classifications some salient point which indicates the identity of a past case with one under observation to-day. It is therefore of fundamental importance to learn the site and nature of the anatomical lesion which produced such a condition and we shall always be grateful to Henschen for his wonderful collection of data. They form a catalogue and commentary to all the pathologically documented cases of aphasia, invaluable to those who attempt to work at this difficult subject.

§2. VON MONAKOW AND DIASCHISIS[4]

It is impossible to appreciate von Monakow's contribution to the problem of aphasia without considering his views on cerebral localisation.

[1] [73 c.], Tafel 1.   [2] [73 c.], p. 161 and [73 b.], p. 206.   [3] [103].
[4] This short summary of the views of Professor von Monakow is the result not only of study of his writings but also of conversations with him in September, 1922, during a visit which I paid to Zürich for this purpose.

After many years spent in unusually careful clinical and pathological investigations, closely associated with physiological experiments on the functions of the central nervous system, he arrived at conclusions which differed fundamentally from those generally accepted at the time. These he put forward as a coherent whole in his monumental work *Die Lokalisation im Grosshirn* published in 1914[1].

The key-note of his position is given by the universally recognised fact that the local symptoms, which immediately follow a non-progressive lesion, are severer, more extensive and often less sharply determined than is the case after the expiration of some days or weeks. Moreover, these initial manifestations may differ profoundly in character from the residual consequences of irreparable anatomical destruction. Thus, an operation upon the cortex and sub-cortical tissues may be immediately followed by a total flaccid hemiplegia accompanied by loss of sensation so gross that it would appear to be the result of a mid-brain lesion. After many weeks or months these temporary signs pass away and the clinical phenomena come to correspond more nearly in form to those consonant with injury of the higher cerebral centres.

Most authors sought to bring these initial manifestations into direct connection with the anatomical changes, which we know to occur in the neighbourhood of a cerebral injury; for every lesion of the brain is notoriously accompanied or followed by circulatory disturbances, oedema and secondary inflammatory changes. Moreover, all operative procedures produce more extensive damage than the surgeon will confess and the mechanical effects of an apoplexy cannot be measured by the amount of the effusion of blood.

As the initial symptoms gradually give place to those which remain as the permanent consequences of the anatomical destruction, they undergo what appears to be a fundamental change in character. At first the affected limbs are toneless and the reflexes may be abolished; a cortical lesion can be followed by defects of function, which are of sub-cortical or even of spinal origin. Goltz and his school laid stress on these phenomena and attributed them to inhibition radiating from the site of the injury. They cannot be explained by anatomical destruction of cortical or adjacent structures alone; for not only is the loss of function extremely gross, but it is transitory, although the lesion may be permanent. Nor, according to von Monakow, is it sufficient to say that the initial symptoms are due to "shock," a term which comprises many different conditions.

[1] [107].

The central nervous system is composed of a series of cell-groups and fibres linked together by synapses and he believes that the symptoms which follow a local injury can only be explained by some temporary solution of continuity or heightened resistance at these junctions. He therefore spoke of this condition as "Diaschisis" (from $\sigma\chi\ell\zeta\omega$, I separate or rend asunder). This he defined as follows[1]:

Die Diaschisis stellt somit eine meist plötzlich eintretende, auf bestimmte weitverzweigte zentrale Funktionskreise sich beziehende "Betriebseinstellung" dar, die ihren Ursprung aus der örtlichen Läsion nimmt, ihre Angriffspunkte aber nicht (wie der apoplektische Shock) im ganzen Kortex (Strabkranz etc.) sondern nur an solchen Stellen hat, wo aus der Gegend der Läsionstelle fliessende Fasern in primär nicht lädierte graue Substanz des ganzen Zentralnervensystems auslaufen. Es handelt sich auch bei der Diaschisis im wesentlichen um Herabsetzung oder Aufhebung der Anspruchsfähigkeit (Refraktärwerden der Durchgängigkeit) der zentralen Elemente (Neuronengruppen) für Reize innerhalb eines bestimmten physiologisch wohl definierten Erregungskreises; dieser Kreis fällt indessen mit dem gewöhnlichen, von der Peripherie und vom Zentrum aus sich ausdehnenden physiologischen Innervationswege nicht zusammen.

The meaning of this passage may be rendered in the following words:

Diaschisis consists of a suspension of activity, which usually arises suddenly, affecting a widely radiating central field of function. It takes its origin in the local lesion, but, unlike apoplectic shock, does not attack the whole cortex; its incidence falls on those parts only where fibres from the site of the lesion terminate in primarily uninjured grey matter of the whole central nervous system. Diaschisis consists essentially of a lowering or abolition of the power of the central elements (groups of neurones) to respond to stimuli within a definite and physiologically definable zone of excitation; this zone does not, however, correspond with the usual physiological paths of innervation, which extend either from the periphery or from the centre.

The local destruction of brain tissue not only destroys or puts out of action directly certain cells and fibres, but the loss of irritability and cessation of function spreads into neighbouring and closely allied neuronal systems. It extends to the termination or to the origin of each system of fibres involved in the local lesion. Those paths of innervation suffer most severely which are physiologically responsible for the more complex activities, or for those which are less organised by practice[2].

Thus, should the cortex be destroyed in the neighbourhood of the precentral convolution, the wave of diaschisis spreads in the direction of

[1] [106], p. 237 and [107], p. 27.   [2] See diagram [107], p. 32.

the injured fibres, through the mid-brain deep into the spinal segments. On the other hand it radiates along the course of the association fibres into other parts of the cortex of the same hemisphere and, by way of the commissural fibres of the corpus callosum, into the opposite half of the brain. Wherever the directly injured fibres enter into connection with grey matter, however far away from the focus of injury, there diaschisis will exert its effect. It is developed along anatomical lines and acts in an elective manner on those parts where fibres make contact with the central elements of the nervous system. In this respect cells must always be thought of as members of a group, which may be influenced alternately both in a centrifugal or centripetal direction.

Such a conception of the direct effects produced by any destruction of cerebral tissue vitiates most of the anatomical conclusions usually drawn from ablation experiments, apoplexies, injuries, tumours, or in fact any but the rarest and most stationary lesions of the brain. For between the rough anatomical trauma and the relatively high-grade disorder of function is interposed the dynamic condition of diaschisis[1].

But von Monakow contends that careful study of the onset and regression of such signs and symptoms throws valuable light on the mode of action of the central nervous system and must precede any attempt at anatomical localisation. Restoration of function depends on three factors[2]; firstly, the recovery from pathological processes of a grossly organic nature; secondly, the passing away of diaschisis and the reappearance of normal activity at synaptic junctions; lastly, the gradual assumption, at a late stage, of compensatory powers by uninjured portions of the nervous system.

Thus, after operative removal of the cerebellum, the recovery of locomotion is not a substitution of new functions, as Munk contended, but is due to the slow resumption of their old activity by extra-cerebellar parts as diaschisis passes away. In other words the final movements of the animal exhibit the functions of structurally uninjured portions of the central nervous system in a form that can never become manifest so long as the cerebellum participates in acts of locomotion.

In the same way, after injury to the cerebral cortex, we can watch the recovery of power step by step as the effects of diaschisis disappear. This reveals not only the topographical order in which the various parts of the body are represented, but also the relative developmental grade of various movements or qualities of sensation. Those which are lower in form, more generalised, and acquired earlier in the life of the individual

<hr>

[1] [107], p. 561.   [2] [107], p. 61.

are the first to be restored. They are little if at all dependent on the functions of the cortex, whereas cortical activity may be a necessary factor for those of higher order or greater complexity. The more a movement is directed towards a definite object, and the later it is acquired in the life of the individual, the greater the probability that it will be represented in the cortex, although the actual forces for putting it into action are of sub-cortical origin.

The only form of anatomical localisation, which can be unhesitatingly accepted, is the relative topographical representation of the various parts of the body[1]. We can confidently assume as the result of physiological experiment and clinical observation that, for instance, the face, hand, elbow and shoulder stand in a definite relation to one another, although the result of stimulating any one point on the surface of the brain may vary from time to time.

We can discover to a limited degree focal centres for certain simple simultaneous muscular actions in some definite part of the body. But, when we attempt to deal with a succession of synergic movements and alternating changes in the limbs or segments, this is impossible; we are face to face with an interrelation of diverse functions. The complete act in its perfect form demands the mobilisation in due sequence of a series of complex procedures; here the time relation, on which von Monakow lays so much stress, is of fundamental importance. A want of chronological exactitude will throw the whole movement into disorder; its "kinetic melody" has been destroyed.

Here there can be no question of a focal localisation of function, even though many of the necessary paths of innervation emerge here and there from definable insular centres. But, on the other hand, all actions which contain a cortical component can be interrupted by a lesion of the surface of the brain, although they cannot be "localised" within its boundaries.

Now of all movements those of expression comprise the largest number of diverse elements. For amongst the complex excitations, which evoke acts of speech, occurs a new factor, the symbol; this is a shortened sign for the widest possible combinations of stimuli, different in aim, origin, significance and feeling. It is therefore obvious that no topographically distinct centre exists for speech or for any such acts as reading and writing. These acts can be interrupted by cortical disease or injury in various situations, because the gross destruction of tissue disturbs their kinetic rhythm in one way or another.

[1] [105], p. 22.

If therefore we wish to understand aphasia, it is necessary to examine the phenomena as manifestations of dissolution of function ("Abbau"). Speech is developed step by step in the life of every individual and a temporal character is impressed upon it from the beginning; some acts of expression are acquired earlier than others and are likely to remain intact after more recent acquisitions have been lost in consequence of a lesion of the higher centres[1].

Thus, although no act of speech can be exclusively attributed to the activity of a definite region of the cortex, destruction of the brain can produce clinical pictures which differ fundamentally from one another according to the parts that have suffered. The discovery of this relation between the morbid phenomena and the site of the lesion is "clinical localisation." To this von Monakow has devoted for years his unrivalled powers as an anatomist.

Clinically speaking the course of a case of aphasia due to an acute non-progressive lesion can be divided into three stages. First, there is the primary period of shock reinforced by the effects of secondary structural changes, such as oedema and inflammatory reactions; this, under favourable conditions, may pass away within a few weeks. Then the phenomena of diaschisis become revealed; these do not express solely the lost physiological activity of the tissues destroyed; both in degree and form they are too severe and they represent a widespread disorganisation of cerebral function. Slowly, after many weeks or months, these may pass away to reveal the residual symptoms, which represent the permanent disintegration, disturbance of rhythm and lowered excitability due directly to the destruction of tissue. Orderly mobilisation of the various components, necessary for certain acts of speech, is prevented and the aphasia assumes some more or less specific form.

If the lesion is not stationary but progressive, as is the case with most tumours of the brain, the diaschisis, far from passing away, increases and may profoundly change the clinical manifestations. This leads to much diagnostic confusion, unless the origin of the new symptoms is recognised.

As the result of studies carried out on these principles von Monakow divides the various forms of aphasia into "motor" and "sensory"; but

---

[1] It is obvious how closely these views approximate in principle to the laws of evolution and dissolution of the nervous system laid down by Hughlings Jackson in the Croonian Lectures for 1884 ([80]). But von Monakow confesses that, like so many continental writers, he was entirely ignorant of this important work until he recently made ample amends by translating these papers into French and publishing them in the *Schweizer Archiv* [108].

he insists that these are only convenient names for groups of symptoms, which may vary greatly in extent and severity not only with every separate instance, but in the same patient from time to time.

"Motor" aphasia[1] comprises a disorder of those components responsible for the higher aspects of articulation and the due performance of movements, external and internal, necessary for acts of speech (articulatory and apraxic disturbances). Internal speech may suffer in consequence and writing become difficult or impossible. The patient is not entirely wordless; he can swear and give vent to expressions, which have become automatic. Similarly he may be able to write his name or single letters and portions of words.

At the same time closer examination shows that the so-called "sensory" components of internal speech, such as the comprehension of spoken and written words, suffer more or less[2]. The patient's powers suffice for ordinary conversation, but he cannot apprehend the significance of a longer logical sequence; this applies in a still higher degree to written or printed matter.

So much for the direct and immediate consequences of the lesion. But, especially in cases of local injury, these symptoms pass away in the following stages[3]. First, internal speech becomes freer and comprehension of spoken or written words may return completely. Then the loss of power to evoke words ("dumbness") yields gradually; the patient learns to utter those in common use and can repeat them to order. But speech is uncertain, the voice monotonous, intonation defective, syllables are slurred and there is a tendency to perseveration. Emotional expressions are uttered with greater ease and certainty. Then follows a period in which short sentences evoked spontaneously and words in common use can be said without difficulty. At this stage the patient may remain for many weeks or months, and sometimes speech never recovers beyond this point.

"Sensory" aphasia[4] consists essentially of a disorder in the perceptive factors of speech. The patient cannot comprehend ordinary conversation or carry out oral commands; spoken words are to him incomprehensible noises, or at any rate he is unable to grasp their full significance. But he is not word-deaf; for he still possesses the power of comprehending the meaning of some isolated words and phrases, such as his name and "How are you?" or similar expressions.

He can talk spontaneously, in sharp contrast to the motor aphasic, and is at times even unduly garrulous. Not infrequently he has command

[1] [107], p. 585 et seq.   [2] [107], p. 588.   [3] [107], p. 591.   [4] [107], p. 594 et seq.

of a relatively extensive vocabulary, although uncertain internal verbalisation constantly leads to errors. He employs the usual forms of speech and his sentences are constructed grammatically, at any rate when using conventional expressions. But his defective powers of speech are betrayed by false intonation and accent, by rhythmic disorder and monotony of voice. The words are badly put together and are confused mainly in accordance with some resemblance in sound. The verbal forms he employs not uncommonly bear some relation to the word he is seeking, but usually consist of ill-composed fragments. Above all things there is a tendency to perseverate; an expression once found, whether right or wrong, tends to recur. Repetition is impossible because he is "deaf" to the meaning of most words.

Complete sensory aphasia invariably leads to some intellectual want of power to manipulate written speech. There is always agraphia combined with alexia; these two symptoms are the most persistent in the clinical picture and usually last longer than the word-deafness[1]. Letters can be appreciated visually and may even be written down correctly, although their sound value and their significance are mistaken. The errors in writing belong to the same category as those of spontaneous speech and of reading. The comprehension of other symbols, such as numbers or musical notes, is also defective and all forms of calculation may be gravely disturbed.

"Sensory apraxia"[2] is another frequent accompaniment of this form of aphasia; the patient is unable to perform a number of acts, such as those connected with his professional work or with the care of his body.

So far we have spoken mainly of complete motor and sensory aphasia. But it is obvious that, according to the principles laid down by von Monakow, these disordered states of activity must appear in many different forms. For, from the onset of the lesion until the final appearance of the residual symptoms, the manifestations are undergoing constant change either in the direction of recovery or ingravescence. This temporary nature is one of the most important characteristics in the life history of an aphasic. Subsidiary or component groups of symptoms may appear as distinct clinical entities during recovery or may form the initial manifestations of the lesion. If so they will either disappear with the passing of diaschisis or be joined by other phenomena as the disease advances.

It is not possible to enter into a description or even to enumerate these different varieties, but von Monakow's treatment of agraphia forms a

---

[1] [107], p. 598.   [2] [107], p. 601; also p. 496.

good example of his attitude towards disorders of speech. There is no
evidence whatever for a "writing centre"; the acts, which go to form
what we term "writing," can be disturbed in three separate ways by
lesions situated in different parts of the brain. This disorder of function
may be produced firstly by defective verbalisation ("word-dumbness"),
secondly by want of appreciation of the verbal significance of sounds,
and lastly by want of recognition of form, due to disturbance of the visual
components in speech.

Everyone is agreed that speech in its various aspects can be affected in
diverse ways by lesions of one hemisphere, and all pathological investigation aims at establishing a relation between the morbid symptoms and
the site of the structural injury; this is "clinical localisation." On the
other hand, search for a strictly local "speech centre" is entirely vain.

Now the phenomena, which have been grouped together as "motor
aphasia," can be evoked most readily from those parts of the brain comprised within the following regions[1]: the whole distribution of both
anterior branches of the Sylvian artery, that is to say the 3rd frontal
convolution (pars opercularis, triangularis and orbitalis), the front
portion of the island of Reil, the operculum together with the sub-cortical
white matter, the corona radiata and the central white matter in the
region of the Broca-Rolandic segment. To this must probably be added
the neighbouring parts of the putamen, a region through which pass the
cortical projection fibres. The "locus minoris resistentiae" or most
favourable situation for the production of morbid manifestations of this
class is the area between the posterior portion of F. 3 and the operculum,
including the deeper white matter. The greater the extent and depth of
the lesion in this area, the more certainly will the disorder of speech
assume this form. But, should the injury remain stationary and the rest
of the brain be healthy, these manifestations gradually pass away in a
characteristic order and may even disappear completely, although a
definite lesion is subsequently found post-mortem. Conversely, if the
organic injury is slight, but the onset acute, death may occur from some
other cause before the effects of the diaschisis have worn off; little may
be found even on careful microscopical examination to account for the
obvious disorder of speech.

"Sensory" aphasia[2] can be produced by a lesion anywhere within the
temporal lobe, more particularly the first temporal and angular gyri. This
area corresponds closely to the supply of the third to the fifth branches

---

[1] [107], p. 767.   [2] [107], p. 822 et seq.

of the Sylvian artery. But the order in which the symptoms disappear is less easily determined than with motor aphasia and von Monakow confesses to considerable doubt with regard to the subsidiary forms.

Affections of the visual sphere, if sufficiently acute or severe, tend to produce on the lowest level some variety of hemianopsia accompanied occasionally with want of ocular orientation. Amongst the manifestations of a higher order are all those forms of amnesia, which depend on defective visual recognition, such as agnosia, asymbolia, and defective spacial appreciation.

In conclusion, the phenomena of aphasia must be considered not only as direct manifestations of the physiological activity of the damaged area, but also from the point of view of the acuteness and duration of the lesion. This is von Monakow's great contribution to our knowledge of the subject, and it matters little if we speak of "diaschisis" or "shock," so long as this fact is firmly grasped during the attempt at any one time to interpret the symptoms and the appearances found after death. From this fundamental generalisation springs the whole of his ideas on cerebral localisation and his doctrine that functions and aptitudes can be destroyed by a lesion of the cortex, but are not localised within centres definable on its surface.

§3. LIEPMANN AND APRAXIA

It is a common experience that a patient with a cerebral lesion, told to protrude his tongue, may be unable to do so, although he licks his lips with ease, if the movement is initiated spontaneously. In the same way he cannot close his eyes, wrinkle his forehead, or show his teeth to command; yet there are no signs of facial paralysis.

Closer analysis shows that this want of power to execute such movements to order may be due to two demonstrably different causes. If the patient is suffering from aphasia and does not understand what is said to him, he is obviously unable to execute a command, however simple; but this will not prevent him from imitating movements made by the observer, provided they do not require some act of verbal or symbolic formulation.

On the other hand, in some instances the power of making these movements of the face and tongue is not only defective to oral commands, but mimicry is impossible. The patient either fails entirely to respond, or tends to perform some totally different action. Evidently this is a disturbance of function, which cannot be classified under any form of "sensory" aphasia.

This condition was described by Hughlings Jackson[1] in 1866 in the following words: "In some cases of defect of speech the patient seems to have lost much of his power to do anything he is told to do even with those muscles that are not paralysed. Thus a patient will be unable to put out his tongue when we ask him, although he will use it well in semi-involuntary actions, e.g. eating and swallowing. He will not make the particular grimace he is told to do, even when we make one for him to imitate. There is power in his muscles and in the centres for the coordination of muscular groups, but he, the whole man or the 'will,' cannot set them agoing. Such a patient may do a thing well at one time but not at another. In a few cases the patients do not do things so simple as moving the hand (i.e. the non-paralysed hand) when they are told."

Many observers recognised this condition more or less completely and offered various explanations of its nature and origin. Thus, in 1882 Westphal described a patient who showed loss of appreciation of posture and passive movement in the right upper extremity with a peculiar clumsiness in using it even with the eyes open. This he attributed to loss of kinaesthetic memories. Unfortunately this peculiar loss of function was not distinguished from agnosia and its attendant manifestations, and Wernicke's conception of asymboly, a term adopted from Finkelnburg, laid stress on want of recognition as the cause of these defective movements.

Liepmann[2] in 1900 was the first to subject the clinical manifestations to comprehensive analysis and to classify them under the term "apraxia." This he defined as inability to act or to move various parts of the body in a purposeful manner, although the power of movement is intact. There is no paralysis and the patient understands what is required of him; yet he cannot execute the action he wishes to perform. The apraxic possesses a sufficient sensori-motor apparatus, but he cannot employ it at will in certain directions, and the forms of activity which suffer are more particularly those acquired by experience, example or instruction.

The phenomena produced by a disorder of this nature are best illustrated by those rare but striking cases of unilateral apraxia of the upper extremity unaccompanied by motor paralysis of any part of the body. Suppose the affected limb is the right arm, it is usually kept motionless against the side, slightly flexed at the elbow, and does not participate in the general movements of the body as a whole. Any object presented to the patient is taken by preference in the left hand and he cannot use a

---

[1] [81], p. 48.   [2] [88], see also [94].

knife, a brush, or a pair of scissors with the right. This is not due to want of recognition of the significance of these objects, for they can be employed correctly by the left hand. The patient is unable to manipulate a lighted match placed between his fingers with sufficient skill to prevent burning himself, and fails to bring his right arm into the correct position to blow it out, when told to do so. Complex acts, such as tying a knot or lighting a cigarette, are impossible, or are carried out without participation of the right hand. Even simple movements, such as closing the fist, are performed slowly and the patient may find difficulty in relaxing his grasp to command. Acts of mimicry, such as touching the nose or the forefinger of the opposite hand, may be impossible with the affected limb, though performed easily with the normal one.

Even in the most demonstrative cases of unilateral apraxia, both sides of the face are equally affected. There may be no paralysis of any kind, but movements of the eyes, lips and tongue cannot be imitated and are badly executed in response to an order of any kind; for all such movements normally require simultaneous activity of both sides and are consequently affected bilaterally in the various forms of apraxia.

Now it is obvious that apart from all theoretical considerations the existence of such a condition must have a profound effect on most of the tests employed to investigate aphasia and kindred disorders of speech. Spontaneous utterance, repetition, reading aloud and writing all suffer more or less gravely; yet it is possible in most cases by detailed examination to discover whether the disturbance of function should be classed as an apraxia, or belongs more properly to some form of aphasia.

Sometimes, if the apraxia is very severe, the patient makes little or no attempt to speak spontaneously. More often he utters a series of articulate sounds consisting of words mispronounced, mutilated or wrongly employed. He insists that he knows what he wants to say, but cannot find the means of expression. Asked to name an object placed before him, he usually replies with some term of cognate meaning or with the correct word badly articulated; it is not the power of naming so much as the higher mechanics of verbal formation that are at fault. Repetition is equally defective and shows exactly the same faults as spontaneous speech.

When an apraxic attempts to read aloud, the sounds he utters are even more defective than those of spontaneous speech. But with care it is frequently possible, especially in the so-called unilateral cases, to show that he understands what he reads to himself; for he may be able to select a series of objects to printed commands and to carry out simple orders correctly, if he is made to employ the less apraxic or unaffected limb.

Writing shows the profoundest changes and may be entirely abolished. The patient cannot hold a pencil or pen in his hand, nor guide it with sufficient skill to make coherent marks upon the paper. Even if he can still write his name, each letter is badly formed, the strokes are uncertain and wanting in firmness, whilst the whole is liable to terminate in an incomprehensible scrawl. Here the so-called unilateral cases are of the greatest value in betraying the nature of the disturbance. For a patient with uncomplicated aphasic defects of language, who cannot write with one hand, is equally unable to do so with the other. He lacks the power of finding words and translating them into written symbols; the disturbance of function is general and bears no relation to any part of the body. But the apraxic, unable even to hold a pen correctly in one hand, may be able to write at any rate to a certain extent with the other. He has not lost words, but the power of formulating the complicated and acquired movements necessary to place them on to paper. Moreover, he may be able to write down with one hand the name of an object shown to him, whilst he fails even to produce a scrawl with the other. The act of copying is affected in the same manner and the patient cannot even reproduce exactly letters placed before him in the form of printed capitals. It is the mechanics of writing which suffer and the defects bear no direct relation to any true verbal activity.

Drawing is usually impossible, at any rate with the more apraxic limb, and there is no difference between the capacity to draw from a model or to copy an outline figure. Here again it is the act itself which is disturbed and not its intellectual content.

In some instances even comprehension of spoken or written commands may appear to be affected. But in suitable cases this defective response can be shown to depend on loss of expression rather than on want of understanding; for an order, which cannot be obeyed when the right hand is employed, may be executed more or less correctly with the left. The movements are at any rate sufficiently appropriate to show that the patient has understood what is demanded of him.

For a similar reason Liepmann's famous Regierungsrat appeared to be unable to subtract five from eight or to multiply two by three, if he was asked to carry out the operation with matches laid on the table before him, even though he employed his less apraxic left hand[1]. Yet he could not only solve these simple arithmetical problems but others of much greater complexity, if he was allowed to point to numbers on a board. Had his left hand been a little more apraxic, it would have been impossible,

[1] [91], p. 73.

owing to his lack of means of expression, to prove that he had not totally lost the power of calculation.

When we remember that apraxia rarely occurs alone and is often accompanied by loss of sensation, agnosia, or aphasia, profound difficulty must often arise in deciding whether some particular manifestation belongs to one or other of these disorders of function. But, if the case is looked at as a whole, there are certain differentiating characters which serve to reveal the presence of apraxia. Asked to imitate a simple movement made by the observer, such as touching the nose or scratching the head, the patient is unable to do so or may fail with the one hand, although he succeeds with the other. On the contrary the aphasic, particularly if he belongs to the "motor" type, can imitate even complex movements made before him, provided they do not necessitate the employment of some formula of internal speech, such as the differential designation of right and left. Thus, he can usually copy movements of the observer reflected in a mirror, although he may fail to do so sitting face to face. Provided he understands what he is expected to do, he can imitate movements of the face and gestures of the observer. On the other hand, the apraxic fails more particularly in all forms of mimicry. Sometimes in so-called unilateral cases, every movement whether of the right or left hand is copied with the less affected limb; should the patient recognise his mistake, he may then proceed to execute the movement with both hands simultaneously. Occasionally he does not respond to gestures indicating that he is to seat himself or to rise from a chair, but simply attempts to copy the actions of the observer.

Given an object, such as a brush or a match-box, the apraxic fails to carry out the natural actions of brushing his hair or lighting a match. He cannot evoke the sequence of movements necessary to attain his object. He may be able to name a pair of scissors placed in his hand, although he cannot use them; or he explains that an envelope and a sheet of paper are "to send through the post," and yet fails to put them together and fasten the flap correctly. Shown a pencil he says it is "to make marks with"; but told to use it, he replies holding it aimlessly in his hand, "That's what I can't manage."

Liepmann classified the various forms assumed by apraxia under three headings corresponding to the relative complexity of the disturbance of function[1]. The first, called by him "limb-kinetic apraxia" ("Gliedkinetische Apraxie"), is due to uncomplicated loss of kinaesthetic memories of a definite part of the body. The limb is not paralysed, but

---

[1] [91], pp. 79–80; also [94], pp. 524–526.

the patient has lost the power to execute certain combinations of acquired movements. Delicate movements are impossible and even the coarser ones are carried out awkwardly and with want of skill. One limb or portion of the body only may be involved and so gross can be the loss of function that the affected part appears to be paralysed.

In the second form, which he calls "ideokinetic apraxia" ("Ideo-kinetische Apraxie"), the kinetic mechanism of the limb is intact, but, owing to the position of the lesion, is dissociated from the total conception of its purposive movements. Ideational and kinaesthetic processes are separated from one another; this is "motor" apraxia in the full sense of the term. Simple movements are at times perfect; at others, when the patient wills to carry them out, they are not forthcoming. Even the power of imitation and mimicry is grossly disturbed.

The third and highest form of disturbance of function is "ideational apraxia" ("Ideatorische Apraxie"). The mechanical kinesis of the limb and the conception of the movements to be performed are intact, but the primary or initiating idea is at fault. The intention or aim of the act is not correctly formulated and the patient cannot execute spontaneously some complex series of adjusted actions, although he is capable of making the necessary movements under other conditions. This is a general disturbance of function affecting the body as a whole and becomes evident if the task to be performed demands the orderly manipulation of a series of objects. Thus, when one of Liepmann's patients was given a cigar and a match-box, he opened it, inserted the tip of the cigar and shut the box as though to cut off the end. Then, taking out the cigar, he rubbed it on the box as if it were a match. All the movements required to execute the complex task were present, but they were not performed in the correct sequence; the general conception was imperfect. In the same way, if a patient is given a tooth-brush, he uses it to brush his hair or clothes and puts a match into his mouth instead of a cigarette.

Apraxia has been described as inability to perform certain purposive movements or complex actions, although motion, sensation and co-ordination are preserved. Such a definition would include many morbid manifestations usually classed under aphasia, particularly its "motor" forms, and in 1900 Liepmann spoke of the aphasia of his Regierungsrat as "apraxia of the speech muscles." Aphasic disorders, in as far as they assume an expressive form, are of an apraxic nature in the wide sense of the term[1]. For instance, motor aphasia is a particular form of apraxia of

[1] [94], p. 540.

the glosso-labio-pharyngeal apparatus; the unparalysed muscles cannot be innervated in such a manner that the sounds of speech come into being.

In his paper before the International Medical Congress[1] in 1913 he spoke in a somewhat more guarded manner:

What holds good in *general* for the movements of our muscle apparatus is valid for the special functions of a part, the laryngo-pharyngo-glosso-labial muscles. This muscle apparatus has besides its *visible* effect, e.g. mimic movements, a special one, that is an *audible* effect, *speech*.

Speech also has its sensori-motor executive apparatus. This is the apparatus, which moves the larynx, palate, mouth and tongue, with its sensory regulations. If this executive apparatus is injured we then have *anarthria* or *dysarthria*.

Since speech as I formerly pointed out, is as it were a parasite which has made use of a sensori-motor apparatus preexisting for other purposes, principally feeding, it is impaired by injuries which affect this apparatus. The speech of the dysarthric patient suffers however only in proportion as his instrument suffers. ... A mnestic-associative apparatus is superposed on this executive apparatus. By means of it one learns to produce sounds, syllables, words, which in turn differ largely according to place and time. ... Just as the limb-centre of the hand must receive directions from the rest of the brain in order, say, to ignite a candle, the "limb" centre of the speech muscles, i.e. the well-known motor speech centre (principally the opercular part of the third gyrus frontalis and the gyrus centralis anterior), obtain directions as to what to speak.

He then insists[2] that in most persons the "motor word" is not directly revived by the idea to be expressed but by way of its auditory components. "In order that the action of speech may take place properly the acoustic sketch must influence the kinematic of the speech muscles just as in an apraxia of the extremities the visual sketch influences the kinematic of the extremities."

Slight affection of this mechanism causes mutilation of letters and syllables with great slowness and difficulty of articulation, which resembles at first sight a dysarthria. But the gross defects of writing show that we have to deal with something more than a disturbance of the executive apparatus governing articulation. Thus, anarthria and apraxia must be strictly distinguished from one another.

But "*in principle* physiologically and psychologically and therefore also pathologically the expressive-aphasic disturbances belong to the more general large sphere of apraxia. This of course by no means excludes

---

[1] [92], pp. 100–101.   [2] [92], p. 102.

a special treatment adapted to their specific kind[1]." The analogy, he adds, must not be carried to extreme lengths and all aphasic manifestations cannot be classed as forms of apraxia.

In 1921 this cautious attitude was further developed in a letter written to Professor Henschen[2], who had asked the meaning of the earlier statement that "Motor aphasia is a particular form of apraxia of the glosso-labio-pharyngeal musculature." Liepmann replied as follows:

Not all motor aphasics suffer from apraxia, that is to say apraxia of the extremities. Apraxia of the face muscles, inability to whistle, to wrinkle the forehead, to make a grimace, etc., is frequently combined with motor aphasia. Apraxia of the hands, though common, is less often present. There are motor aphasics, especially those with so-called "pure word-dumbness," without apraxia and conversely I have observed apraxic patients, not only without motor aphasia, but without any form of aphasia. Graver degrees of apraxia appear occasionally with sensory aphasia, probably owing to the proximity of the temporal and parietal lobes.

It is evident therefore, although apraxia and motor aphasia often occur together, they do not stand in direct causal connection with one another. Thus, there are three forms of executive disorders of speech, aphemia or "motor" aphasia, apraxia, and anarthria. These may appear alone or in various combinations, but are essentially different.

Some observers have taken Liepmann's earlier statements literally and hold that the executive varieties of aphasia are forms of motor or ideational apraxia. On the other hand, the receptive or sensory disorders of speech are instances of agnosia in the widest sense of the term.

This view was clearly expressed by Wilson[3] in the discussion which followed my Hughlings Jackson lecture in 1920. He said:

I accept the general division of aphasia into receptive and executive defects. I hold that ordinary motor aphasia is but a part of motor apraxia and sensory aphasia of agnosia. The patient with auditory agnosia hears sounds, but does not recognise them, i.e. does not know their meaning. Among those sounds may be word-sounds, which he hears, but the content, the symbolic meaning, is for him unknown. The same is true of alexia as a variety of visual agnosia. ... On the executive side motor aphasia is a part of apraxia; the patient is not paralysed, but he cannot say what he wants to say, as the apraxic cannot do what he wants to do.

But, as we shall see later, agnosia in the strict sense of the term includes loss of power to comprehend the meaning of auditory and visual impressions far in excess of the manifestations of "sensory" aphasia. The patient is not only unable to understand what is said to him or to read

[1] [92], p. 104.   [2] [73 c.], p. 280.   [3] [44] p. 438, see also [132].

from print, but he cannot appreciate the significance of sounds, or re-cognise objects by sight alone. Had it been possible to prove the existence of pure "word-deafness" or "word-blindness," as isolated groups of clinical manifestations, they might have been included under the com-prehensive title of agnosia. But the phenomena of "sensory" aphasia cannot be comprised under these headings and it is unwise to throw into one class two sets of symptoms which show such obvious differences. Both agnosia and aphasia are simply names applied to certain morbid states discovered by clinical observation and, since they are in no way identical, it is useful to retain the two independent terms, bearing in mind that they are descriptive only.

In the same way "motor" apraxia, whether of the local or general type, comprises manifestations not only more extensive, but of a different nature from any which can possibly be included under aphasia. Nothing is gained by attempting to equate executive disorders of the use of language in terms of high-grade defects of movement. Anarthria, verbal apraxia and "motor" aphasia are purely descriptive terms for three different forms of abnormal speech, which can occur separately or in combination and there is no advantage in classifying any form of aphasia as a variety of apraxia.

In some cases, which belong to the category of what I have called "semantic" aphasia, the patient experiences difficulty in executing a complex series of actions, because he cannot formulate the intention or goal of some task he is asked to perform. Judged purely by the test of behaviour, this might be attributed to "ideational" apraxia; but closer examination shows that the disturbance of function is due to defective use of symbols, rather than to loss of conception of movements. Such patients find no difficulty with the simpler actions of daily life, so long as they hold the necessary tool in their hands. They drink out of the cup and not out of the jug, they use a brush correctly, extract a match from a box and can blow it out before it burns their fingers. Their difficulty consists in thinking out beforehand how the table should be laid for breakfast, or a stroke at billiards can be made off the cushion; having made the pieces of a box or a door, they cannot put them together. In the same way, when telling a story heard or read, they are liable to miss its logical conclusion or implication. Moreover, articulated speech and the mechanical aspect of writing are not affected in this form of aphasia. A high-grade disturbance of function of this order obviously belongs to defects of symbolic formulation and is not due to lack of ideas of move-ment, however general.

Liepmann looked upon apraxia as disturbance of a definite function called "praxis," and attempted to discover "eupraxic" centres by close anatomical examination of the site of the lesions in those who had suffered from these morbid manifestations. But he experienced extreme difficulty in finding any part of the brain where a strictly limited lesion would of necessity produce apraxia. He concluded[1] that the left hemisphere exerts a preponderating influence over the higher aspects of movement on both sides of the body and that in this the fibres of the corpus callosum play an important part. A lesion situated anteriorly, especially in the cortex of the central convolutions and adjacent parts, is liable to produce a local disturbance, which affects the kinesis of one limb. "Ideo-motor" apraxia is more likely to appear, when the central convolutions are cut off from the visual, auditory and tactile regions of both hemispheres, more particularly the left. On the other hand, "ideational" apraxia, a more general disorder of function, is associated with lesions in the parietal and parieto-occipital regions. Thus, the further back the focus in the left hemisphere the more definitely do the manifestations assume an "ideational" form, whilst more anterior lesions tend to be associated with "motor" apraxia.

Gross destruction of the left "hand area," or of deep parts in the region of the central convolutions, paralyses the right upper extremity and makes the left dyspraxic. A similar lesion of the internal capsule produces paralysis of the right half of the body and no apraxia. A sufficiently grave focus in the left parietal region causes severe apraxia of the right side with slighter manifestations on the left half of the body. On the other hand, "ideational" apraxia is a general disturbance of function and can be evoked in right-handed persons by a lesion in the parieto-occipital region of the left hemisphere only.

But, although these rules with regard to the lesions capable of producing apraxia are roughly correct, it must not be forgotten that the destruction of tissue is always severe and the brain usually shows in addition widely diffused changes. The disorder of function may be distinctive in character and occupy certain definite parts of the body, although the anatomical changes are not confined to a single focus.

Moreover, as von Monakow[2] pointed out and Liepmann himself confesses, apraxia is in many cases a transitory manifestation. It may be present to a striking degree shortly after the stroke, but tends to fade away with time, to recur in the same or some other form with another cerebral attack. It is in fact a common accompaniment of the condition

[1] [94], p. 529 et seq.   [2] Cf. Brun R. [3].

called by von Monakow "diaschisis." In this way it resembles true visual and auditory agnosia, which with the lapse of time give place to some less extensive and specific loss of function.

Thus, in conclusion, the term apraxia must be reserved strictly for loss of power to execute purposive movements or complex acts, in the absence of paralysis and with perfect comprehension of the meaning and ultimate intention of commands, whatever form they may assume. This implies that the loss of function is not secondary to any variety of agnosia or "sensory" aphasia. Granting these conditions, certain distinctive defects of speech, ranging from slight articulatory abnormalities to almost complete mutism, may be due to apraxia. They are accompanied by lack of mimicry and are frequently associated with some loss of power to write and to carry out movements of one or more limbs in a normal manner.

Applied to disorders of speech, apraxia, like anarthria and aphasia, is descriptive of a peculiar form of abnormal behaviour. Each set of clinical manifestations must be carefully scanned and investigated to discover to which class they rightly belong; for the three groups of morbid phenomena differ in kind and correspond to various levels of functional integration. We must, however, be on our guard against assuming a corresponding set of normal functions which can be localised in different portions of the brain. There are no centres for "eupraxia" or "euphasia," although there are regions where a lesion of sufficient extent and severity can disturb normal acts of speech in a way that can be designated "apraxia" or "aphasia."

§ 4. IMPERCEPTION OR AGNOSIA

If a man is blind or deaf he cannot read printed words or understand those spoken in his presence; but no one could class these defects amongst the phenomena of aphasia. In the same way, before it is possible to determine the behaviour of a supposed aphasic to tests which depend on reading or the comprehension of spoken words, we must be certain that he is capable of appreciating the significance of sights and sounds. For if, when shown a knife, the patient not only fails to name it, but cannot indicate its use or match it with its duplicate on the table, he is obviously suffering from something more than "visual aphasia." Similarly, should his inability to understand spoken words be accompanied by want of power to recognise the meaning of other sounds or familiar melodies, he is certainly not an uncomplicated instance of "auditory aphasia."

In 1876 Jackson[1] defined for the first time a state produced by a gross cerebral lesion in which the patient was unable to recognise objects and persons, although her vision was apparently unaffected. He summarised the condition as follows: "The first symptoms were those of what I call Imperception. She often did not know objects, persons, and places. To the statement that there was only 'confusion of mind,' I do not object, for I should say that her mental confusion showed itself in inability to recognise objects, persons and places. Nor do I object to its being called 'only loss or defect of memory'; it was a loss or defect of memory for persons, objects, and places....There was what I would call 'Imperception,' a defect as special as Aphasia. The case did not correspond however to *loss* of speech, but to defect of speech. There was partial Imperception."

These views, together with Jackson's description of apraxia, were put forward in Journals difficult of access and remained entirely unnoticed. They were out of harmony with current ideas and produced no impression on the literature of the time[2].

But as soon as Munk discovered that by removing a portion of the occipital lobes on the two sides he could produce a condition which he called "Seelenblindheit" or "Mind-blindness," this conception was eagerly accepted by clinicians. Munk's dog avoided obstacles and was certainly not blind, but it showed no reaction to threats with a whip and did not respond, when tempted with meat placed within sight. Munk explained this as a psychical condition in which the power of receiving optical impressions remained, but perception was grossly defective in consequence of bilateral destruction of the visual centre.

He also showed that, by removing on both sides what he took to be the auditory centre in the temporal lobe, he could cause an analogous loss of function; this he called "Seelentaubheit" or "Mind-deafness." The dog could hear sounds and, if they were loud or unusual in character, started or pricked its ears; but it no longer responded to words or to the crack of a whip. Here again it seemed as if perception of the meaning of sounds rather than crude hearing was at fault.

These experiments had a profound effect upon clinical medicine. Wernicke applied them to the study of aphasia and spoke of destruction of memory images. "These patients," he wrote[3], "apparently see, since they avoid obstacles and to judge from their facial expression they can hear; they also feel what they hold in their hands, but all these impres-

[1] [79], p. 437.
[2] Pick [114] alone mentioned them in his "Studien" in 1905.   [3] [130], p. 553.

sions are strange and useless, for they have lost the power thereby to recognise objects."

Now it is obvious that such manifestations must represent a disturbance on a lower functional level than those of any form of aphasia or amnesia; they are primarily defects of perception. Even if the lesion were strictly confined to the surface of the brain, it might presumably cause a loss of function which belonged to several different levels. Firstly, it might destroy the receptive centre for visual, auditory or tactile impressions and so cause gross loss of any one or more of these senses. Secondly, although the patient could see or hear, he might be unable to recognise the use or spoken names of common objects and show other signs that he could not utilise certain sense impressions. Finally, he might suffer from a pure "sensory" aphasia either "visual" or "auditory." Henschen[1] went so far as to postulate in the temporal lobe three different centres associated with hearing, the primary acoustic centre, the word-sound centre and the word-comprehension centre; these psychic centres lie above one another, are of different value and separate situation.

Freud had already employed the term "agnosia" for a state where sensory impressions could be received, but their significance was no longer recognised, and Liepmann's well-known studies brought this convenient term into fashion. Now it is obvious that want of power to appreciate perceptual meaning might affect independently the impressions produced by sight, hearing or somatic sensations; agnosia falls naturally into "visual," "auditory" and "tactile" forms. Of these the first two only would materially affect the use of language. For inability to appreciate the meaning of things seen must affect the power to read, whilst want of recognition of sounds would diminish the capacity to understand spoken words. But such defects alone have no bearing on the phenomena of any variety of aphasia; as Jackson pointed out, imperception and aphasia may exist independently, and had this conception been adopted at an early stage in the history of the subject, much subsequent confusion might have been avoided.

Visual agnosia in the strict sense of the term postulates the following condition. The patient can see an object shown to him, but fails to appreciate its character and meaning. Not only is he unable to name it or to demonstrate its use but he does not remember ever to have seen it before. As soon, however, as an appeal is made to his understanding through another sense such as touch, he can find the approximate name

_____

[1] [70], p. 442.

and employ the object correctly. Such a state cannot be justifiably classed as a form of "sensory" aphasia; for words can be employed more or less accurately provided the nature of the object can be perceived and the loss of verbal aptitude is secondary to lack of perceptual recognition.

In the same way a patient suffering from pure auditory agnosia should be unable to appreciate the significance of sounds, although there is distinct evidence that he can hear them. He cannot appreciate music and fails to execute oral commands, but carries out the same orders correctly if they are given in writing.

Such are the fundamental symptoms which should characterise a pure case of visual or auditory agnosia. Everyone is agreed that these disorders are psychical and, although they are produced by gross lesions of the brain, the manifestations can be classified in functional terms only. If one aspect of perception is disturbed, the clinical phenomena must express the response of the organism to the new situation. Signs and symptoms will therefore both exceed and fall short of those that might have been predicted on purely theoretical grounds, and it is impossible to deduce the morbid manifestations from a point to point examination of the extent of the anatomical destruction.

It is therefore of fundamental importance to examine the actual records of those cases, which have been brought forward as examples of visual or auditory agnosia. Unfortunately, in the majority of instances the clinical observations are lamentably defective, although extreme care may have been expended on the details of the pathological examination. Moreover, many of the patients showed considerable loss of intellectual capacity; in some, hearing or vision was so grossly defective that it was questionable how far the loss of functional ability was due to this cause. In many instances the lesions were progressive and it might be doubted to what extent the post-mortem findings corresponded to the clinical manifestations during the period when it was possible to subject the patient to detailed examination. There are, however, a few admirable reports to be found in the literature of the subject and it is on these that I shall rely to discover the manifestations which actually accompany lack of visual or auditory perception.

(a) *Visual Imperception*

One of the best examples of this condition was reported in 1913 by von Stauffenberg[1] in his monograph on mind-blindness and is summarised shortly by von Monakow on pages 473-4 of his *Die Lokalisation*

[1] [123].

im Grosshirn. Not only are the clinical observations fuller and more extensive than in most instances of this condition to be found in the literature, but the anatomical site and distribution of the lesion was determined with the greatest accuracy. Moreover, in this interesting study the author reviews the whole question of "Seelenblindheit" (mind-blindness) in the light of all the cases that justly fall under this appellation.

The patient B. was a woman, who in January, 1904, at the age of 61, suffered from her first stroke. This was followed by some defect of vision, slight loss of speech and want of memory but no paralysis. She returned to work in three weeks complaining of her eyesight, but otherwise apparently normal. A year and nine months later she was admitted to hospital with left hemiplegia, some disturbance of sensibility and hemianopsia on the same side. The paralysis passed away, sensibility was almost completely restored, although the loss of vision remained. In July, 1907, she began to have further attacks, associated with headache and mental confusion and followed by paresis of the left half of the body. These became more frequent and she died in 1912 of pulmonary tuberculosis, accompanied by general atheroma of the vessels.

Thus, as in all these cases of imperception the disease was not stationary. It was associated with recurrent attacks followed by an increase of morbid signs and symptoms many of which gradually passed away in the intervening period. But for six years, during which she was under observation, there was profound visual agnosia; she could not recognise with certainty people, objects or pictures and yet her intelligence and memory remained fairly good throughout.

She showed permanent left hemianopsia with maintenance of central vision. At first her visual acuity was undoubtedly diminished; but in spite of considerable recovery of sight, her power of recognising objects remained grossly affected.

When first she came under observation, she avoided objects placed in her way and appreciated them by their size and luminosity, but could not say what they were. Later she learnt to recognise them, although she was unable to point to the legs or back of a chair and thought the straw seat was made of wood.

Shown some common object she at once asked to be allowed to handle it. She complained, "I see that something is there, I see it quite clearly to catch hold of and afterwards I don't see anything." Thus, unable to recognise a sponge held in front of her she did so at once when she touched it with her hand. In the same way she named a cigar correctly after putting it into her mouth. Whenever it was possible she called in the aid of hearing, touch, smell or taste to help her out of her difficulty in visual perception. Amongst objects of daily use a spoon was occasionally recognised and less often a knife or a fork. She failed to indicate the use of a wash-hand basin, a sponge, a key or a pocket knife. After looking for a long time at a watch, she recognised the numbers on the face and told the time correctly.

She did not apparently distinguish people readily by sight alone. She said she knew the nurses from the doctors because the former wore white head-dresses, white aprons, black frocks and they walked silently. The latter had long white coats and "boots which you hear when they walk." Sounds played a profound part in this recognition; for it occurred much less certainly if the particular person stood still and remained silent. As a matter of fact she learnt by practice to distinguish a number of people she met habitually. At first sight this appeared to be due to immediate visual perception; but closer investigation and the patient's own statements showed that some movement, mode of salutation, gesture or peculiarity of gait helped in the identification. Recognition occurred, however, with astonishing promptitude and certainty if they spoke.

At first colours were matched according to their luminosity and she put together bright red, blue and yellow. She soon regained the power of sorting wools correctly, although to the last she was liable occasionally to make the grossest mistakes.

A striking feature of the condition was her uncertain behaviour with regard to the simplest objects, both during testing and spontaneous action. Sometimes she scarcely recognised a single article by sight, whilst on other days she succeeded with a whole series of familiar objects. The certainty of her answers also varied greatly. It was often easy to lead her to a false conclusion, such as that a sponge was a brush; on other occasions she would deny this energetically. She undoubtedly acquired the power of appreciating sufficiently for use many objects she saw daily. Thus she employed a knife, fork and spoon correctly in eating and a towel, soap and comb, when she washed herself. She could often use articles spontaneously which she could not employ to command.

She showed no capacity to register her experience for subsequent action. If, for instance, she had succeeded with the help of touch in naming an object, the impression passed away so rapidly that, when it was placed before her again, she failed to recognise it and did not remember that she had ever seen it before.

Hearing remained intact and, except at the very beginning, auditory perception was unaffected. She reacted to the slightest sound, recognised running water and, when she heard whistling, said it was like the noise made by the tramcar and locomotive. She could sing well-known melodies correctly and finally her hearing became so acute as to form a valuable aid to recognition in daily life. Taste and smell were unaffected.

During the first few weeks there was tactile agnosia and she recognised a lemon by its smell, bread by its taste, a watch and a match-box by hearing. But she gradually regained her powers of appreciating objects by touch and could name them, when they were placed in her hands, although she could not do so by sight alone.

Spontaneous speech was unaffected except for slight difficulty in finding words to express her meaning; when in doubt she either used some allied term or a descriptive phrase. So fluent was she that on one occasion she delivered on behalf of the patients an address of thanks to the doctors for the Christmas entertainment. She could repeat anything said to her and there was no trace of agrammatism.

Throughout the whole period of observation she was totally unable to describe with certainty common objects placed before her, and yet she occasionally indicated correctly the conditions of their use. Thus, unable to name a fork, she said, "I want it when I eat," but added, "I can also cut with it." Even when the object was placed in her hand, she did not always recognise it at once. After some tests with money she was given a pocket-knife which she called "something to open, a purse"; when handed the same knife again she said, "A purse; you put money into a purse, in order that you can put it into your pocket and pay people." Then she opened the knife and exclaimed, "That is a knife and no purse." She said that a riding boot was "something belonging to soldiers," but added "a knapsack."

The profoundest disturbance was in the power of naming objects and colours. Sometimes she could indicate in words the use of some article in sight, but could not name it unless it was placed in her hand; on other occasions even this was impossible. She had slight difficulty in finding names during spontaneous speech, yet her descriptive powers were very defective not only if the object was in sight, but also in response to a name said to her by the observer. Mingled with confused or contradictory terms were expressions which revealed some conception of the signification of the word she had heard. Thus a bell was "round, half round and four cornered so round and large, when I hear it then I know it"; in response to the word "scissors" she said, "Please give me them otherwise I don't know them, you use them when you sew." She could not describe a cat, but made the sound of mewing. Asked the colour of the sky and the grass, she said that both were yellow and the oak was white.

As might have been expected, she could not read even her own name with certainty. She was unable to decipher letters or syllables written by herself; but later, on her good days, she recognised some of them, if she made the movements of copying them with her finger. At times she could read a few simple numbers, but those of three figures always puzzled her.

From the beginning she could write her name and a short letter and, if allowed to hold an object in her hand, she promptly wrote its name. She succeeded in writing to dictation, although she appeared to be able to do so better with the eyes closed. The normal control of vision seemed to be gravely diminished and, whether she wrote spontaneously or to dictation, she did not keep to the lines, mixed the words together and produced letters of different sizes. She copied with the greatest difficulty, perpetually referring to the original, and did not understand a word of what she had written.

Only after much urging could she be persuaded to draw spontaneously, and the results were poor. She copied a simple drawing with great difficulty and many errors.

At first she was completely unable to find her way, even to the lavatory, which was directly opposite to her bed. But, within a month of her admission, she could go in and out of the ward and along the corridors. She seated herself on a chair, made her way to her bed and found her handkerchief, when asked to do so; yet from time to time she made considerable mistakes. Finally, although she was able to move with astonishing precision in familiar surroundings, she failed to discover the way out of a strange room by the road she had entered. When she was re-admitted to hospital after a year's absence, she showed an accurate recollection of the position of the bed she had previously occupied and of the passages. Taken to the lecture room she indicated correctly the places occupied by the professor, the students and herself during a previous clinical demonstration.

She died in 1912 and the post-mortem examination showed somewhat severe arterio-sclerosis of the basal arteries with diffuse changes in the vessels of the brain, which must have produced some diminution of its total functional capacity. There was extensive softening in the substance of both occipital lobes and all the appropriate paths on the right side and most of those on the left were affected. The right temporal lobe was totally destroyed, whilst on the left side all but the first convolution must have been thrown out of function. Every connecting tract between the occipital and temporal lobes was completely destroyed and there was considerable degeneration of the splenium and anterior commissure.

As the result of critical examination of all the cases of this condition reported in the literature, von Stauffenberg arrived at the following conclusions: Mind-blindness is a symptom which can never exist alone, but is always associated with permanent or transitory defects of a higher order, such as those of memory, intelligence, speech, etc. This forms a "syndrome" and is never a pure and isolated loss of function.

In all characteristic examples the main manifestation consists of inability to recognise objects with certainty and to appreciate their use by sight alone. Details may be described correctly, as for instance the shape and appearance of a pencil without knowledge of how to use it. Unusual objects suffer most, whilst those which make a more personal appeal are least affected, and recognition is always easier when the patient is amongst familiar surroundings. Extreme variations occur from time to time; there may be a sudden uprush of power to appreciate the use of objects and to name them correctly, whilst on other occasions the whole process may be slowed down materially. The power of visual recognition was never destroyed without bringing in its wake other more severe intellectual manifestations. Thus, orientation in space suffered almost constantly at one time or another, but it was remarkable how often the patient regained a knowledge of familiar surroundings and power to find the way unaided. Letters of the alphabet were recognised with difficulty and reading was defective in twenty-one out of twenty-two instances. Numbers, on the other hand, were relatively well appreciated. Writing was often more or less disturbed and "agraphia" was reported eight times in twenty cases. In nearly half the patients spontaneous speech was normal, but ten out of twenty-two showed some want of facility in finding words. Naming and description were always difficult and sometimes almost completely impossible. Cerebral activity and functional capacity were always diminished and the patient tended to become apathetic towards events in the world around.

Visual imperception rarely occurred alone throughout the whole course of the disease; some lowering of tactile appreciation was frequently associated with mind-blindness, but hearing, smell and taste were affected six times only in twenty-nine cases.

The anatomical basis for this condition cannot be discovered in any one strictly localised portion of the brain. There is not a single instance where a pure traumatic lesion of one or even both occipital lobes alone, in an otherwise normal cerebrum, led to permanent visual imperception. In the majority of cases the lesion was bilateral, extensive and was associated with general arterial degeneration[1].

(b) *Auditory Imperception*

Those sensory impulses which form the basis of hearing pass to the posterior portion of the temporal lobe and impinge primarily on Heschl's gyrus, which forms their receptive centre. Bilateral destruction in this region is liable to be associated with deafness of a gross character and severe degree[2].

But apart from this crude loss of function, there can be no doubt that organic disease of the brain may lead to a condition mainly characterised by auditory imperception or agnosia. In many of the cases reported in the literature, which seem to belong to this category, the clinical description is sadly lacking in fulness. Sometimes this was due to the impossibility of exposing the patient to systematic and repeated examination; in other instances the full importance of the case was not recognised until the autopsy revealed the situation of the lesion.

But in order that we may obtain some idea of the actual defects of function, which are liable to be associated with manifest auditory imperception, I shall consider in detail two examples of this condition where

---

[1] [123], p. 157 and pp. 168, 169.   [2] Cf. v. Monakow [107], p. 811.

the clinical investigation was sufficiently extensive and the patient was under observation for a considerable period.

First let us take the case reported by Dejerine and Sérieux under the misleading title "Un cas de surdité verbale pure terminée par aphasie sensorielle[1]."

The patient was a woman of 51, who was admitted to the Asylum of Vaucluse on March 11th, 1891. For six years she had suffered from increasing difficulty in understanding what was said to her, although she could hear sounds. In December, 1892, she had a stroke after which her symptoms increased progressively until her death in March, 1895. The following account of her condition is abstracted from observations made between her admission and the attack at the end of 1892.

The right ear was deaf from otitis media, but the hearing of the left was good. She certainly heard sounds and distinguished the voice of a man from that of a woman, or the blow of a hammer on the table from the tapping of a knife on a glass. But she had difficulty in appreciating the difference between whistling, the song of birds and the human voice. She mistook the birds for the voices of women in church and complained that she did not hear the words. She could neither recognise nor sing certain popular airs and said "Au clair de la lune" was a funeral march.

She failed to comprehend most of what was said to her and was unable to carry out oral commands. She complained that, although she heard the words, she could not understand them. Certain words in common use, such as "bottine," "chapeau," "table," were, however, recognised and she frequently picked out some part of a phrase, appreciated its meaning and gave an answer, which bore some more or less appropriate relation to the question.

She talked volubly, replacing one word by another, reversing the order and frequently changing a letter or a syllable; there was evidently slight "paraphasia." She could not name objects shown to her and suffered from some "verbal amnesia."

Repetition gave inconstant results; some words were repeated, which she could not say spontaneously, but on other occasions this was impossible, although she could utter them if she read them from print. Names she repeated with difficulty.

She read aloud better than she talked, but many words were not understood. Her comprehension of written questions was better than if they were asked orally and the only mode of communication with her was in writing.

When she wrote spontaneously, she reproduced the faults of articulated speech and a short letter composed by her unprompted was comprehensible in part only. To dictation certain words alone were heard and transcribed correctly; the passage as a whole was unintelligible.

She seemed to be able to recall vividly certain visual images and talked accurately of the appearance of the streets in her quarter of the town. But her intellectual

[1] [120] and [39].

powers were enfeebled and her attention was fixed with difficulty; memory was retained to a fair degree.

On December 28th, 1892, she suffered from a cerebral attack and from this time onwards her symptoms progressively increased. She became completely "word-deaf." She could still read aloud but without understanding. Speech and writing grew more and more incorrect and what she wrote to dictation was completely incomprehensible.

When she died in March, 1895, both temporal lobes were found to be atrophied symmetrically as a whole and reduced to half their size. All the convolutions were affected, the first temporal to the greatest degree, then the second and the third to the least amount; the wasting diminished from before backwards extending to the gyrus supra-marginalis and the base of the insertion of the gyrus angularis, which appeared to be intact. Microscopically the destruction affected exclusively the cellular elements and tangential fibres; those of Türck's bundle were much diminished in number. The remaining portions of the brain were unaffected.

The second case I have selected to illustrate auditory imperception was reported by Henschen[1].

A woman of 54 years of age was admitted to hospital in April, 1902, with the following history: In 1883 she became infected with syphilis from nursing a child of another family and developed characteristic manifestations of the disease. In May, 1901, she was seized with twitching in the right half of the body and face, followed by indistinct utterance and some defect of memory. In March, 1902, her left hand suddenly became numb and cold; she did not lose consciousness, but the hand was paralysed and the left leg weak. On April 3rd, she had another attack of twitching in this arm and leg followed by loss of power, and she was admitted to hospital next day with left hemiplegia unaccompanied by aphasia or hemianopsia.

On April 12th, 1902, she suddenly became agitated and confused and from this time onwards was "word-deaf." Fuller examination next day showed that crude hearing was not lost, although she did not answer questions or understand what was said to her. Speech was on the whole fluent, but she found difficulty in pronouncing some words and phrases. She seemed to have forgotten her husband's name and, although she recognised objects and their use, she could not name them. She neither understood the contents of a newspaper nor obeyed written commands. It was impossible to test her powers of writing, for she could not be persuaded to make the attempt and refused to take a pen into her hand.

This severe and characteristic set of symptoms gradually diminished and she regained her capacity to read aloud with understanding and to obey written commands. At times she appreciated what was said to her, at others she failed altogether to do so; her "word-hearing" was variable though generally defective.

---

[1] [69], [70] and in abstracted form [73 a], p. 3.

Further systematic examination at the end of 1904 showed that she was not deaf and could then appreciate all tones from the highest to the lowest. She recognised common melodies, gave the names of the songs and could repeat them if they were sung to her. She was able to appreciate the difference between voices and, although she was "not completely word-deaf to a certain kind of words," she had great difficulty in understanding what was said to her. Even when she could not see the mouth of the speaker, she sometimes understood and answered questions; for instance, asked her age she gave both the day and year of her birth. Told to put out her tongue, she repeated the order aloud and then executed it correctly. She seemed to understand what was said to her more readily if she had asked the question herself. She was talkative, humorous and fond of telling stories; at times there was slight "paraphasia," at others her speech was clear. She could repeat words said to her and named objects correctly. Printed and written matter was now understood and there was no "alexia." She wrote spontaneously and to order, but she failed with certain words and paid no attention to small errors or defects of letters and syllables.

Death occurred on June 6th, 1904, and the autopsy revealed profound destruction in both halves of the brain. In the right hemisphere it occupied the operculum, the whole of the insula and the greater part of the temporal convolutions including the gyrus transversus (Heschl). The disorganisation extended deeply to the lenticular nucleus and frontal portion of the internal capsule. On the left side the softening occupied an area beginning in the occipital lobe and extending forwards over the first and second temporal convolutions together with part of the gyrus transversus.

These two cases form characteristic examples of the morbid manifestations associated with auditory imperception; for, although the gravity and incidence of the symptoms differed in the two instances, they showed certain main features in common. They were not deaf, but failed to understand what was said to a degree far in excess of anything found in a pure aphasia[1]. Sérieux's patient was also unable to distinguish sounds such as whistling, the song of birds and the human voice. Speech was voluble though slightly "paraphasic" and both patients were unable to name objects, at any rate in the early stages of the affection. In the same way neither could read perfectly at first and writing reproduced the faults of articulated speech. Henschen's patient showed the greatest amount of recovery between the two principal examinations and evi-

---

[1] In Henschen's patient the description of hearing in the early stage (April, 1902) is unsatisfactory. He records that "she could hear a 'Hallo' in the neighbourhood of her ear. She paid little attention to the ticking of a watch, but on the other hand was more affected by the rattling of a bunch of keys close to her ear." ([69], p. 326.)

dently regained some comprehension of spoken words and power both to read and to write.

Study of the literature reveals all grades of such defects, ranging from almost complete deafness with considerable intellectual loss to perfect recognition of the significance of musical and other sounds with comparatively slight difficulty in understanding spoken words. But the cruder the loss of auditory perception the more extensively will the power of reading and writing be affected. Conversely, should the organic disease remain stationary, these are the first acts to recover, even though capacity to comprehend what is said or to execute oral commands still remains gravely defective.

Thus we are justified in recognising a group of symptoms ("syndrome"), which for want of a better name may be called "auditory imperception" or "agnosia," with the clear reservation that this is a purely empirical term. The actual phenomena differ from the manifestations of aphasia or amnesia in the comparatively profound loss of comprehension of the meaning of the non-verbal aspect of auditory impressions. Any disturbance of articulated speech, reading and writing, that may be present at first, tends to be relatively less severe than in those higher disorders classed as aphasia or amnesia.

(c) *Conclusions*

Critical study of cases to be found in the literature shows that we are justified in recognising certain groups of clinical manifestations, which can be termed empirically imperception or agnosia. These belong to a lower functional order than those of aphasia or amnesia. They do not correspond exactly to any definite category of psychical activities, but comprise a variable number of abnormal responses of which the most insistent and severe centre around defects of visual or of auditory perception. The nature and degree of these morbid reactions must be determined by examination in each particular instance and cannot be anticipated or strictly defined from a priori reasoning. With some notable exceptions, most of the observations in the past have been of a comparatively perfunctory character and much fuller and more extensive methods of examination are necessary to establish the true symptomatology of visual and auditory agnosia. Tests must be applied systematically, which are adapted to reveal not only the expected defects but also those which would not have been anticipated from a priori consideration.

Yet, in spite of the sparsity of the clinical data, imperception obviously differs from any disorder of speech which can justifiably be classed as "sensory" aphasia or amnesia in the fact that at one time or another the patient had difficulty in recognising the significance of sights or of sounds.

This is of necessity associated with some want of capacity to read or to comprehend spoken words; but this want of verbal appreciation is secondary to a more fundamental disorder of sensory perception. The disturbance of function comprises more than a defective use of language and affects a lower grade of intellectual activities. Should the imperception be severe, higher forms of mental activity suffer massively; there is not only gross inability to read and write, but the patient's intelligence is usually distinctly lowered. Articulated speech remains however relatively unaffected compared with that of a severe example of "sensory" aphasia.

Provided the lesion remains stationary, the symptoms diminish in severity and amplitude. In fact the condition tends to be transitory and in this the clinical manifestations correspond with the results of physiological experiment. Most of the more striking examples of imperception passed through a period in which the symptoms were severe, followed by a varying degree of recovery; this gave place to further degradation of function as the disease progressed to a fatal issue.

No single local lesion can produce imperception. The destruction of tissue must be severe, extensive, and in most of the best reported cases was bilateral. Sometimes, however, a widespread unilateral lesion, accompanied by general cerebral changes due to arterial degeneration, may be responsible for the appearance of this "syndrome."

Should the destruction of tissue, though widespread, more particularly affect the supra-marginal, angular and occipital gyri, the imperception tends to assume mainly a visual form, whilst affections of the temporal lobes are more likely to be associated with inability to recognise the meaning of sounds and spoken words. But there is no strict point to point connection between the detailed nature of the symptoms and the site of the anatomical lesions.

§5. THE WORD AS A UNIT OF THINKING AND SPEAKING
(a) "Word-deafness" and "Word-blindness"

Bastian's views on disorders of speech were founded on two false assumptions, which have haunted the work of neurologists ever since. He begins his first paper in 1869 with the statement that we think in words, a doctrine prevalent at the time, which bound pathologists to antique theories of parallelism between speaking and thinking and rendered their observations useless to the psychologist and grammarian.

As a corollary he postulated that words were revived as sound impressions in the auditory perceptive centres of the cerebral hemispheres and, when thought has to be expressed articulately, impulses arising from these revived impressions must be transmitted to the more immediate motor centres for speech. "In amnesia there is an inability to recall words, i.e. they cannot properly be revived in the auditory perceptive centres, and there is an almost proportional impairment of the thinking power."

"In the same way, when the individual attempts to write, the revived sound impressions call up visual impressions, which are transmitted to the motor centres for the hand." "Where the individual cannot read, I am inclined to think that this must be owing either to some lesion of the afferent fibres of the visual perceptive centre itself or of the communications between the cells of this centre and those of the auditory perceptive centre. No meaning would be conveyed by the hieroglyphic marks of the printed or written pages. They would be mere meaningless strokes."

Bastian was the first to postulate two forms of "sensory" disorders of speech to which Kussmaul subsequently gave the names of "word-deafness" and "word-blindness." Here we see the outlines of a theory, which has dominated more or less every attempt to explain the clinical manifestations of aphasia. Perfect use of language depends on the normal activity of receptive and executive centres, which can be disturbed independently of one another by an organic lesion of the brain. On the "sensory" side locally distinct areas of the cortex are the seat of "memories of words" or "verbal images," and the after effects of past experiences are stored up in these foci like photographic plates or, according to another simile, are stamped on the cells of the brain as the impressions of a seal upon wax. Words, the basis of thought, are built up out of auditory and visual elements, which stand revealed in consequence of organic lesions of the brain. Perfect use of language demands the exact combination of auditory and visual "word-images" and their translation into motor "word-images" for the purposes of speaking or writing. This theory, which was subjected to numerous modifications at the hands of various observers, rested fundamentally on the a priori assumption that acts of speech were composed of verbal images, generated in distinct areas of the cortex and separable by disease.

With the discovery of "mind-blindness" and "mind-deafness" further impetus was given to such hypothetical conceptions. But closer investigation of the phenomena of imperception in man showed that these morbid states differed profoundly from any variety of aphasia.

A patient with auditory imperception might not understand what was said to him, but he also failed to appreciate the meaning of many sounds other than words. Similarly, in a case of visual imperception, inability to read, or to comprehend verbal symbols, was always associated at one time or another with want of power to recognise objects by sight. The symptoms of "mind-deafness" or "mind-blindness" were obviously in excess of any that could rightly be attributed to "sensory" aphasia; they affected a range of activities far wider than verbal meaning or the power of recalling words.

Recognition of these clinical facts led to the further hypothesis that, in addition to primary cortical receptive centres responsible for appreciation of the significance of sights and sounds, there were others of a higher functional order concerned with the meaning of words, syllables and isolated letters. These were locally distinct from the lower receptive areas and could be affected independently. Henschen went so far as to postulate the existence of several such separate centres both on the auditory and visual side, each of which was responsible for some specific aspect of memory word-images. "The corticality for vision." he says[1], "is locally separated from the superior psychical centre for the memory of words. There are therefore relatively to vision at least two cortical centres; an inferior, which immediately receives the impression of light and a superior, which is the corticality of memory or of representation." He makes similar statements with regard to auditory impressions, erecting a whole series of separable centres, each of which exercises a higher function than the one beneath it in complexity[2]. He insists that "mind-blindness and deafness" are fundamentally different from "word-blindness and deafness" and can be "localised" in independent areas of the cortex[3].

Hypothetically a patient with uncomplicated "word-blindness" cannot read aloud or execute printed commands, although he shows no other defects of visual perception. He sees the printed design on the paper without appreciating the meaning of the verbal symbols and recognises letters and syllables but not words; nor can he read what he has written. "Word-deafness," on the other hand, is shown particularly by inability to understand spoken words. Like a person in a foreign country, the patient hears the sounds, distinguishes one from another, but they convey to him no meaning. He reads to himself but not aloud and can write freely.

[1] [70], p. 424, see also [71], p. 95 et seq.
[2] [70], pp. 442–443.   [3] [73 b], p. 192.

But all attempts to demonstrate the existence of primary, uncomplicated "word-deafness" or "word-blindness" have failed completely. For in every instance where the clinical records are sufficiently detailed, either there was some want of perceptual capacity beyond that for words, or the patient was a straightforward example of "sensory" aphasia unable to execute both oral and written commands of a certain difficulty.

Auditory and visual imperception are definite disorders of function usually evoked by extensive or bilateral lesions of the brain. However gross the symptoms, they are more or less transitory and vary greatly in degree at different stages of the disease. At one period the patient may have recovered, or may still retain his power of appreciating the meaning of sounds and sights, although he cannot understand spoken words or read printed matter. But complete records of the case show that it was essentially an example of imperception and not one of primary "word-deafness" or "word-blindness."

Want of care in distinguishing such partial states of imperception has been responsible for many supposed examples of defective "word-imagery." The observer concentrates his attention on the fact that the patient either cannot understand what is said, or is unable to carry out printed commands, and reports the case as one of "word-deafness" or "word-blindness," oblivious of the grosser defects in perceptual appreciation. Dejerine actually describes the two main forms of imperception as "surdité et cécité verbale *pure*," reserving the terms "surdité et cécité verbale" for varieties of sensory aphasia. Though an ardent upholder of the importance of verbal images, especially for internal speech, he warns his readers that in practice disturbance in one of the sensory elements in the use of language is liable to upset the normal flow of speech, and so induces accessory defects, especially on the expressive side.

Moreover, the whole conception of the importance of verbal images in acts of speech is contradicted by the clinical facts of "sensory" aphasia. Many observers, from Wernicke onwards, have pointed out that in this condition the defects cannot be classed strictly as isolated loss of auditory or visual word-images. In typical examples there is want of comprehension of both spoken and written words; certain commands are badly executed in whatever form they are given. Moreover, the loss of appreciation is rarely if ever complete; should the task be made easier, it can be performed without error. It is absurd therefore to say that the patient is "word-deaf" or "word-blind"; for his power of appreciating spoken or written words depends more on the nature and severity of the problems to be solved than on the particular sense to which it is presented. The more careful and detailed the examination, the less can cases of "sensory" aphasia be classified as "word-deaf" or "word-blind."

Evidently the hypothesis that the normal use of language is built up out of auditory and visual word images is unsupported by experience, and fails to explain the phenomena of so-called "sensory" disorders of speech.

(b) *The word as a unit of speech*

Apart altogether from the fact that "word-deafness" and "word-blindness" do not correspond to distinct and separable clinical phenomena, the selection of the word as the unit of speech has been one of the most disastrous errors in the classical theories of aphasia.

As early as 1866 Jackson wrote[1]: "Of course we do not either speak or think in words or signs only, but in words or signs referring to one another in a particular manner....Indeed, words in sentences lose their individual meaning—if single words can be strictly said to have any meaning—and the whole sentence becomes a unit and not a word-heap." Moreover, he pointed out that the whole question of the forms assumed by an aphasia was essentially a psychological one. Only after determining the nature of the phenomena could we proceed to connect them with organic lesions of the brain tissues.

We neither think nor speak in combinations of verbal units. In order to understand the morbid phenomena of speech they must be considered as a disturbance of progressive acts, which cannot reach their proper conclusion. They are not due to disintegration of isolated words strung together in sequence. Not only is it impossible to break up a word into auditory and visual elements, but disease does not analyse a sentence into its verbal or grammatical constituents. We cannot even assume that a sentence is strictly a unit of speech. Speech, like walking, is an act of progression. It is impossible to obtain a satisfactory conception of how a man walks from a single instantaneous photograph; before we can give the impression of motion, the pictures must pass in an unbroken series as through a cinematograph.

Grammarians, who had long ago deposed the word from its pre-eminent position as the unit of language, could make no use of the data yielded by pathology. They ceased to pay attention to the ideas of the clinician and gave up all attempt to reconcile them with modern doctrines of the nature of normal speech.

[1] [81], p. 56.

Nothing is more absurd or less consonant with the facts than the statement that in some forms of aphasia nouns, in others verbs, are more particularly affected. Defects of language cannot be adequately expressed in terms of parts of speech; the total manifestations may be conveniently designated by a name culled from grammar, because it most aptly describes what is happening. But no variety of aphasia can be dissected into grammatical elements.

Equally false is the idea that letters, syllables or words suffer specifically and independently of one another. For, as soon as we attempt to translate disorders of speech into literal or verbal elements, we are at once met by psychological factors outside the range of purely grammatical structure.

The view that the word is the unit of speech fails to take into account the importance of silent pauses in speech. Nothing is more striking in the phenomena of aphasia than the way in which speech is either slowed or quickened by changes in the frequency and length of these pauses. Thus, the last remains of what I have called a verbal aphasia are to be found in shortened phrases and prolonged pauses; every word may be appropriate and correctly pronounced, but the rhythm is distinctly abnormal. On the other hand, the stormy utterance of a patient with syntactical aphasia is due as much to disorders of rhythm as to defects in the grammatical structure of his phrases.

No test can ever exactly resemble one which has preceded it, however closely we may attempt to reproduce the conditions. Suppose a set of colours are laid before the patient and he is asked to choose green, he may fail to do so, although he is successful with blue. This does not of necessity signify that he is totally ignorant of the meaning of the word green, but recognises blue. For on the next occasion, when these two colours recur in the series of tests, his conduct may be the exact reverse and he points correctly to green, but fails to indicate blue.

Looked at from the point of view of a set of single momentary responses, we can only conclude that his behaviour was untrustworthy and erratic. From the psychological aspect, on the other hand, we learn the important fact that, with a sequence of tests of this kind, he once failed and once succeeded in selecting both the colours named. We are face to face with reactions which vary, not only with the mode of giving the command, but with the situation at the moment. Thus, the result is modified both by the sequence of the tests and by the fact that the same individual task has been set and executed on a previous occasion. The response obtained at any one moment is profoundly influenced by past events.

The nature of the response also varies profoundly with the attitude of the speaker, both to the task set him and to his auditor. In forming his words and phrases much depends on his efforts to express what he wants to say in terms which can be understood. He is debarred by his disability from the use of verbal forms natural to him and, like a man talking a foreign language, seeks some other and less difficult mode of conveying his meaning.

Moreover, a word has all sorts of secondary meanings, which cannot be expressed in grammatical terms. This it shares with pictures and every act in which symbolic significance plays a part. Semantic changes, or defective appreciation of ultimate as opposed to immediate significance, cannot be accounted for on any of the classical theories. For it is not the word, the phrase, or even the sentence that is at fault. The patient fails to recognise the aim or meaning of the whole act as a progressive series; he misses the humorous intention of a joke or of a picture and fails to see exactly how the various utensils should be arranged on the table for breakfast.

§ 6. THE CLINICAL PSYCHOLOGISTS

Marie rejected the whole hypothesis of verbal images and attributed aphasia proper to intellectual defects. Moutier says[1]:

Il existe, chez tout aphasique un déficit intellectuel général et un déficit intellectuel spécialisé pour le langage. Général, le déficit porte sur la mémoire, la mimique descriptive, l'association des idées, les connaissances professionnelles. Spécialisé pour le langage, il porte sur la lecture, l'écriture, la compréhension de la langue orale ou écrite. Les altérations du calcul participent tout spécialement à la fois du déficit général et du déficit spécialisé. Les altérations de ces facultés surviennent, évoluent, régressent conformément aux lois ordinaires des désordres intellectuels en général.... L'aphasie n'est pas une démence[2]. Elle différera toujours de celle-ci par un déficit spécialisé pour le langage.

There are no specific varieties of aphasia; the so-called "sensory" symptoms are a myth and "word-deafness" and "word-blindness" are no more than an intellectual disturbance of the power to comprehend language. When Wernicke's zone, which comprises the gyrus supramarginalis, angularis and the first two temporal convolutions, is affected, the patient exhibits intellectual changes of a high order, which vary in severity with the gravity and extent of the lesion. On the other hand, the "motor" manifestations are due to anarthria and are not in themselves accompanied by any intellectual changes.

[1] [110], p. 248.   [2] [110], p. 249.

At first sight it might seem as if Marie, with his insistence on the importance of intellectual defects in aphasia, had adopted a psychological view. But his attitude differs fundamentally from that of the modern psychologist, for his doctrine postulates the identity of speaking and thinking. Disorders of verbal formation are not distinguished from those of thought and the use of the symbol is mistaken for what it symbolises. Moutier says, "Chez l'homme, la pensée se conduit uniquement par les mots[1]."

Moreover, the view of Marie and Moutier is essentially anatomical. When a certain area of the brain, called Wernicke's zone, is affected, the intellectual aspect of language and intelligence as a whole are more or less disturbed; internal speech suffers as part of these general defects. On the other hand, when speech is affected by a lesion in any other part of the brain, the disorder of function is not accompanied by any want of intelligence, general or special, and the processes of internal speech remain intact.

Such a conception reduces executive speech to a high-grade articulatory act and makes all other faults of expression secondary to some form of intellectual failure. But closer examination shows that there are forms of disordered speech, commonly classed as "motor," which show psychical defects in the use of language akin to those found in other varieties of aphasia. They exhibit changes of a higher order than any which can rightly be included under the term "anarthria" or even "aphemia." Speaking has a psychology of its own, which is not co-terminous with that of thinking.

Patients with aphasia and kindred disorders of speech come under the care of the neurologist or general physician as an incident in the practice of his profession. On the other hand, the psychologist, who is acutely interested in the phenomena, is compelled to accept a statement of the facts at second hand, based as many of them are on antiquated theories of speaking and thinking.

Pick was one of the first clinicians to adopt a frankly psychological attitude towards the morbid manifestations of speech. In 1905, after the publication of much admirable work on conventional lines, he recognised the fallacy of attributing "sensory" aphasia to destruction of verbal images, auditory or visual. He saw that the use of language comprised a series of progressive actions, which could be thrown into disorder by disease; by assuming this point of view he was able to free the subject from those doctrines based on sensation and association, which had dominated the theoretical conceptions of the pathologist.

[1] [110], p. 239.

He chose for closer study that peculiar disorder of speech known as "Agrammatism[1]," in which the syntax of the sentence is more particularly affected. Speech is rapid and stormy; many words, which serve to unite the phrase into a coherent and logical whole, are omitted and at times utterance may become incomprehensible jargon.

The selection of this particular morbid manifestation has several distinct advantages. Speech is not abolished, as in so-called "motor" aphasia, but exhibits profound loss of control, which can be recorded and tested systematically. Not only is the production of words and phrases disturbed, but the rhythm of speech is gravely affected and these disorders of grammatical structure throw light on the manner in which language as a whole breaks up under the influence of disease. Finally, the disturbance of speech in its pure form can be attributed with certainty to a lesion of Wernicke's zone, more particularly the temporal convolutions; yet it is not "sensory" in the classical sense and cannot be explained in terms of auditory word-images, or any supposed elements of verbal memory.

Having chosen a disorder of speech, which was of interest both to the psychologist and to the grammarian, Pick devoted the first volume of *Die agrammatischen Sprachstörungen* to a voluminous account of any work in whatever field of knowledge, which could shed light on this group of abnormal phenomena. Throughout he alludes to cases observed by himself and others, but he reserved their systematic consideration for the second volume. Interrupted by the war, this was unfortunately never completed and we are left with a theoretical and historical introduction only. The work remains a torso, incomplete, but definite in outline and intention.

Yet in spite of these lamentable defects, Pick's attitude is clear and differs fundamentally from that customary amongst clinicians. He looked upon "agrammatism" as the result of disturbance of a purposive and orderly procedure, the use of language. The form assumed depended on adaptation by the patient to the new situation and could not be expressed in static terms, such as a destruction of component verbal images. All aphasic phenomena must be looked at in this way, not as it were in cross section, but in longitudinal progression. We cannot say that the memory of words is lost, or that memory images are stored up in different centres of the brain. This departmental theory of memory, against which Hughlings Jackson uttered a warning, has long been given up by psychologists.

[1] [115].

Pick showed a remarkable knowledge of and sympathy with Jackson's ideas and accepted the view that, on the intellectual side, these disorders of speech were due to failure to produce a propositional statement. Even a name has no reality in living language, except when referred to its place in some part of a proposition.

He separated the formulation of thought, a preliminary to the use of language, from the formulation of speech, a necessary part of the executive process; thus he distinguished a psychological schema, which comprised the thought, from the grammatical schema, which preceded its formation in words.

He divides the processes on the way from thinking to speaking into intuitive thought, the proposition, the grammatical schema and the explicit verbal formula. The first phase is the mental attitude; here thought is still undifferentiated. The second is consciousness of psychological differentiation; ideas are distinguished, but are still without verbal expression. The third comprises the schema of the phrase. The fourth is the stage of the choice of words. These are not elements, which unite to form a normal act of speech, but stages in the development of a mode of behaviour, which can be interrupted or disturbed at any point in the process. What is spoken is a manifestation of the whole psychical activity of the individual and is not an isolated phenomenon produced by the loss of some single constituent faculty.

In agrammatism some of the most important changes are due to defects of rhythm and yet pathology has almost entirely neglected the tonality of speech. The use of language consists of far more than can be put down in black and white. Every phrase may be considered from the point of view of material content and of syntax, which is its form. Both aspects suffer in agrammatism, the latter more profoundly than the former.

Pick also laid stress on lack of inhibition as an important factor in the production of this variety of disordered speech, a statement which is amply confirmed by the cases I have cited as examples of syntactical aphasia. The patient cannot check and regulate his words and phrases; he dashes on in the hope that he will be understood. Asked to repeat what he has said, he may be unable to do so and his utterance then becomes confused and incomprehensible.

A closer study of agrammatism and similar perverted forms of speech compels us to record, not only the exact utterances of the speaker, but also his attitude to the response of his hearer. This feature in aphasia has been habitually neglected by clinicians with the notable exception of Pick.

He was deeply imbued with Jackson's ideas on "Evolution and Dis-solution of the Nervous System[1]" and insisted on the necessity for closer examination of the lower forms of speech produced by organic lesions. The higher intellectual aptitudes are the first to be lost in the order of their difficulty, whilst emotional forms of speech suffer later, to disappear just before mimicry, the ultimum moriens of expression. In this con-nection he lays stress on the occurrence of modes of thought which are not strictly logical. Robbed of the power to evoke a predicative state-ment at will, speech may be reduced to a form resembling in certain ways that of a child. This may depend less on executive faults of word pro-duction than on more primitive methods of unformulated thinking.

By his choice of the phenomena of agrammatism Pick was able to determine the site of the lesion capable of evoking this distinctive dis-order of function. He insists[2] that we are not dealing with the loss of independent psychical elements, but with disturbance of a highly organised process. When therefore he states that syntactical defects are caused by a lesion of the left temporal lobe, he does not mean that "grammatism," or the correct use of syntax, is centred within this region. He implies solely that a lesion, situated in this part of the brain, can disturb the processes of normal speech in such a way that the phenomena of agrammatism become apparent.

Unfortunately in this introductory volume he does not give in detail the observations on which this localisation was based. He alludes, however, in passing to cases recorded by himself[3] and others in favour of this view, which subsequent investigation has tended to support.

In this book the first attempt was made to consider an unmistakable disorder of speech from every point of view, psychological, grammatical and anatomical. The work was unfortunately never completed; but it remains a storehouse of knowledge, necessary as a preliminary to any attempt to deal scientifically with disorders of language. Moreover, as Pick pointed out, the time had come to revise the current ideas of aphasia, agnosia and even apraxia in the light of newer conceptions of speaking and thinking[4].

---

[1] [80].   [2] [115], p. 35.   [3] [115], pp. 123, 150 etc.

[4] Whilst this book was passing through the press I received, owing to the kindness of Dr Otto Sittig and the editors of Bethe's *Handbuch der Physiologie*, the proof sheets of Professor Pick's article on Aphasia, written just before his death in 1924. [117].

This is a systematic attempt to present the clinical facts under headings corresponding in the main to disorders of function, such as affections of spontaneous speech, want of power to understand or to repeat what is said, defects of internal verbalisation, inability to read, to write, or to execute tasks demanding the use of numbers. Certain distinct groups of abnormal symptoms, for example agrammatism, paraphasia and perseveration are treated as syndromes, are subjected to analysis, and an attempt is made to determine the various lesions responsible for their appearance.

From the beginning Pick lays down that all these morbid manifestations must be considered dynamically as disorders of a normal process. Our present knowledge does not permit us to found a comprehensive explanation of the phenomena of aphasia on anatomical and physiological facts. We can simply record what happens with a clear understanding that the abnormal responses do not reveal the elements out of which speech is built up. But, from the lowest to the highest centres, the products of disintegration assume the character of "formed structures" ("gestaltete Strukturen").

By a "centre" Pick does not mean strictly definable portions of an anatomical system, nor the seat of some distinct physiological function, but a portion of the nervous system where some normal process can be most easily affected.

In this article he not only repeats in a summary form all the points on which he laid stress in *Die agrammatischen Sprachstörungen*, but attempts to associate the various manifestations with lesions in definite parts of the brain. The conclusions to which he arrives correspond closely with those of other pathological anatomists.

For the purposes of localisation he divides acts of speech into expressive and impressive, corresponding roughly to "motor" and "sensory" of other observers. Of these two groups of functions the former is disturbed by a lesion in the frontal portion of the cortical field, whilst the latter suffers with structural changes in the temporal area.

The frontal defects in the use of language correspond to Broca's aphasia; they comprise gross loss of articulatory speech, including the power to repeat what is said or to read aloud together with occasional inability to write spontaneously and to dictation. Internal speech is also liable to be somewhat affected. The fault lies in the mechanism for converting thought into words. Such "expressive" aphasia is the result of a lesion situated somewhere in the neighbourhood of the opercular portion of the third frontal gyrus. But the nearness of this area to the precentral motor centres for the articulatory apparatus is liable to lead to additional dysarthric complications.

"Impressive" or "sensory" aphasia comprises inability to understand the verbal aspects of the use of language with consequent paraphasia and disturbance of reading and writing. This disorder of speech is produced by a lesion of those parts of the posterior portion of the first temporal gyrus, which lie in front of Heschl's gyrus. The close approximation to this centre for hearing frequently causes confusion between auditory aphasia and true cortical deafness. "Word-deafness" is a misnomer, because there is no isolated affection of words, letters or syllables; but "speech-deafness" is of temporal origin.

Passing to the various syndromes of disordered speech, Pick states that there are at least two forms of agrammatism, which can be associated with lesions in different portions of the cortical field. The temporal variety is characterised by defective syntax, false verbal inflexions, wrong prefixes and suffixes; the tempo of speech is not slowed, but is rather quickened and hurried. On the other hand, in that of frontal origin, articulation is slow, the pauses are lengthened and the words are juxtaposed as in a telegram.

In view of the many functions employed in reading there can be no definite correspondence between any cortical area and loss of power to read. But the junction point of all these various capacities seems to lie in the gyrus angularis and it is here that a lesion is most likely to produce alexia.

Clinically pure cases of agraphia are rare. This condition seems to exist in two forms,

By far the most fruitful application of the methods of psychology to the problems of disordered speech is due to the members of the Frankfurt school of neuro-pathology. In 1910 Kurt Goldstein[1] published a paper on aphasia, in which he assumed an attitude towards the defective use of language differing fundamentally from that of his contemporaries. He pointed out that cortical "motor" and "sensory" aphasia never occurred in a pure form. Both, moreover, are accompanied by disturbances of reading and writing and there is no isolated "alexia" or "agraphia." In most instances no one function is totally lost and it is therefore of the first importance to consider the individual difficulty of each task set to the patient.

When all the symptoms which can be attributed to "motor" or "sensory" aspects of speech are subtracted, there is always something over; speaking psychologically, this consists of defects of verbal representation. For it must not be forgotten that either speaking or thinking, or the association between them, may be affected. Memory images exist as part of a psychical act and never in isolated forms. Appreciation of an object demands not only summation of the single processes on which it is based, but their combination to a single unity.

Only after investigating some form of disordered speech psychologically can we pass to questions of anatomical localisation; we must

one of which is due to affection of the visual aspects of speech; this is evoked most effectually by a lesion of the gyrus angularis. The other variety occurs as part of an "emissive" or "motor" aphasia and is due to destruction in the neighbourhood of the foot of the second frontal gyrus.

Failure to manipulate numbers belongs to the intellectual affections which follow temporo-occipital lesions, in association with defective perceptions and comprehension of "shape" ("Gestalt Auffassung"). When it consists mainly of inability to count, the disturbance may be occasionally of frontal origin.

All such localisation of the various clinical manifestations must be of the widest general character. At present there can be no consensus of opinion, because of the impossibility of bringing any single defect of function into satisfactory connection with the nature and extent of a lesion determined microscopically. Moreover, profound clinical differences may arise between the effects produced by destruction in the same area of the brain in consequence of diaschisis.

Here we find a serious attempt to associate various defects in the use of language treated dynamically with the facts of pathological anatomy. But Pick recognised that this presentation revealed our ignorance of the nature of the phenomena rather than our knowledge. Vast gaps must be filled in both clinically and anatomically before it will be possible to correlate disorders of the psychical mechanism of speech with cerebral physiology.

[1] [59].

first know what we have to "localise." The fundamental problem will always remain a psychological one. Since there are no single foci for separate elements of speech, and aphasic disorders are the product of lesions in a single large association field, the question of centres and conducting paths loses in interest compared with investigation of the form assumed by the phenomena.

The war produced a multitude of problems in neuro-pathology, which could only be solved by the combined observations of a neurologist and a psychologist. Goldstein therefore joined with Gelb to found in Frankfurt the "Institute for Research into the Consequences of Injuries to the Brain." Here patients with head wounds were examined exhaustively from a psychological point of view. The results were published in a series of papers of the greatest interest and value, which can be summarised here in so far only as they touch directly the phenomena of aphasia and kindred disorders of speech.

Their first communication[1], which appeared in 1918, was an enquiry into the processes of visual perception and recognition based on a case of "mind-blindness." The patient was a man of twenty-four years of age, who had received two deep wounds in the occipital region, the one in the middle line, the other to the left "about 3 cm. above the border of the hair." The lateral and median portions of the occipital lobe were injured and probably also the cerebellum, to judge by certain signs of incoordination. The fields of vision were profoundly restricted both to the right and to the left, but central vision was preserved and acuity was normal.

Yet in spite of the fact that the patient could see, visual perception and recognition were gravely disturbed. He could appreciate colours and colourless patches which fell within the intact area of his fields; he recognised that a particular patch was higher or lower, more to the right or left, nearer or further away, larger or smaller, but nothing more. The separate patches gave rise to a confused impression and were not appreciated as a whole. Although he retained his elementary sensations, he could not recognise the simplest shapes and the disturbance might be described as "total form-blindness" ("Gestaltblindheit"). This was the underlying cause of all his symptoms and abnormal reactions.

He could appreciate the use of familiar objects and both recognised and named many of them so quickly that at first sight no obvious fault could be discovered. But he was often slow in arriving at a fully correct answer and, if the time of exposure was reduced, he tended to become

[1] [55] and [56].

uncertain. Although he could draw objects spontaneously, he failed to do so when they were placed before him.

He was entirely unable to recognise words, letters, figures or pictures exposed for a definite period in the tachistoscope, and excused his want of comprehension by the complaint that "it was too quick." But, when the words were placed before him in the ordinary way, he could read them after long consideration; he seemed to depend for their comprehension on coincident writing movements of the hand. He traced the lines of a letter or diagram, or made minute movements of the index finger before he could arrive at a conclusion; if he depended on vision alone, he was "word-blind."

Such in short were the main symptoms of this remarkable case of "apperceptive mind-blindness." The general intellectual state and reactions of this patient formed the subject of a further report by Benary[1]. He came to the conclusion as the result of exhaustive tests that it was impossible to state categorically whether "general intelligence" was or was not affected. Systematic psychological examination alone could reveal in what way the mental activities of the patient had suffered. His symptoms were not due to defects of attention, want of concentration, or loss of memory; for, although at times his memory failed, it usually served amply for the solution of problems that were not unduly complex. Nor could the abnormal manifestations be explained by lack of association. He often went to work in a roundabout manner and his mental operations tended to become mechanical and wanting in mobility. But so long as a problem was not in principle impossible, he brought the most diverse intellectual aptitudes to bear on its solution. He possessed considerable "logical" capacity, especially in appreciating "relations" and even "relations of relations." His power of comprehension and of judgment were not materially diminished and he could define the characteristics of some object or quality named as easily as might have been expected from his education.

It is certain that gross general defects of visual perception and recognition could not account for his condition. Qualitative differences were certainly appreciated; but the spacial character of optical impressions, in its widest sense, was distinctly affected and for this reason Gelb and Goldstein termed the condition "form-blindness" ("Gestaltblindheit"). To this fundamental disturbance can be attributed the patient's difficulty in dealing with groups of signs as a whole, even those remotely based on visual impressions. It is not the sensory elements of perception that are

1 [10].

defective, but rather the power of evoking that general "shape" to which they should normally give rise.

It has long been known that certain patients with amnesia have difficulty in naming colours, although there is no reason to suppose that they are colour-blind. Lewandowsky[1] described such a case in 1908 under the title "Ueber Abspaltung des Farbensinnes." A man of fifty suddenly developed "sensory" aphasia with right homonymous hemianopsia. When the more severe symptoms had passed away, he was found to be unable to name colours or to choose them to oral commands, although his colour sense was intact. After an extensive and unusually complete examination, Lewandowsky came to the conclusion that the morbid phenomena were due to a severance of the normal association between representations of form and colour.

Sittig[2] took up the whole question in the light of a personal experience of three examples of this remarkable condition. He gave a critical account of all the cases to be found in the literature and confirmed in the main Lewandowsky's description. One of Sittig's patients, who had been wounded in the left parietal and occipital region, showed the usual difficulty in naming familiar objects, reading, writing and drawing. Tested with Holmgren's wools, he was unable to name them with certainty and could not select a given colour to oral commands. Asked to give the colour of well-known objects, his answers were slow and uncertain, although he could often select the skein of wool of the required tone. When the test required the acceptance or rejection of a pair of matched colours, this patient behaved like a normal person, although he could not select from a set of wools the one which corresponded in tone to a given sample.

Sittig debates the possibility that this form of amnesia may be due to defective powers of naming, but tends on the whole to reject this explanation. For, in addition to the obvious disorders of speech, functions of a higher psychical order on the way between thinking and speaking are also affected.

In their tenth communication, entitled "Ueber Farbennamenamnesie," Gelb and Goldstein[3] carried the investigation of this condition considerably further. The patient, a man of twenty-three, was wounded by a shell fragment in the left parietal region. At first he suffered with paralysis and loss of sensation in the right arm, but two years later, when he came under examination at the Frankfurt Institute, this was reduced to a slight weakness only.

[1] [84].   [2] [122].   [3] [57].

There were no gross defects of speech except the amnesia. He had, however, extreme difficulty in naming colours and in choosing them to oral commands. It was this aspect of the case which Gelb and Goldstein selected for minute and extended examination by modern psychological methods.

Shown a series of colours, the patient was unable to name them correctly, and as a rule neither accepted the right name nor refused a wrong one, if the words were said to him by the observer. But he often indicated the tone accurately with the help of a simile or concrete example; thus, red was "cherry colour," green "grass colour" and orange was described as "like an orange" ("wie eine Apfelsine"). He also had extreme difficulty in choosing a colour to oral commands. There was evidently a severe disturbance of the relation between perception of a colour and its nominal symbol.

When tested, however, by methods of comparison, which require the acceptance or rejection of a pair of colours only, he behaved like a normal person; his colour sensations were certainly unaffected. But, told to select from a number of skeins of wool those which corresponded in tone to a sample placed before him, he carried out the test slowly and was as often wrong as right; not infrequently, having taken up the right one, he would lay it aside again. His choice might be governed by the luminosity of a colour rather than by its tone and many of his responses were inexplicable.

But, if he was given two sets of colours identical in tone and luminosity, he succeeded in matching them perfectly. This he did by holding one colour against another; he was not satisfied unless they corresponded exactly. A normal person gathers together all those which contain the same basic tone, whilst this patient failed to make any selection unless the two colours were identical.

He was certainly not colour-blind and could carry out the act of matching in a concrete, but not in a more abstract form. Evidently some change in the method of sorting must underlie this peculiar behaviour. His conduct was less rational than normal; he seemed to have no principle of arrangement, but made his choice according to the more primitive method of concrete likeness or congruent experience. These defects can be explained by a definite lowering of categorical capacity.

This patient also showed considerable loss of power to name familiar objects, although he knew their use and never failed to select them in response to oral commands. But Goldstein and Gelb[1] came to the con-

1 [58].

clusion that amnesic aphasia is not primarily a disorder of speech. Not only the abnormal behaviour of the patient, when naming, selecting or sorting colours, but also all the other characteristic defects are due to a diminution of conceptual power, which compels him to act in a less logical and more concrete manner. He does not possess names for abstract use, but he can designate a colour by comparing it to some concrete object, such as blood, grass or the sky.

The defects of speech stand out in the foreground, but are not primary; the fundamental change is one of categorical behaviour. Words are there for use, but they cannot be employed demonstratively. Categorical behaviour and the possession of signs for ideas are the expression of one and the same function, a definite form of cerebral activity. A lesion of the brain can therefore diminish this power and reduce the conduct of the patient in certain directions to a more primitive level.

It is impossible to give in a short compass the full trend of these researches. Enough has been said to show that the whole conception of "amnesic" or "sensory" forms of aphasia has undergone a profound change, especially under the influence of recent developments in psychology. The older views, based on theories of combination and synthesis of elementary functions, have given place to the idea of a single unitary reaction in response to multiple factors. This principle underlies what I have called the "psychological attitude." It was foreshadowed by Hughlings Jackson more than fifty years ago and is gaining adherents day by day as aphasia and kindred disorders of speech come to be considered as manifestations of the mental processes, thinking and speaking.

CHAPTER VII

HISTORICAL RETROSPECT

IN the preceding pages I have not attempted to give a complete history of the views propounded at one time or another concerning the nature and causes of aphasia and kindred disorders of speech. A century and a quarter have elapsed since it was first suggested that a local injury to the brain could disturb the use of language and the evolution of our knowledge is one of the most astonishing stories in the history of medicine. During this period current philosophy, physiology and medicine have undergone profound modifications, and many of these changes have reacted, not only on the theories, but also on the clinical observations made under their influence.

These developments formed the subject of my historical sketch and I therefore selected certain epochs and men as representing some definite aspect of thought. But I have been unable to notice or to give due weight to the admirable work of many observers, who supported the ideas of more prominent protagonists. Moreover, since I hold definite views of my own, such a historical summary cannot be an unprejudiced account. For it is intended to prepare the way for fresh facts and new theories and, whilst I have striven to give due credit to my predecessors in this vast field, I could not divert the narrative to deal adequately with hypotheses, which have no direct bearing on my observations.

Ever since interest in the question was first aroused, the phenomena of aphasia have been presented for investigation in the same forms and under identical conditions; there has been no change in the problem to be solved. Every generation has examined the manifestations afresh, armed with different general conceptions and dominated by prejudices arising from the ideas of the day. The knowledge transmitted to subsequent workers in the field has thus been a mixture of theory and fact, and it has frequently happened that the theory has survived, whilst the new observations have been forgotten. Many an hypothesis, based on pure conjecture, has been handed on from one authority to influence his successors, whilst the luminous clinical investigations of the same author have been entirely neglected, or have been absorbed into the general bulk of knowledge. The world clings to theories, for they are easier to remember, can be reproduced with effect and lead to a clarity of exposition foreign to a description of the crude experimental facts. There is in consequence a tendency to carry over the conceptions of one age on to the observations of the next. New wine is poured into old bottles with disastrous results.

The persistent tendency to localise a centre for normal speech in the frontal convolutions is one of the most striking examples of the influence of a theory, deduced from certain a priori considerations, upon observations of an entirely different character.

Gall pointed out that injuries to the head showed that the normal activities of the mind were dependent upon the integrity of the brain, which consequently serves as the organ of intellectual life. The nervous system of man was therefore the physical instrument of his moral attributes, for the nerves were the conductors by which the will was transmitted to all parts of the body. At that time man was supposed to be endowed with certain "faculties" and these moral and intellectual qualities Gall attempted to localise in different parts of the brain. There were six different forms of memory, each of which he placed in a different "organ," or, as we should say, "centre." There was the memory of things, the memory of locality, the name-memory, the verbal and grammatical memory and the memory for numbers. All of these "organs" were situated in those portions of the brain which were in relation with the posterior part of the orbital cavity.

He appears to have taken no precautions to verify this localisation, which was based on pure speculation dating back to Gall's childhood. For as a boy he noticed that his companions who had prominent eyes had a gift for languages and an excellent memory for words. When his admirable anatomical investigations led him to believe that the brain was not a uniform mass but consisted of a number of specialised organs, he was led by his fantastic preconceptions concerning verbal memory to place the centre for this "faculty" in the frontal lobes and particularly on the under surface in contact with the roof of the orbit.

Bouillaud, rejecting the conception of "moral faculties," carried on and developed the doctrine that certain functions were dependent on the activity of certain areas of the brain. He attempted to show from clinical evidence, checked by post-mortem examination, that affections of motion and sensation were due to lesions in different parts of the brain. Many of his observations were accurate and the interpretation he set upon them acute. He was, however, obsessed by the hypothesis that the seat of the "faculty of speech" lay in the "anterior lobes." As he lived to a remarkable age and reached a position of great power in the medical world, he was always able to insist upon this view, whenever the question arose.

Thus, when Broca saw his first case of aphasia, he was familiar with the idea that the "faculty of speech" was thought to reside in the anterior lobes and he called in Auburtin, Bouillaud's son-in-law, to examine the patient with him at Bicêtre. It was agreed between them that the autopsy would form a test of the rightness or not of this theory.

The brain showed destruction of the posterior part of the second and third frontal convolutions, the inferior portion of the Rolandic area and the first temporal convolution. Marie subsequently pointed out that the lesion also occupied the supra-marginal gyrus, a part which at that time was not considered of any importance from the point of view of speech.

This was followed by a second case in which the situation and nature of the lesion was acknowledged to be more doubtful; there seems to have been some wasting at the foot of the second frontal convolution, such as is not uncommon in a senile brain.

Broca had discovered and described with perfect accuracy a definite clinical condition, which he called "aphemia," and he believed that he had found the seat of the faculty of articulated speech in the third frontal convolution. As autopsies increased in number, he began to appreciate that this crude conception did not cover all the facts.

He divided affections of speech of central origin into "aphemia" and "amnesia verbalis," laying down clearly the difference between them. The aphemic patient has a profoundly reduced vocabulary and may be speechless, except for some monosyllables, oaths and words that do not seem to belong to any language. His ideas are intact, as shown by gestures, and he can understand what is said to him, recognising the meaning of words and phrases, which he cannot pronounce or even repeat. On the other hand, the amnesic patient no longer appreciates the conventional associations established between ideas and words. He can pronounce them, but they do not seem to have any bearing on the ideas he wishes to express. He is able to show by gestures that he has not lost all kinds of memory, but it is the special memory, not only of spoken but of written words, that is lost.

So far Broca's statements were admirably clear and consonant with fact. When, however, he tried to determine the site of the lesions responsible for these clinical manifestations, he became confused and indefinite. He saw clearly that the larger number of cases did not correspond to these two clean-cut divisions. In practice, both states can exist together and this greatly hampered determination of 'the site of the responsible lesion. But he insisted that "aphemia" was caused by destruction of the third frontal convolution.

Marie attempted to eradicate this doctrine by totally denying that the third frontal convolution had any direct bearing on speech. True aphasia was produced by a lesion of Wernicke's zone, whilst destruction within a wide-spread sub-cortical area, which he called the "quadrilateral," was responsible for loss of the higher articulatory aspects of speech. He did not deny the validity of Broca's clinical observations, but rejected his anatomical conclusions.

In spite of the vast amount of excellent work expended on this question, many still place a centre for normal speech in the third frontal and one for writing in the second frontal convolution. Gall's young friend with the "yeux à fleur de tête" still exercises a subtle influence on the problems of aphasia. Long vanished ideas of "human faculties" have been carried over into more modern theories of cerebral localisation. I hope to show later that there are no cortical centres for normal mental activities, but that there are certain areas within which destruction of tissue produces a disorder of some particular mode of behaviour.

Moreover, the only anatomical localisation, in the strict sense of the term, is topographical, corresponding to the parts of the body or to their projection in space. Thus the "motor centres" are arranged according to the contiguity of the segments of the limbs and trunk. The so-called "sensory zone" represents the spacial arrangement of somatic sensibility, whilst the area striata is in reality the central reproduction of certain aspects of the projected field of vision. The older conceptions of "centres" for normal functions is an anachronism in the light of modern physiology.

That we think in words was a widely prevalent hypothesis, which still exercises its influence on the theories of aphasia, long after it has been abandoned by the philologists. Bastian based his views on this dictum and postulated that words were revived as sound impressions in the auditory perceptive centres, whence they were transmitted to the more immediate motor centres for speech. In amnesia there is an inability to recall words, associated with an almost proportional impairment of the thinking power. Similarly, when the patient is unable to write, the revived sound impressions cannot call up the necessary visual impressions of words.

These views rapidly led to the doctrine that all forms of aphasia and amnesia could be attributed to lesions of a "motor," "auditory," or "visual word-centre," or of the fibres which connected them with one another. But this whole conception is contradicted by the facts of "sensory" aphasia. The defects discovered on examination cannot be classed as an isolated loss of auditory or of visual word-images, and it is absurd to speak of one patient as "word-deaf," of another as "word-blind."

We no longer believe that we think in words, and the whole doctrine of the importance of verbal images has gone by the board. These phenomena form part of the mechanism of internal thinking together with a multitude of other modes of psychical activity. Like all forms of imagery, they may suffer or not in disorders of speech according to the use to which they are put.

On the other hand, certain clinical manifestations can be justifiably grouped under the terms auditory and visual imperception or agnosia. The patient suffers from much more than "word-deafness" or "word-blindness." The disturbance belongs to a lower order of functional disintegration than aphasia and amnesia. For, at one time or another, the patient has difficulty in recognising the meaning of crude sounds or sights. This is of necessity accompanied by some want of verbal appreci-ation, or inability to read and to understand printed symbols. But all such lack of comprehension of language is a secondary consequence of the gross imperception. Should this loss of function be severe, higher forms of mental activity tend to suffer gravely and the patient's intelli-gence is usually distinctly lowered.

Much confusion has arisen from failure to distinguish between methods of unrestricted thinking and internal speech. This latter term should be confined to acts of complete verbalisation, which have not passed over the articulatory apparatus. The patient remains completely silent, although not infrequently his lips move as if he were forming the words. This is a common accompaniment of writing; we express to ourselves what we wish to convey before putting it down. Every word is in place, every phrase fully formed and we may even have the impression that we hear the words "in our head," although no sound is uttered. This is not "thinking in words," but consecutive thought clothed in complete verbal terms. If it were articulated, it would remain identical in form and content; in fact, as expressed in writing, it is often more perfectly grammatical than if it had been spoken aloud.

Most of the work on aphasia has been vitiated by a far more subtle and deep-seated error. It was almost universally assumed that the phenomena revealed by analysis could be treated as elements, which were independent and had entered into combination. Thus, speech was made up of the direct products of articulatory, visual and auditory activities, which united to ensure the normal use of language. As the result of disease or injury, this could be resolved into the elements out of which it had been built up. All conscious processes were reduced to sensory or motor presentations and laws of association. Mental activities were not considered from the dynamic point of view, but as a static synthesis of constituent factors.

It was assumed that for every mental element there was a neural element, either identical or in exact correspondence with it. Such a conception made it possible to postulate regionally distinct centres for diverse aspects of speech. Any one of these could be destroyed independently and the result would be manifested in terms of one of the constituent factors, motor, auditory or visual. From such a priori principles it was possible to deduce in turn the defects of function, which must follow destruction of each centre or internuncial path, and the form assumed by the manifestations of organic disease could be confidently explained by an exact study of the site of the lesion.

But these attempts to explain a vital process in terms of dead-house anatomy were bound to fail. All the morbid manifestations are more or less transitory; symptoms change or pass away, although there is no reason to suppose that the site or extent of the lesion has altered materially. On the other hand, an acute exacerbation of the disease may be followed by defects too profound and wide-spread to be associated with the functions of any single localisable group of cortical centres.

Hence the difficulty in classifying cases in tabular form, either by symptoms or according to the site of the lesion. For patients with destructive changes in approximately the same area of the brain presented during life astonishingly different symptoms, and in most of the clinical records there is little or nothing to show that at the time of death the functional defects were those which existed at an earlier stage in the case.

Tables are almost as fallacious as diagrams. For the abnormal manifestations are not susceptible of arrangement under such headings as speaking, comprehension of spoken words, reading or writing. These acts may be possible under certain conditions, but not under others, and the facts of observation cannot be summarised dogmatically. Nor is accuracy increased by substituting "word-blindness," "word-deafness," "motor disorders of speech" or similar abstract terms of a priori origin.

Applied to disorders of speech, aphasia, amnesia, apraxia and agnosia are names for certain forms of abnormal behaviour, which must be determined by observation. They are descriptive terms only, representing certain distinct varieties of morbid activity due to structural changes in the brain, but they have no validity as criteria for anatomical localisation of normal functions. Since they are an expression of a disorder of function, they must be described in terms of the process itself and not in categories deduced from a priori analysis of the activities of the normal mind. There are no "centres" for the use of language in any form, but solely certain places where an organic lesion of the brain can disturb speech in some specific manner.

Hughlings Jackson laid down these principles more than fifty years ago, but his teaching gradually sank into oblivion. From the first he emphasised the psychical nature of the loss of speech. These changes are associated with material destruction to the cerebrum, but it is fallacious to attempt to localise in various parts of the cortex the diverse activities into which speech can be analysed by introspection or by the phenomena of disease. "To locate the damage which destroys speech and to locate speech are two different things[1]." "It is well to insist," he says[2], "that speech and words are psychical terms; words have of course anatomical substrata or bases as all other psychical states have ... a psychical state is always accompanied by a physical state but, nevertheless, the two things have distinct natures." "A method which is founded on classifications which are partly anatomical and physiological, and partly psychological, confuses the real issues[3]."

When I reprinted Jackson's papers in 1915, the medical world was more prepared to adopt a psychological attitude towards the problems of aphasia and kindred disorders of speech. Pick had already published his voluminous work *Die agrammatischen Sprachstörungen*, in which he described the fruitful researches of philologists and psychologists unknown to the majority of medical workers in this field. The war was producing a series of cases unique in the history of the subject. Young men with local wounds of the brain, but otherwise in perfect health, anxious to be examined and interested in their own condition, presented material for investigation that had never before passed through the hands of the neurologist.

Unfortunately most physicians and surgeons were ill prepared to deal with these opportunities. Time and energy for long-continued examination were lacking and the methods in general use were too

[1] [81], p. 81.   [2] [81], p. 114.   [3] [81], p. 108.

crude to provide satisfactory records. The admirable work along psychological lines, carried out by Gelb and Goldstein and their associates in the Frankfurt Institute for war neurology, forms a notable exception.

In 1920 I was able to bring forward the first-fruits of my observations on disorders of speech due to limited wounds of the brain. The following chapters of this book are devoted to an attempt to develop these views and to describe in fuller detail the cases on which they are founded. The results I have obtained are of little direct practical value to the physician, but they form a fascinating example of the interaction of body and mind, one, moreover, capable of experimental investigation.

PART II

INTRODUCTORY

THE power to make use of words was developed at a late stage in the evolutionary history of man. Before he learnt to formulate his thoughts and desires in speech, he was capable of a wide range of accurate discrimination, which could express itself in action only. Progressive development of the cerebral centres led to increased discriminative powers, and speech, one of the highest and most recently acquired functions, was from the first concerned with formulating and expressing man's relation to the world around him for the purposes of action.

The association between certain sounds and consequent behaviour was enormously widened until he was able to express the significant bond between himself and some external object in the form of a direct proposition. He not only called the white substance which covered the ground in winter "snow," but formulated the sensory impression made upon him in the phrase "snow is cold." In this way he became capable of manipulating words for the purposes of constructive thought and thereby shortened or avoided the wasteful procedure of learning by trial and error. Moreover, he was not only able to register his own impressions and experiences, but could convey them to others.

Speech is a highly discriminative form of behaviour capable of fine degrees of adjustment; it is essentially an intellectual mechanism. But there always remain elements in thought which are not associated with words. The more nearly a mental state approaches pure feeling, the less readily can it be expressed in words alone, apart from gesture and the tone of the voice. Even in the gravest cases of aphasia the patient is evidently fully aware of his emotions and can manifest them clearly in his conduct and gestures. Under the influence of emotion he may be able to say "yes" and "no" or utter phrases such as "Oh! dear me," "I know it," "I can't tell," although he is entirely unable to evoke these words voluntarily or to command. Such emotional and stereotyped forms of speech are the equivalent on a higher plane of the growl or purr which can occur in the decerebrate cat. Words employed in this manner are useless for the purposes of constructive thought; in order that they can subserve intellectual activity, they must be mobile and capable of manipulation at will.

Even amongst higher-grade processes of thought there are many forms of behaviour which at one time demand verbal formulation and at another are carried out independently of words. If, for instance, I select from amongst a set of colours on the table the one which corresponds to that I have just seen, I can do so without preliminary formulation; I recognise the similarity immediately. But should I be asked to name the colour shown to me and then to point out the one which matches it, I am compelled to evoke some appropriate word before making my selection. In the operations of daily life verbal and non-verbal methods of thought are intimately associated and the study of aphasic disorders of speech is a valuable means of investigating this complex relation.

At first sight it might seem difficult to understand how gross destruction of the brain could produce loss of so complicated a form of behaviour as speech without reducing the patient to a state of dementia. But we are familiar with the high-grade defects of sensation produced by injuries of the cerebral cortex; the qualitative and affective aspects are not materially affected, whilst the power of estimating the spacial relations, graduated intensity and similarity or difference of external stimuli may be gravely disturbed. All these changes occur without reducing the patient's intellectual capacity, apart from his power to appreciate sensory differences. Speech is a more complicated psychical aptitude acquired during the life of the individual. It can be disturbed without of necessity producing grave intellectual defect, except for the loss of those functions which demand for their existence the perfect use of language.

The fact that speech can be thrown into disorder by a local lesion of the brain is one of the most wonderful means placed in our hands for investigating the relation of mind and body. But unfortunately most of the elaborate and careful work expended on this fascinating problem has been vitiated by certain fallacious conceptions.

It has been almost universally assumed that the diverse defects of speech which constitute aphasia reveal the elements out of which the use of language is composed. A salt can be broken up chemically into an acid and a base; by analogy it was supposed that the morbid manifestations corresponded to the functions which had been combined to produce normal acts of speech. This fallacy led to the classification of the clinical phenomena under such categories as " motor " and " sensory," " auditory " and " visual " or some analogous terminology.

An even more disastrous error consisted in the attempt to correlate anatomical changes in definite regions of the brain with " speech," " reading," " writing " and the " memory for words." These are purely verbal descriptions for certain human actions. There is no reason to suppose that these convenient terms correspond to any distinct and separable group of psychical or physiological functions and we should as soon expect to find centres for "eating" and "walking" as for "speaking" and "writing."

Any lesion gravely disturbing speech affects activities which are not usually classed with the use of language; the more carefully the patient is examined, the less certainly does his disorder correspond to any pre-conceived category. I shall therefore devote the following chapters to describing the forms assumed clinically by aphasia and kindred affections of speech and shall attempt to express these morbid phenomena in terms drawn directly from the act itself.

CHAPTER I

METHODS OF EXAMINATION

A<small>N</small> inconstant response is one of the most striking results produced by a lesion of the cerebral cortex. During our studies in sensation, we found that a stimulus, exerting a constant physical force well above the normal threshold, was sometimes appreciated and at others evoked no reply. Moreover, a graduated increase of intensity did not of necessity lead to an equivalent improvement in the answers given by the patient.

Bearing in mind this characteristic want of certainty in the reaction to measured stimuli, it seemed probable that disorders of speech due to cerebral injuries would reveal the same tendency. This is notoriously the case. It is not a sufficient test to hold up some object, and ask the patient to name it; at one time he may be able to do so, at another he fails completely. No conclusion can be drawn from one or two questions put in this way; his power of responding must be tested by a series of observations in which the same task recurs on two or more occasions.

Not only is it necessary to arrange the tests in sequence, but each set must be placed before the patient in several different ways. For example, six common objects are laid on the table in front of him, and he is asked to point to the one which corresponds to a duplicate placed in his hand out of sight. This is repeated for eighteen or twenty-four observations, so that the choice of any one object recurs three or four times in the course of the series. He next gives names to the various objects one by one, indicates each one in turn as it is named by the examiner and makes his selection in answer to printed words set before him on a card. Finally, he writes down the names without saying anything aloud. The order in which each single test follows another in the series remains the same throughout the various methods of examination; this alone makes it possible to draw any conclusion from the inconstant responses which are so disconcerting, unless the answers are recorded in this manner. Moreover, this method enables us to learn how the patient responds to the same sequence of tests presented to him in different ways.

It is also important to graduate the severity of the task before concluding to what extent the patient can speak, read or write. For instance, he may be able to touch his eye or his ear correctly to oral or printed commands, although he fails entirely to do so if the right or left hand is specified. Similarly a man can write his own name and address, but not that of his mother with whom he lives, and the hands of a clock may be set to an order given in figures, but not when it is expressed in words.

Before we pass on to consider these tests more in detail, it is necessary to say something of the character of the patients on whom this research is mainly based. In civilian practice many of those who suffer from aphasia are old, broken down in health and their general intellectual capacity is diminished. Most of them are affected with arterial degeneration and in many the blood tension is greatly increased. Such patients are easily fatigued and are obviously unsuitable for sustained examination.

But the war brought under our care young men who were struck down in the full pride of health. Many of them were extremely intelligent, willing and anxious to be examined thoroughly. As their wounds healed, they were encouraged and cheered by the obvious improvement in their condition. They were euphoric rather than depressed, and in every way contrasted profoundly with the state of the aphasic met with in civilian practice.

Moreover, with gun-shot wounds of the head the symptoms tend to clear up to a considerable extent, provided there are no secondary complications, even though the effect produced by the initial impact of the bullet may have been extremely severe. Some aspects of the disordered functions of speech recover more rapidly than others and the clinical manifestations assume more or less characteristic forms. In the end the patient may recover his powers to such an extent that he no longer fails to carry out the rough and simple tests which can be employed in clinical research; or on the other hand some aptitude may remain permanently defective. By this means we are enabled to trace the various steps by which the defective functions are restored, whereas in civilian practice any change in the clinical manifestations is usually in an opposite direction. Even if the vascular lesion is stationary, the symptoms rarely disappear, whilst in most cases the condition of the patient gradually deteriorates.

There is still another difference between the results produced by gunshot injuries of the head and those vascular lesions which are usually responsible for disorders of speech in the old. The missile strikes the skull from without, and even if it penetrates the brain, tends to cause the greatest damage on the surface. Vascular lesions, on the other hand, destroy the substance of the brain where the fibres are diverging or converging on their path to or from the cortical centres; a small haemorrhage may in consequence be followed by a profound and wide-spread disturbance of function. But structural changes produced by a local injury to the external surface of the skull not only cause less severe and extensive manifestations of cerebral injury, but give greater opportunity for the appearance of loss of function in more specific forms.

Before proceeding to describe the actual tests used in this research, I wish to lay stress on certain general rules necessary for their success. The patient must be examined alone, in a quiet room, apart from all distracting sights and sounds. It is of fundamental importance to record not only what he says or does, but also every remark or question of the observer. As soon as it is certain that the patient understands the task he is asked to perform, each series of tests must be carried out in silence; should this rule be broken, both sides of the conversation must be recorded. It is particularly important to write down at the moment any statement which throws light on the ideas or feelings of the patient with regard to the test, or to the difficulties he experiences in carrying it out. If it consists in executing some choice to oral commands, the observer must say the words once only in the simplest and most direct manner. Should it be necessary to repeat the order at the request of the patient, the fact must be noted, so that we may learn in how far his subsequent conduct is influenced by the repetition. Between any two series of tests, it is well to permit the patient to rest or to talk freely; but as soon as a fresh set of observations has been started, all conversation should be confined to the task in hand, and every word spoken on either side must be recorded.

It is extremely important to avoid all causes of fatigue or loss of temper. Some patients, especially the older aphasics, become depressed or angry, when they fail repeatedly to carry out tests which are childishly simple. The sequence of the various sets of observations must then be rearranged, so that the next series belongs to a group that can be carried out easily. It is remarkable how quickly this restores the patient's equanimity. In all work of this kind fatigue and disappointment must be avoided by every possible means, if necessary even by terminating the sitting.

For it must be remembered that we are dealing with a general disorder of function and there are no normal parts that can be used as an indication of the patient's aptitudes and condition, as was the case when we were investigating the sensory defects produced by a lesion of the cortex. It is not a question of local loss of attention; the functions which are disturbed in disorders of speech form part of the general activities of the mind.

10—2

This opens up another difficulty, which was not present in our previous researches. Much in the character of the patient's answers depends on his previous aptitudes, which are entirely unknown. When testing sensation, this was of little importance, because every observation made on affected areas of the body could be compared with the response from equivalent normal parts. Since it is impossible to discover how the patient would have responded before he became aphasic, I have depended mainly on the reactions of young men wounded in the war; for, especially in the case of officers, it was possible to estimate with considerable accuracy the extent of their education, and the ability with which they had carried out the more exacting of their military duties. At the same time the profession or occupation exercised before the war frequently showed that they must have possessed faculties which were subsequently found to be grossly affected. Thus, in one case, an accountant could no longer carry out simple arithmetical operations, and a bank clerk had lost the power of adding up a column of figures with certainty.

The tests I am about to describe vary greatly in the difficulty they present to persons of normal understanding. Most of them, such as selecting or naming common objects and colours, the man, cat and dog tests, the coin-bowl tests are childishly simple and can be carried out perfectly by the stupidest individual. But many normal men are liable to hesitate or make mistakes over the hand, eye and ear tests, when attempting to imitate the movements of an observer sitting face to face. This is also true for pictorial commands, if the card is held in the patient's hand. But the normal individual and the majority of aphasics find little difficulty in copying these movements, when they are reflected in a mirror. Instruction in signalling, through which all officers were compelled to pass before obtaining a commission, seems, however, to improve the capacity to perform these tests in their most complex form.

All the tests in any one group are not of the same order of severity. Some can be carried out with greater ease and rapidity, even by normal persons, and these differences may become greatly exaggerated in pathological cases. This is particularly evident, when the command requires choice between two or more courses of action. Moreover, words conveying an order always set a harder task than those which indicate an object. Told to put out his tongue, the patient may point to it, but be unable to protrude it; and yet he can do so perfectly to lick his lips.

Throughout these observations it is important to record the rapidity as well as the nature of the response. Frequently the number of erroneous answers is sufficient to show that the power to carry out some particular series of tests is defective. But occasionally every actual reply may be correct, and yet it is evident from the patient's statements and demeanour that he has difficulty in carrying out the task he has been set. A bare record of the number of times he has been successful in his choice would not reveal this defect. In many cases, therefore, it is necessary to time the interval between question and answer. Speaking roughly, it will be found that the majority of rapid replies are correct, and any task performed with ease is carried out quickly.

Moreover, on the termination of a series of tests it is important to enquire of the patient whether he found them easy or difficult; by this means, if he is intelligent, we can often obtain much illuminating information.

The order in which these serial tests are applied must be varied to suit the circumstances of the case. It is a mistake to begin with those which present the greatest difficulty and the length of the series must be adapted to the patient's capacity. For instance, the names of common objects can be written in printed capitals only, it is a mistake to insist on the whole eighteen tests; these may, however, be usefully employed in full to discover the extent to which the patient can make a choice to oral commands. With the older and more debilitated aphasics of civilian practice it is sometimes necessary to reduce the number of tests in the series throughout the whole of some particular examination, so as to avoid the disastrous consequences of fatigue or depression.

§ 1. SERIAL TESTS

(a) *Naming and recognition of common objects.*

Six objects of daily use, such as a pencil, a key, a penny, a match-box, a pair of scissors and a knife, are laid on the table[1]. Before starting the observations it is well to record the actual position in which they lie to one another from the patient's point of view. They are then screened from his sight, and a duplicate of one of them is shown to him; the screen is rapidly withdrawn, and he is asked to point to the object on the table which corresponds to the one he has just seen. Eighteen observations are carried out in this manner, and patient and observer remain completely silent throughout. The power to carry out this form of the test

---

[1] Sometimes with highly educated patients these familiar objects were replaced by wooden blocks cut into the form of geometrical figures such as a cube, a sphere, a pyramid, a cone, etc. The tests were then carried out systematically exactly as with the articles of common use.

is not affected by any of the disorders of function which are the subject of this research; but it is well to begin with a task that can be performed without difficulty by the patient in order to encourage him, and at the same time to gauge his general powers of comprehension.

This is followed by a series of observations to test his power of naming each familiar object in turn as it is shown to him. Then he is asked to point to the one which corresponds to the name said aloud by the observer. Next, he is given cards one by one, each of which bears in printed characters the name of an object on the table in front of him, and he is told to make his choice accordingly.

Table A[1].

	Pointing to object shown	Naming object indicated	Oral commands	Printed commands	Duplicate placed in hand out of sight	Repetition	Writing name of object indicated	Copying from print
Knife	Perfect	Correct	Correct	Correct	Perfect	Correct	rib	Knive
Key	,,	,,	,,	,,	,,	,,	Beeg	Gey
Penny	,,	,,	,,	,,	,,	"Punny"	penney	Tenny
Matches	,,	"Matcher"	,,	,,	,,	Correct	Mahickes	Mahickes
Scissors	,,	Correct	,,	,,	,,	,,	Secissors	Ssuccoors
Pencil	,,	,,	,,	,,	,,	,,	peicel	Penceil
Key	,,	,,	,,	,,	,,	,,	Bey	Key
Scissors	,,	"Key"; corrected	,,	,,	,,	,,	Sicissors	Scissors
Matches	,,	"Match-ox"	,,	,,	,,		Martchs	Matchers
Knife	,,	Correct	,,	,,	,,	"Knive"	Bnife	Knife
Penny	,,	"Pea-ny"	,,	Pencil	,,	Correct	peinny	Penny
Matches	,,	"Match-ōz"	,,	Correct	,,	,,	Matches	Mahches
Scissors	,,	Correct	,,	,,	,,	,,	Scissars	Ssissors
Pencil	,,	No answer	,,	,,	,,	,,	pencel	Penceil
Penny	,,	"Pence"	,,	Pencil	,,	,,	penny	Penney
Knife	,,	Correct	,,	Correct	,,	,,	Knife	Knife
Key	,,	,,	,,	Knife; corrected	,,	,,	guey	Key
Pencil	,,	"Knife; no, pencil"	,,	Correct	,,	,,	pencel	Pencel

Each series is carried out in exactly the same order as the first and all subsequent observations. But I am accustomed to vary the relative order in which the different forms of test follow one another according to the nature of the defects of speech. Thus, after assuring myself that the patient can indicate an object he has just seen, I not infrequently begin the subsequent observations with oral followed by printed commands, before testing his power of naming.

These three forms of test may give him considerable difficulty; I am therefore accustomed to follow them up by placing a duplicate in the

[1] See No. 20, Vol. II, p. 300.

normal hand, out of sight, and asking the patient to choose the corresponding object from amongst those on the table. This can be carried out perfectly in all cases of uncomplicated disorders of speech.

He is then asked to write down in turn the name of each object indicated by the observer. This must be carried out in silence; but it is impossible to prevent many persons from moving their lips soundlessly during the act of writing. After carrying out the test in this way, it is often useful to make the patient name the objects aloud and then designate them in writing, to discover if he is helped by articulating the words. Occasionally he is asked to write the names to dictation and to copy them from print in cursive script.

At some period in this group of tests he is made to repeat the words one by one as they are said by the observer.

When the patient is almost wordless it is sometimes possible by the following method to show that he can still recognise the name of an object shown to him. Cards bearing the printed names are laid on the table and he is asked to point to the one which corresponds to the familiar article placed before him; this he can frequently do, showing that he appreciates its name, although he has not words in which to express it.

(b) *Naming and recognition of colours.*

This test is carried out in the same manner as the one I have just described, except that coloured silks are substituted for the objects of common use. Eight strips of different colours are laid in a row and hidden from the patient by a sheet of cardboard; he is then shown an exact duplicate of one of the pieces on the table and, when the screen is removed, is asked to indicate the one which corresponds with it. Should there be hemianopsia or any defect of the visual field, it is important to make sure that the whole gamut of colours is visible to the patient from the position in which he is sitting. Provided this source of error is avoided, the test in this form could be carried out correctly in all the cases of unilateral lesion of the brain comprised in this research.

The patient is then asked to name each colour as it is shown to him and to make a choice in response to oral or printed commands read silently and aloud.

He then writes down the name of each colour in turn as it is shown him, or to dictation by the observer. Sometimes he is required to copy these words from the printed cards in cursive script.

Finally, he may be set to select one of these cards which corresponds in nomenclature with a colour he has just seen.

Table B¹.

	Pointing to colour shown	Naming colour shown	Oral commands	Printed commands	Printed commands read aloud and colour chosen		Writing name of colour shown	Writing name to dictation	Copying name from print in cursive script	Choosing card bearing name of colour shown
					He said	He chose				
Black	Correct	Correct	Correct	Correct	Correctly	Correctly	Correct	Correct	Correct	Correct
Red	"	"	„ Violet	Correct; slow	"	No choice	"I can't think of it"	"	"	Violet
Blue	"	"I don't know what colour it is; there is blue in it"		Correct	"	Blue; then correctly	Black	"	"	No choice
Green	"	Correct; very slow	Correct	"	"			"	"	"
Orange	"	"Red...No, it's yellow"	Yellow	"	"	Yellow	Yellow, bit of red	"	"	
White	"	Correct	Correct	"	"	Correctly	Correct	"	"	Correct
Violet	"	"It's got a lot of blue in it. It wants a bit of red and blue"	Blue	"	"	Blue; doubtful	Blue	Violate	"	No choice
Yellow	"	"It's got yellow in it. I can't tell what colour you'd call it"	Orange	Correct; very slow	"	Correctly	Correct	Correct	"	Correct; very slow
Red	"	Correct	Correct	Correct	"	"	"I can't"	"	"	Correct
White	"	"I've forgotten...a warm tint...yellow"	Red; then white; then orange	"	"	"	Correct	"	"	"
Yellow	"	"It's got blue in it"	Violet	"	"	"		"	"	"
Blue	"			"	"	Correctly; slow	Violet	"	"	Correct; slow
Green	"	Correct	Correct	"	"	"	Correct	"	"	Correct
Black	"	"Red"	Correct	"	"	"		"	"	Correct
Orange	"		Yellow	Yellow	"	"	Red"	"	"	Yellow. "It's too red to be yellow"
Violet	"	"It's got blue and a little red"	Correct	Blue	"	"	Violate (correct)	Violate	"	Correct; very slow

¹ See No. 22, Vol. II, p. 345.

On superficial examination, some aphasics have been thought to be colour-blind on account of their difficulty in naming colours. But this is excluded by the rapidity and correctness with which they match colours in the first series of observations. The defect in such cases is one of names and the gross errors are due to want of nominal recognition. Even though the printed words can be read aloud accurately, the consequent choice of a colour may be defective.

(c) *The man, cat and dog tests.*

Table C[1].

	Reading aloud	Writing from dictation	Writing from pictures	Reading from pictures	Repetition	Copying
The cat and the man	"Dē...carnt... art...that... mart"	tat the Man	the Cat the Man	"A cat...the mand, man, mant"	Correct	Correct
The dog and the cat	"Dē...god...and the...cat"	the dog the cat	dog cat	"Got...a god... cat"	"The cat...the cad and the man"	,,
The man and the dog	"The...māt... and...these, the ...gone, gone, got"	the ca	the man the dog	"Mand...got, the gone, dog, dog"	Correct	,,
The cat and the dog	"Dē...gāt, gone, cat...and...ee ...dot"	the cat and the god	the cat the dog	"Cat...god, dog"	,,	,,
The man and the cat	"Thēte...mat, mant, mand... and...then... cad, cat"	the man and the cat	the man the cat	"Man...cat"	"The man...the man and the... cat" (correct)	,,
The dog and the man	"The...gond... and...the... mem, man"	the god and the man	the dog the man	"Dog...mant, mand, a man"	"The dog...the dog...the dog and the...and the man" (correct)	,,

This test is designed to investigate the power of reading and writing in its simplest and most elementary form. Every word employed comprises three letters only; the patient is, therefore, precluded from guessing at the constituents of the phrase by their length, a fallacy which is otherwise liable to vitiate all observations of this class. But, on the other hand, the task set is childishly easy, and the defect in speech must be severe, before it shows traces on so simple a test.

On the other hand, if the power of reading and writing is diminished, these observations may become both fatiguing and disheartening. Usually the series consists of ten or more tests, but in the one chosen as an illustration (Table C) they were reduced to six only.

The various forms assumed by the examination are as follows. The patient is asked to read the simple monosyllabic phrases aloud. He is shown two pictures of the series and translates them into words; this

[1] See No. 7, Vol. II, p. 99.

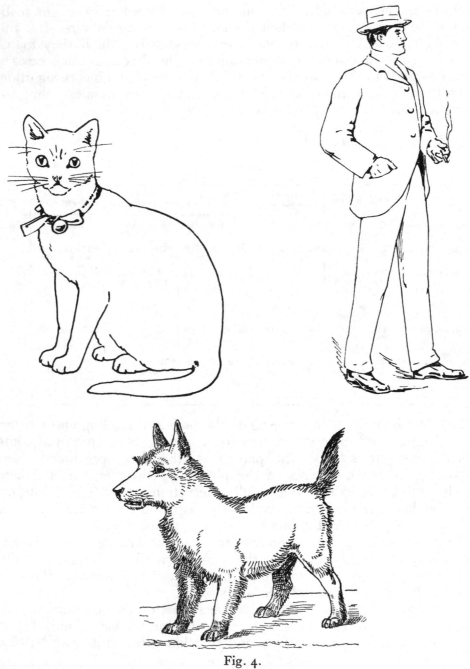

Fig. 4.

is called "reading from pictures" (Fig. 4). He repeats the phrases after me one by one. He writes them down from pictures or to my dictation and finally copies them from print in cursive handwriting. Occasionally I ask him to choose from amongst a set of printed cards on the table the one which corresponds exactly to the pictorial combination placed before him. Sometimes, when incapable of writing, he attempts to put together out of block letters the names of the two pictures he has seen.

(d) *The clock tests*.

Table D[1].

	Direct imitation	Telling the time	Clock set to oral commands	Clock set to printed commands	
				Ordinary nomenclature	Rail- way time
5 minutes to 2	Correct	Correct	Correct	Correct	Set 12.40
Half past 1	,,	,,	,,	,,	Correct
5 minutes past 8	,,	,,	,,	,,	
20 minutes to 4	,,	"Quarter to 4; 5 and 20 to; 10 minutes to 4"	,,	,,	Set ,, 2.40
10 minutes past 7	,,	Correct	,,	Set 10.10	Correct
20 minutes to 6	,,	,,	,,	Correct	Whispered "5.40" Set 4.50
10 minutes to 1	,,	,,	Set 10 minutes past, but hour hand before 1	Set 10 to 10	Correct
A quarter to 9	,,	,,	Correct; slow	Correct	,,
20 minutes past 11	,,	"5, 10, 15, 20 past 11"	Correct	,,	Set 10.40
25 minutes to 3	,,	Correct	Set 20 minutes to 3	,,	Correct

Two clock faces are prepared, about twelve centimetres in diameter, fitted with metallic hands, which are adjustable. On each, the figures of the hours are clearly marked in arabic numerals[2]. One of these clocks is given to the patient, and he is asked to place the hands in an exactly similar position to that of the other one, set by the observer. This direct imitation can be carried out correctly, unless the power of comprehending the nature of the task is considerably diminished.

Next, the patient is told to set the clock to oral and then to printed commands, and in each instance the sequence of tests is the same. The hands of the clock are now moved by the observer into various positions

[1] See No. 20, Vol. II, p. 303.
[2] I wished to avoid the complication of roman numerals, especially in view of the fact that the wrist-watches in use during the war were usually marked in arabic numerals.

and the patient tells the time aloud, or without speaking writes them on paper.

In many cases it is advisable to present the printed commands not only in the ordinary nomenclature, but also in numbers, so-called "railway time." For instance, in one series of observations the patient is handed a printed card bearing the legend "20 minutes to 6" and in the next the same order appears in the form "5.40."

The erroneous answers to these tests assume many different forms[1]. The patient may confuse "to" and "past" the hour, setting twenty minutes *past* four instead of twenty minutes *to* the hour. Or he may place the short hand exactly opposite the figure 4 on the clock, whilst the long hand is set correctly; this is a most confusing mistake, for it is impossible to discover whether this signifies 4.40 or 3.40 without questioning the patient. Again, he frequently confuses the significance of the two hands, setting the long one at the hour, the short one to mark the minutes.

(e) *The coin-bowl tests*.

Four bowls or saucers are set upon the table and in front of each is laid a penny. The patient is told to count them from left to right; he is then shown the nature of the task he has to perform, which consists in placing a coin into one of the bowls according to a series of numerical commands. First, the order is given orally, or by means of a printed card, which is read silently. Then the patient is asked to read it aloud, and to carry out the action demanded under the influence of words spoken by himself.

This is so simple a test that no normal person fails to carry it out correctly; but in some instances of aphasia and kindred disorders it may cause considerable difficulty, as seen by the example given in Table E. In this case both oral and printed commands were poorly executed, even if the patient was permitted to read the order aloud.

It is sometimes useful to make two sets of observations with the printed cards under somewhat different conditions. First, the orders are given in numerals only, e.g. "1st into 3rd"; then the whole phrase is set out in full, as for example, "First penny into third bowl." In some cases of aphasia the second form of this test presents greater difficulty to the patient, and may reveal defects, that do not appear when the command is given in numbers only.

[1] Compare Table 5, p. 26; Table 4, p. 161, and many others in Vol. II.

Table E[1].

	Oral commands	Printed commands (not read aloud)	Printed commands read aloud	
			He said	Movement executed
2nd into 3rd	Correct, slow	Correct	"Two, three"	Correct
1st into 3rd	„	Correct; slow	"Won, tree"	„
2nd into 1st	2nd coin..."I forget which one" (repeated) correct	1st coin...2nd coin... No further action	"Two, won"	1st into 1st
3rd into 2nd	3rd coin..."I forget" (repeated) correct	2nd into 3rd	"Ree, tree, two"	3rd into 3rd
1st into 4th	1st coin; (repeated) correct	Correct; slow	"Won, four, four"	1st coin..."Was it four?"; did nothing
4th into 3rd	3rd into 2nd	3rd into 4th	"Four...one, ree, tree"	3rd into 3rd
2nd into 4th	Correct	Correct	"Two, four"	Correct
4th into 1st	4th coin..."I forget" (repeated) correct	„	"Four, won, won"	1st into 4th
3rd into 1st	Correct	3rd coin..."I forget which one I've got"	"Tree, won, tree"	Correct
1st into 2nd	2nd into 1st	Correct	"One, two, two"	„
3rd into 4th	Correct, slow	3rd coin..."I forget which one to put it in"	"Three, four"	3rd into 3rd
4th into 2nd	"I forget which it was" (repeated), 4th into 1st	Correct	"Four, taw"	Correct

(f) *The hand, eye and ear tests.*

First of all the patient, seated opposite the observer, attempts to imitate a series of movements which consists in touching an eye or an ear with one or other hand. Before beginning these tests it is well to make sure that he knows his right hand from his left, and understands the nature of the task he has to perform. He is asked, therefore, to name each hand as it is raised by the observer, and then to lift the one which corresponds to it, bearing in mind the face to face position. When we are certain from these preliminaries that he appreciates the action demanded of him, the observations are begun.

Some normal persons find difficulty in performing these movements correctly over a series of from sixteen to twenty-four tests; many, however, can carry them out perfectly, especially if they are young and intelligent, and belong to the class from which so many of my war patients were drawn. There is at first a natural tendency to select the hand opposite to that used by the observer; this error is in most instances checked consciously and the movement is carried out correctly. But none of the normal men I have examined failed to recognise that, when the left hand was in contact with the right ear, it had crossed the face;

[1] See No. 7, Vol. II, p. 99.

and yet this want of appreciation of crossed movement was one of the commonest pathological mistakes. Moreover, in certain cases, I have been able to watch a steady improvement in the records, resulting finally, after a considerable lapse of time, in a perfect series of answers (No. 20, Vol. II, p. 319; No. 7, Vol. II, p. 107).

Table F[1].

	Imitation of movements made by the observer	Imitation of movements reflected in a mirror	Pictorial commands	Pictorial commands reflected in a mirror	Oral commands	Printed commands (not read aloud)	Printed commands read aloud and executed	Writing down movements made by the observer	Writing down movements reflected in a mirror
L. hand to L. eye	Correct	Correct	Reversed	Correct	Correct	Correct	Correct	Left left eye (correct)	Correct
R. hand to R. ear	L. hand; then correct	,,	L. hand to R. ear	,,	,,	,,	,,	Correct	Left hand right ear
R. hand to L. eye	Correct	,,	L. hand to R. *ear*	,,	,,	,,	,,	,,	Correct
L. hand to R. eye	L. hand to L. eye	,,	Reversed	,,	,,	,,	,,		,,
L. hand to L. ear	Correct	,,	Correct	,,	,,	,,	,,	Left hand ("I forget which it was")	
R. hand to R. eye		,,	Reversed	,,	,,	,,	,,	Correct	
L. hand to R. ear	L. hand to L. ear	,,	,,	,,	,,	,,	,,	,,	Left hand right
R. hand to L. ear	R. hand to R. ear	,,	,,	,,	,,	,,	,,	,,	Correct
L. hand to L. eye	Correct	,,	Correct	,,	,,	,,	,,	,,	,,
R. hand to R. ear	,,	,,	Reversed	,,	,,	,,	,,	Right hand ("I think it was the same side")	,,
R. hand to L. eye	R. hand to R. eye	,,	L. hand to R. *ear*	,,	,,	,,	,,	Correct	,,
L. hand to R. eye	R. hand to R. eye; then reversed	,,	Reversed	,,	,,	,,	,,	,,	Left hand left eye
L. hand to L. ear	Correct	,,	Correct	,,	,,	,,	,,	No response ("I've forgotten")	Correct
R. hand to R. eye	,,	,,	,,	,,	,,	,,	,,	Correct	,,
L. hand to R. ear	,,	,,	Reversed	,,	,,	,,	,,	Left hand right *eye*	,,
R. hand to L. ear	L. hand to L. ear	,,	,,	,,	,,	,,	,,	Correct	,,

Then the patient is placed in front of a large mirror, and is asked to imitate the reflected movements of the observer standing behind him. In all normal persons and in most of those suffering from disorders of speech, this can be carried out perfectly; it is an act of direct imitation uncomplicated by considerations of right and left. But, if the aphasia is severe and especially when it assumes the variety I have called "semantic," the patient is liable to become confused even over this simple task (No. 10, Vol. II, p. 162).

The next form of this test consists in handing the patient cards, each of which represents a human figure carrying out one of the desired movements (Figs. 5 and 6). These drawings are simplified to the highest degree consistent with their significance, and a line is drawn down the centre to separate the right and left halves of the body. Most patients,

[1] See No. 4, Vol. II, p. 61.

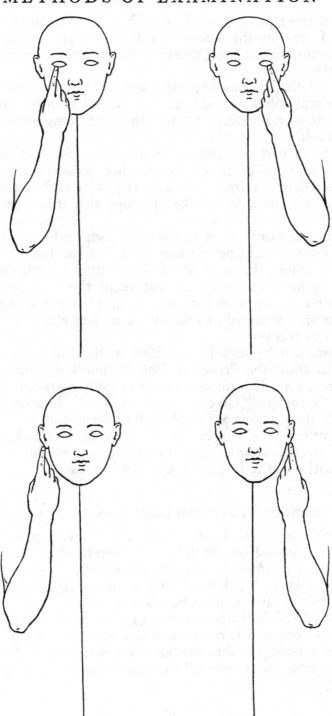

Fig. 5.

when shown these pictures, make exactly the same kind of mistakes as when seated opposite the observer. But as soon as they are allowed to see the reflection in the glass, every movement may be executed rapidly and correctly.

Then the patient is made to carry out the same series of actions in response to oral and to printed commands read silently. Next he reads aloud each order and executes it under the reinforcing influence of words said by himself.

Finally, he is told to write down in silence the movements of the observer sitting opposite to him or, in other instances, the same movements reflected in a mirror. Occasionally, where the crude power of writing is in question, he is asked to copy the orders printed on the cards.

This is the most difficult of all the serial tests and the only one where the answers of a normal person may be defective. But, if we bear this possibility in mind, this method of examination is capable of yielding valuable evidence concerning the nature of the various disorders of speech. Moreover, in many instances, I have been able to compare the defective records obtained at first with a perfect series of answers at a later period of recovery.

These tests can be usefully modified in the following manner and graduated to show the degree of loss of function. First, a series of observations are made with commands requiring a single choice only; the patient is told to "Give me your hand," "Shut your eyes," etc. Then two of these orders are combined, as for instance "Give me your hand and put out your tongue," or "Shut your eyes and give me your hand." From such simple combinations it is possible to work up to the complexities of the full hand, eye and ear tests.

§2. FURTHER TESTS EMPLOYED IN THIS RESEARCH

These serial tests carried out with discretion give a good indication of the character assumed by the defects of speech. But I am accustomed to employ other methods of examination which, although they are not arranged in serial form, depend on the same principles and must be carried out in the same systematic manner.

The alphabet. If the patient is asked to say the letters spontaneously in their proper order, it is remarkable how often he fails to execute this childishly easy task. He then repeats them one by one after me. Next he is told to write them down silently unprompted. This is followed by

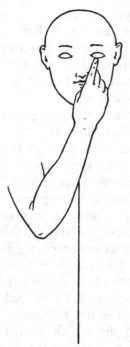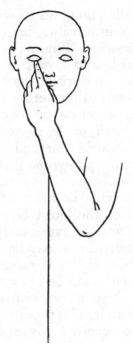

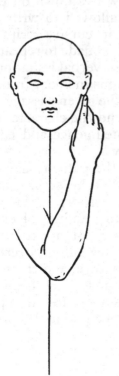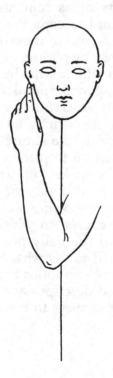

FIG. 6.

writing to dictation and copying the printed alphabet in cursive script or, if this is impossible, in printed capitals, an act of little more than imitative drawing. Finally, he is given the twenty-six letters printed on separate cards and is told to arrange them in due order ("the block letters"); it is surprising how frequently even highly educated patients find difficulty in discovering their correct sequence.

A similar set of observations may be carried out using as a basis the *days of the week*, or the names of the *months of the year*.

Another valuable method of examination, belonging to this order, is to choose some *paragraph* from a newspaper or book and to use this as a test of the capacity of the patient to understand and formulate in different ways what he has read silently or aloud. Sometimes I select a description of the latest boxing match, at others he is given a short coherent account in typed script of his own daily activities. More highly educated individuals may be allowed to select some passage of greater literary value; but it is essential that the chosen piece should not be long or obscure and be of interest to the patient. This he reads through silently as often as he wishes and then attempts to say what he has gathered from it. The paper is handed to him again, he reads the passage aloud and a record is made of the form of the words he utters. After reading the passage once more silently, he writes down on paper what he remembers of its contents. He is then allowed to write the words to dictation and to copy the printed matter in cursive script. At some period in the course of these observations, he is made to repeat the whole after me phrase by phrase, to test his power of verbal imitation. Finally, he is asked to tell me what he has retained in his memory from the many occasions on which he perused or listened to the given passage. The order in which these observations are carried out and the character of the task selected must be strictly adapted to the intelligence and education of the patient and to the nature of his disability.

It is my custom to place a *picture* before the patient, and to ask him to describe in spoken or written words what he sees. Sometimes a combination of this pictorial test with the comprehension of printed matter, in the following way, makes a useful method of examination. A picture is chosen to which is attached a short printed description, so common in the daily press. At first the legend is covered up; the patient is asked to say what he sees in the picture, and the manner and nature of his observations are carefully recorded. Then he is allowed to see the printed description; after reading it silently to himself, he writes down what it conveys to him, reinforced by the pictorial representation.

He then reads it aloud and writes it to dictation. Finally, he is told to fix his attention on the picture, and to say what it conveys to him. An excellent example of this combined test is given in Vol. II, p. 202.

Numbers. The patient is asked to count, if possible unaided, up to a hundred and particular attention is paid to the verbal form of the numerals and any tendency to confusion on reaching a fresh decade. He then writes them down as a series of figures in due order. Much valuable information can be gathered from the coin-bowl tests with regard to his capacity to comprehend the significance of single numbers for the purpose of executing an oral or printed command.

To be of any value *arithmetical tests* must be simple and carried out systematically in the order of their progressive difficulty. I am in the habit of beginning by asking the patient to add two numbers of three figures each, such as 231 and 356, which do not necessitate carrying over. This is followed by a couple which require one act of carrying over from one column to the next and then in turn by a sum where it is necessary to perform this operation twice. From this he passes to the subtraction of one number of three figures from another where no carrying over is required and the difficulties of the problem are then increased progressively in exactly the same manner as with addition. The importance of this method of testing the patient's arithmetic powers by graduated tasks of this kind is shown by such records as those obtained from No. 10 (Vol. II, p. 177). This officer, who was an accountant in civil life, could solve the first two additions and the easiest subtraction sums, but failed to bring out a correct answer to all the others. Had he been set one example of addition and one of subtraction only, he might have been thought to be capable or incapable of carrying out arithmetical operations, according to the nature and severity of the task. All these tests are absurdly simple to the normal man, provided he is not entirely illiterate.

A complete set of *coins* in current use, including a note for ten shillings and one for a pound, is laid upon the table and the patient is asked to name them one by one. Whenever he shows the slightest difficulty in doing so, the series is repeated twice or more to exhibit the customary uncertainty of response.

Then two pieces of money are selected with the request that he would state how many of the one " go into " the other of higher value. Many patients, who can name coins correctly, fail completely to carry out this test; and yet they can pile up accurately its equivalent from amongst the various pieces of money on the table. In such cases it is not the recognition of value that is at fault, but the power of formulating it as a definite proposition. Incidentally in this connection, questions are asked as to any difficulties experienced with regard to the monetary transactions of daily life.

The power of *drawing* must be tested in a more systematic manner than is usually the case. First, the patient is asked to draw from a simple model, such as a jug or a vase. If he is fond of drawing and naturally intelligent, I put before him a glass spirit lamp, because of the difficulties presented by the wick; for the parts above and below the collar must be shown as a continuous structure interrupted by the metallic neck of the lamp. This forms a useful problem in significance.

Then both model and drawing are removed and, after ten minutes, an attempt is made to reproduce it from memory.

Another valuable test, which has been used by Marie and others, is to ask the patient to draw an elephant. Fortunately most of my patients were familiar with the appearance of these animals and many had seen them in India during their military service. The salient features of an elephant, especially its trunk and tusks, are so obvious that their omission from the drawing clearly indicates defective powers of formulation.

Finally, I suggest to the patient that he should draw anything that comes into his mind unprompted; it is remarkable how often a man, who has failed grossly to reproduce the figure of an elephant, can draw spontaneously something of interest to himself.

To test his power of formulating at will relations in space, he is asked to sketch roughly from memory a *ground-plan* of some familiar room, such as that in which we worked together or his ward at the hospital. In some instances this can be carried out with ease whilst in others it is entirely impossible. Yet, if I draw a quadrilateral figure in the centre of a sheet of paper to represent the position of his habitual seat at my table or of his bed in the ward, he may be able to point to the position of windows, doors, furniture and other salient features with absolute correctness. He knows their position with regard to himself, but is unable to represent their relation to one another, not only diagrammatically but even in words.

This test with an intelligent patient forms a useful preliminary to an enquiry concerning *visual imagery*. Most of those who formed the basis of this research evidently employed visual images to a considerable extent in the processes of thought and many of them were able to give me valuable information on this subject.

The power of *orientation* and capacity to find the way along some familiar route can usually be gathered from the statements of the patient, his friends or the nurses. But I am accustomed, whenever possible, to make my own observations, accompanying him once or more on his way to my house or on his return to the hospital. By this means many abnormalities of behaviour can be detected that escape the notice of an ordinary companion or relative.

Great stress will be laid on the patient's ability to play *games*, such as dominoes, draughts, chess, cards and billiards. Many who succeed with the first three cannot play cards. Billiards, demanding as it does ability to calculate the path of a ball rebounding from the cushion, forms a valuable test for capacity to appreciate the intention of an act anticipatory to its performance.

A favourite amusement during the war was the putting together of jigsaw puzzles. A large picture was affixed to a thin sheet of wood and then sawn into a multitude of fragments of the most diverse shapes, and the art consisted in fitting them together again accurately. This formed a splendid test; for many aphasics were entirely unable to appreciate the particular piece that would fit a certain gap in the picture.

So far all the tests I have described are new or, if in common use, have been employed by me in an unusual manner. They are in no way complete and are capable of profound improvement. Moreover, they must be strictly adapted to the capacity of the patient and should not be applied in a routine way. But I have set them out in detail to show the methods actually employed to reach the conclusions enunciated in the following pages.

CHAPTER II

CLINICAL EXAMPLES

GROSS injury confined to one cerebral hemisphere can disturb the power of speaking, reading and writing without producing any general loss of intellectual capacity. Evidently there must exist a group of functions indispensable for language in its widest sense, but not equally essential for all intellectual performance; it is these functions which are the subject of this investigation, in so far as they can be affected by destruction of certain parts of the brain.

An organic lesion can only cause a disorder of speech by disturbing underlying physiological processes; the structural changes prevent the orderly performance of certain cerebral acts and speech suffers in consequence. These abnormal reactions are apparent to the external world in terms of a disorder of language, just as some defect in the mechanism of a clock is manifested by failure to keep correct time. Capacity to make use of language in a normal manner requires the perfect exercise of physiological activities in certain portions of the brain; when they are imperfectly carried out, from whatever cause, the acts of speaking, reading and writing become more or less disturbed.

Before we can determine anatomically what parts of the brain are responsible for these manifestations, it is essential to discover the nature of the disorder itself. Unfortunately the actual phenomena have usually been dismissed in a very summary manner, and none of the conceptions put forward to explain them are in harmony with the facts presented by these disorders of language. For any satisfactory generalisation must be capable of explaining why the patient succeeds in reading or writing under certain conditions, although he fails entirely to do so, when the task is presented to him in a different manner. All attempts to summarise the actual disabilities of the patient under any categories, formulated up to the present time, have failed lamentably; they succeed approximately in those cases only where the clinical examination leaves much to be desired, and the will to believe is manifest on the part of the observer.

Let us then consider the actual phenomena elicited by the methods of examination I have described in certain typical examples of disordered speech. I will begin with an ordinary case of so-called "aphasia" with "alexia" and "agraphia."

Example I. (Case No. 21.)

On the evening of May 13th, 1911, a man of 56 suddenly lost all power of speaking naturally; next day he was drowsy and the disorder of speech increased. On May 17th he came to my out-patient department and was admitted to the wards, suffering from severe aphasia without hemiplegia or hemianopsia. He was discharged a month later and remained constantly under supervision until his sudden death on January 6th, 1920. His condition throughout this period of nearly nine years remained unchanged; I was able to make an extended series of observations in November 1919, and it is on these that the following conclusions are based.

Articulated speech. He was almost completely speechless, but could reply "Yes" and "No" correctly; asked to say "Yes" he answered, "No, I can't," and told to repeat "No," he usually shook his head, but once said, "No, I don't know how to do it." He could at times use the expression "Thank you" appropriately, and when puzzled would exclaim "Can't get it," "I know what it is," "I don't know what it says," etc. Once, when excited by a request to draw an elephant, he said, "Yes, I've been all over; seen lots. I've got some on my what you call it," alluding to figures on the mantlepiece of his sitting-room.

He was unable to repeat anything said to him, even the expressions he used spontaneously.

He could not name a single object, although he showed clearly that he knew its use; he scrawled with the pencil, turned the key in an imaginary lock and struck a match in pantomime. In the same way, although he could not tell the time aloud, he occasionally made signs that he understood the significance of the position of the hands. Thus, when they were placed at 1.30, he held up one finger bisecting it with the other hand, and for 1.55, he extended five fingers and then two more to indicate "five minutes to two."

Understanding of spoken words. But, in spite of this almost complete lack of words, there was no doubt that he understood what was said. He could choose correctly an object or colour named by me from amongst a group lying on the table. He was able to set a clock to oral commands, although he tended to mistake the significance of the two hands. As soon, however, as the order demanded for its perfect execution more than one propositional act he failed grossly. He could not carry out the various movements of the hand, eye and ear tests to oral commands, and failed in twelve out of fifteen attempts to place the right coin into the correct bowl.

Reading. He could not read anything aloud and, given a printed command, such as to touch one eye or ear with either the right or left hand, he made no effort to carry out even the slightest movement. He shook his head saying "I can't," "I know what it is, I don't know what it says." In the same way, with the coin-bowl test, he did not attempt to execute an order given either in printed words or numbers.

But in spite of his inability to carry out these printed commands there was no doubt that he could read. He was able to point correctly on seventeen out of eighteen occasions to an object named in print. With colours he was less certain; but such mistakes as the selection of yellow for orange showed that he understood the meaning of printed characters. He was able to carry out an even more severe test on the following lines. Eight cards, each of which bore the name of a colour, were laid on the table in front of him; shown a certain colour, he picked out the corresponding card correctly in nine out of sixteen attempts. Two of his errors again consisted in confusing yellow and orange, which in itself showed that he understood the printed words.

In the same way, his power of understanding simple words in print was shown in the course of the man, cat and dog tests. Six printed cards were laid on the table, each of which bore one combination of the series. Then he was shown pictures of one pair, for instance the man and the dog, and he picked out correctly, ten times in succession, the card which corresponded to the combination he had seen. Once he chose the inscription "The cat and the man," but rejected it for "The man and the cat," the correct order from left to right in which the figures had been presented to him. Later in the same series, he again chose a card with the right names in the reverse order, but immediately corrected his mistake. Thus, he was not only accurate with regard to the verbal significance of the card he selected, but also paid attention to the order of the words in print.

Writing. His signature was reduced to the one word "Beadon" (instead of Beaton) and he was totally unable to write the alphabet spontaneously. Attempts to write the name of an object indicated, ended in the production of a group of badly formed letters, which bore little or no resemblance to the name he was seeking. When he was shown any two pictures of the man, cat and dog series, he usually wrote down two incomprehensible groups of letters. All power of spontaneous writing was completely lost.

He succeeded fairly well in writing the alphabet from dictation, but tended to substitute wrong letters for those said to him. Copying was carried out better and, although the formation of the letters was poor, he made fewer actual mistakes. Asked, however, to write from dictation and to copy the names of common objects, the results were equally bad. On the other hand, with the man, cat and dog series, he found greater difficulty in copying the printed legend than in writing from dictation; for, when the words were said to him, he eliminated all but the two nouns and wrote something that occasionally bore a relation to the essential content of the phrase. But, on attempting to copy the printed cards, he was puzzled by the smaller words, the articles and conjunctions, and wrote an incomprehensible combination of ill-formed letters.

Numbers and coins. He could not name a single coin, but indicated the relative value of any two of them by holding up the exact number of fingers. Thus, when a penny and a shilling were laid on the table, he raised his right hand with all five fingers extended; he then said "Nover" (another), held up his hand again and then added two more fingers; making twelve in all. He even indicated the relation between a penny and a half-crown, raising his hand six times in succession; and yet he could not count beyond nineteen and was unable to carry out correctly simple addition and subtraction on paper. Moreover, he failed to execute the coin-bowl tests, even when the command was given in numbers orally or in print.

Imitation of movements involving choice. He had also lost the power of executing orders, which demanded formal choice, although they were expressed in ways not usually associated with speaking or reading. Asked to imitate my movements, when I touched the right or left eye or ear with my right or left hand, he failed grossly sitting face to face; for under such conditions our actions were apparently reversed. When, however, my movements were reflected in a mirror, he never made a mistake nor did he show the least hesitation. An exactly similar result was obtained if the command was given in the form of pictures; holding the card in his hand, he was wrong every time, but, with the picture reflected in the glass, he completed the required action rapidly and without fail.

Setting the clock. Throughout the clock tests he tended to confuse the two hands. He made no attempt to set the time to printed commands in the ordinary nomenclature (e.g. 5 minutes to 2) although he succeeded sometimes in doing so when they were set out in railway time (e.g. 1.55). When he tried to tell the time aloud, he did not make a sound; but he was able to express half-past one and five minutes to two on his fingers, showing that he knew the meaning of the position of the hands on the clock.

Drawing. Asked to draw an elephant, he produced an absurd figure bearing no relation to any living creature. He marked in what appeared to be an eye; asked what it was, he said, "Don't know" but pointed to his own eye. Questioned about a peculiar horn-like projection on the front of the drawing, he caught hold of his own ear; and when I asked "What is this?" pointing to the object hanging down in front, he passed his hand upwards over his face from beneath his nose saying, "Sometimes up this way." This was evidently intended to represent a trunk.

It is obvious that this patient had not lost the power of reasoning and was in many ways highly intelligent. He suffered from a severe form of aphasia in which all power of word-formation, either articulatory or in writing, was destroyed. But the power of responding to verbal meaning was preserved, provided the words did not demand formal choice between expressed alternatives. He could choose the right object or colour, from amongst those on the table, to oral or printed command, but could not carry out the hand, eye and ear or coin-bowl tests; nor could he set the clock correctly, whatever the form of the order.

He imitated movements extremely badly, if I sat opposite to him, or if he held a picture of the required act in his hand; when, however, such commands were reflected in the mirror, they were carried out perfectly. For in the first instance, the words "right" and "left," "eye" and "ear," must be silently interposed between the reception and execution of the order; but, when reflected in the glass, the movements are almost purely imitative and no verbalisation is necessary. Immediate and intuitive recognition caused him no trouble.

His power of drawing some stipulated form, such as that of an elephant was defective, although he clearly attached a definite significance to the marks on the paper, which did not correspond in shape to that part of the animal they were intended to represent.

Example II. (*Case No.* 19.)

My next example is a sergeant of 23, who was bombed from the air on the Salonika front in February 1917. Three years and eight months after the injury he was sent to me as a pure case of "motor" aphasia.

Articulated speech. He could use "yes" and "no" correctly, but was otherwise almost completely without words for voluntary expression; yet his gestures were so surprisingly apt that there was little difficulty in understanding what he wanted to convey. For instance, one morning on arrival at my house he said, "I been good," moving his hands as if manipulating the steering wheel of a motor car, and added "Same come here." I asked if he had driven the car and he answered, "Yes, good. I been good." To a further question "Did you find it difficult?" he replied, "No, no."

He managed to indicate his likes, dislikes and desires by the combination of his scanty vocabulary with expressive gestures. For instance, when testing his sense of taste, quinine was followed by saccharin; he said, "Good, good, no good other." On another occasion he enquired, "Can I you know like this?" placing his hand over the lower part of his abdomen. I showed him the lavatory and he went in to pass water saying, "Yes, thank you." Subsequently he used this gesture without words to express a wish to micturate.

Thus, I was able to elicit from him much more information than would have seemed possible from the few words he possessed for voluntary use. On asking him about his schooling, I found out that he had reached the sixth standard at twelve years of age, the highest class in the elementary school he had attended. He added, "Then was going," lifting his hand into the air, "you see." I asked, "to a higher school?" and he replied, "Yes. He something here," pointing to his chest, "he dead." I then said, "Your father died?"; he answered, "Yes, not enough me go there," and raised his hands again. I summed up his meaning as follows: "You had not enough money to go to a higher school," and he replied, "Yes, yes."

When printed cards were laid on the table and he was asked to choose the one which corresponded to some object shown him or to some movement made by me, he said, "Yes, me good now" (that is easy); "you see, here," pointing to his forehead, "something to get hold of there," spreading both hands over the cards on the table.

In the same sort of way he was able to tell me how he had acquired the power of imitating correctly my movements in the hand, eye and ear tests, which at first puzzled him considerably. He wanted to explain that, as soon as he discovered he must make an apparently opposite movement, the task became easy. He thrust one hand forwards and simultaneously drew the other backwards exclaiming, "I got to go... see?"; then he said, "See...goes, you know," and made similar movements in the reverse direction.

He could not repeat anything said to him except occasionally the word "key" and failed entirely to reproduce even the simple monosyllabic words of the man, cat and dog tests.

Understanding of spoken words. In spite of this almost complete loss of words, he evidently had a clear appreciation of names. He could indicate objects or colours named orally and he picked out from amongst a series of cards the one which bore the name of a colour he had just seen. He even succeeded in putting together out of block letters something sufficiently close to the name of the colour to show he had a definite idea of its name. Oral commands necessitating choice, such as the hand, eye and ear tests, were carried out accurately, though somewhat more slowly than in response to pictures.

Reading. All power of reading aloud was abolished. He was unable to articulate the names of common objects or colours presented to him on printed cards and he failed entirely with the monosyllabic words of the man, cat and dog series. He could not even convert the pictures of this simple test into external speech.

There was not the slightest doubt, however, that he understood much of what he read to himself. He not only chose correctly common objects and colours from printed commands, but he executed the complex orders of the hand, eye and ear tests without fail, although he was unable to read the cards aloud. He could also carry out the reverse operation; when a movement was made by me he selected the card on which it was written. In the same way, he picked out the legend appropriate to the two pictures of the man, cat and dog series, which had been shown him. Although he could not tell the time by any other means, he could choose the card bearing the correct inscription, whether in numbers or words.

Writing. He wrote his name and the address of his previous home in the country; but he failed to complete that of the house in which his wife had lived for a year, although it was to this place that he returned every time he left the hospital on leave.

His power of writing depended on the nature of the task he had to perform. When he attempted to write the name of a colour, he failed entirely. If, however, it was dictated to him, his script bore a distinct relation to what he intended to express and frequently began with the correct initial letter. As soon as he was allowed to copy the printed words, he reproduced them accurately in cursive handwriting. With familiar objects he succeeded in writing something, which corresponded more or less to the name in nine out of eighteen attempts, and dictation yielded a still better result; copying was in every way perfect. Shown any two pictures belonging to the man, cat and dog tests, he wrote the two nouns correctly, coupled by "and" without the definite articles. To dictation he followed exactly the same procedure; but he copied the printed cards in cursive handwriting with accuracy.

When he attempted to write down movements made by me, he simplified the problem by leaving out one term; thus, if I touched my left ear with my right hand he wrote "R—ear." Here the "right" or "left" indicated the hand I used and the side of the ear or eye was left unspecified. He copied these printed commands correctly, but was slow and hesitating, repeatedly consulting the copy and evidently unable to retain the whole sentence in his mind at the same moment.

The alphabet. These various disabilities were particularly evident, when the alphabet was used as a test. He failed entirely to say the names of the letters in sequence; he made a few meaningless sounds and then gave up the attempt. Asked to repeat them after me some were correctly pronounced, but many were unrecognisable. He read the alphabet aloud extremely badly. Told to write it down he succeeded as far as F, but in spite of repeated attempts could go no further; after he had given up, he suddenly wrote O W V Y S Q in order to show me that there were other letters, which he remembered. When, however, they were dictated to him he wrote the whole series correctly.

I then gave him more than enough block letters to make an alphabet and, after mixing them on the table, told him to put them together; this he was unable to do. When each letter was dictated to him one by one, he ultimately succeeded, after many corrections, in building up an almost complete alphabet.

Evidently these difficulties were not due to an isolated defect of speaking, reading or writing. All aspects of verbal expression were affected; even when block letters were given him he failed to construct an alphabet. Words were lacking as symbols for voluntary use in both external and internal forms of speech.

Numbers. Counting also revealed the same want of words associated, however, with perfect appreciation of numerical values. From ten onwards he counted "one one" (eleven), "one two" (twelve), etc.; twenty became "two and oh" and a hundred and ten was "one one no."

He had no difficulty in placing one of four coins into the right bowl, when the command was given orally or in print. Moreover, it seemed to make no material difference to the time required for choice whether the order was printed in words or in figures; in both cases he seized on the essential numbers and executed the task with great rapidity.

Coins and their relative value. He was unable to name a single coin but perfectly appreciated their relative value. He shopped with accuracy and experienced no difficulty with change; yet he failed to carry out even simple arithmetical operations on paper.

The clock tests demonstrated in the clearest manner that he suffered from defective verbal expression and not from lack of names. For he had no difficulty in choosing a printed card corresponding to the time shown on the clock face. He could even write the time correctly if he was allowed to use figures only and, in spite of the paucity of his vocabulary, he was able to tell the time aloud provided care was taken to note exactly what he said. Thus, half-past-one became "one, three and no" (1.30), and twenty minutes to six was "five, four, no" (5.40); he also called twenty minutes to four "four and eight," because the two hands pointed to those numbers on the clock face.

Drawing. Unlike the previous patient he could draw excellently both from a model and from memory and his representation of an elephant showed all the salient features correctly.

He produced an accurate plan of my room full of details correctly related to one another and his orientation was perfect.

He played games well, such as billiards and draughts, and enjoyed putting together jigsaw puzzles.

This patient evidently suffered from lack of power to express himself verbally, although he still appreciated the meaning of spoken and printed words. He named a series of objects correctly, if he was allowed to choose the appropriate printed card, and he told the time by indicating numbers on his fingers. But the disorder of language was not limited to articulated speech. It interfered with internal verbalisation and expression, as shown by his inability to write spontaneously or to dictation. It prevented him from building up an alphabet out of block letters and yet he could copy print perfectly in cursive handwriting. Obviously these defects cannot be classed categorically under the heads of speaking, reading or writing.

Example III. (Case No. 15.)

My next example belongs manifestly to another variety of disordered speech; for there was no lack of words, but they were badly combined and the patient talked a form of jargon.

A private, aged 25, belonging to the regular army, was admitted to the London Hospital on March 2nd, 1915. In the last days of January he had been hit by a rifle bullet, which entered to the left of the inner canthus of the right eye and passed out just above the insertion of the left ear. The entry was represented by a minute white scar and the wound of exit by a small hernia cerebri; this finally healed by June 5th, 1915, three months after his admission to hospital.

Articulated speech. From the first his speech had certain peculiar characteristics, which were still present seven years later. He said little spontaneously, but answered questions readily; once started he talked rapidly and volubly. He tried to "rush" his phrases and not uncommonly was brought to a standstill by pure jargon. It was extremely difficult to hear the conjunctions and articles; for these minor parts of speech, so important for binding together groups of words into a phrase, were frequently omitted or insufficiently stressed. This made it extremely difficult to report exactly what he actually said. Asked what he had done since he came to the London Hospital, he replied, "To here; only washing, cups and plates." Have you played any games? "Played games, yes, played one, daytime, garden."

He did not usually employ wrong words and, if the subject under discussion was known, it was not difficult to gather the sense of what he wished to say. Thus, when I was testing his taste and placed some quinine upon his tongue, he said, "Rotten to drink it. Something medicine or that. Make you drop of water after it, so to take out of your mouth." On a later occasion, wanting to explain to me how he came to develop an inguinal hernia, he said, "I got that rupture, after left hospital, when dark, no lights, when airships came over. Couldn't see, smashed the wall, the house like, smashed into wall, couldn't see. Had a pain, saw doctor, pushed it up. If it should come up, press it up and use what you call 'em. When it do go up, pain inside."

Single words were as a rule perfectly pronounced; but, when they formed part of a phrase, he frequently slurred them. For example, when pointing to the various features of the elephant he had drawn, he said, "Zis-iz-ear" (i.e. this is his ear) and tusks were characterised as "bonezinks" (i.e. bone things). At first he had somewhat more difficulty in finding unfamiliar names of two or more syllables, e.g. orange; but this gradually passed away with time.

He could repeat single words or even simple phrases, such as those of the man, cat and dog series. But, when asked to say after me short sentences, which he had not heard before, his defective syntax became evident. On one occasion he repeated three simple statements separately with fair accuracy; but, asked to say them over again consecutively, he failed entirely to do so, exclaiming, "I can't think." His power to reproduce words grouped in coherent sequence and to repeat consecutive phrases was strikingly defective.

Understanding of spoken words. From the time he first came under my observation he recognised the names of common objects and colours perfectly and could usually evoke a sound, which bore some obvious relation to their usual nomenclature; thus a pencil was called "blacking" and then "blacklead." Occasionally it was perverted, as "volley" for violet and "masses" for matches; but on the whole single words were well articulated and could be used correctly for naming.

In his struggle to produce his phrases he sometimes used a wrong name and if so his understanding was liable to be led astray. For example, when drawing an elephant, he said "irons" and "highons" and added to the picture what were evidently intended for horns.

He understood perfectly what was said to him, provided the order was given in the form of a single word. At first he hesitated somewhat, when setting the hands of a clock to oral commands, and twice mistook "past" and "to" the hour; but on the last examination he was quick and accurate. Throughout, however, he had some difficulty in carrying out the hand, eye and ear tests to oral commands, although this was shown more in slowness and hesitation than by actual errors.

Reading. He was able to read aloud single words on the various combinations of the man, cat and dog series. After this test he remarked, "It's alright, these small words; thick 'uns, can't understand 'em." But groups of words in formal sentences troubled him greatly. Thus, a simple passage about a collecting box for flowers placed on the platform of Snaresbrook Station was read as follows: "This box has placed on the...platform at...can't name either...station...at a...no sir...for flowers for the wounded. Any of the...passengers...can't stand (understand) that letter...nosegay...daily...for the gardens...and those are sent...to the Befnal Green...Infirm."

Such jargon confused him greatly and hindered his comprehension of what he read aloud; he then placed on the nonsense he had uttered some meaning not in consonance with the text. For instance he read, "Mr Lloyd George says Red take must go," instead of "Red tape"; this puzzled him and he explained it by suggesting that Mr Lloyd George was going to pass an Act to restrict the sale of beer, a possibility much discussed at the time.

He was frequently confused by what he read to himself silently, unless it consisted of isolated words. These, however, he appreciated and he was able to choose without fail from among a set of common objects or colours the one mentioned in print. He could even carry out the complex commands of the hand, eye and ear tests with comparatively few errors, though somewhat slowly.

But consecutive sentences failed to convey their full meaning with certainty, whether they were read silently or aloud. Thus, when asked to narrate what he had learnt from the paragraph about the collecting box for flowers placed on the station platform, he said, "Flowers for sale; selling at stations. At Bethnal Green, at Bethnal Green station." Here he converted collecting into selling and transferred the name Bethnal Green from the Infirmary to the station. He was puzzled by the jargon both of his internal and articulated speech.

Writing. He wrote his name and address rapidly and correctly; but at the earlier examination he was unable to write that of his mother with whom he lived. I said to him, "Now write your mother's address"; he hesitated and asked, "What her name before?" To this I replied, "No, her name now, as if you were going to direct a letter to her." He wrote "S"; then after a pause "Sams" and, saying "Susie," gave up the attempt. Urged to try again, he wrote "S. Sams, 203," the number of the house, and said, "No, I can't; you mean her address, no I can't." Evidently the need for substituting one new word at the beginning prevented him from carrying out an act, which he could execute perfectly if he was writing his own name and address.

Single words, though badly spelt, gave a definite indication of the name of an object or colour shown to him; the articulated sound corresponded even more closely to the true nomenclature than the written word.

When writing from pictures he omitted the definite articles and shortened the phrase to "man and dog," etc. Moreover, he tended to transpose the order of the pictures; for instance, shown the cat and the man, he wrote "man and cat," although in his previous answers he had recorded the figures accurately as they stood from left to right. Even in the latest examination there were four such inversions out of twelve tests, although he was never in doubt as to which pair of pictures he had seen. Evidently he found it difficult to retain the exact order of short phrases, even when they were expressed solely in silent speech.

Spontaneous writing was also spoilt by the confusion produced by internal jargoning. He wrote to his sister, "My dear Sister, I now write to you that I hame geting the best of hearl and I am getting to walk to the garden to play a lot of game and I hame the all of." This he read aloud in the following manner as if it was perfectly written, "My dear Sister, I now write to you that I am getting the best of health and I getting to walk to the garden to play a lot of games and I have the whole of...I've forgotten now what I was going to say."

Numbers and coins. He could count perfectly and solved with ease the six arithmetical problems set him. He found no difficulty with money, or with the names and relative value of coins.

The clock tests. He told the time correctly; but, asked to write it down without saying it aloud, he tended in the earlier stages to use a curious nomenclature. Thus, after writing correctly "20 minutes to 6" he wrote "45 to 9" and "30 past 2."

Drawing. He drew excellently from a model and from memory, representing the various parts of a spirit lamp with remarkable accuracy. During his first attempt to draw an elephant he said aloud "mouth" and then "irons," "highons"; misled by these words he added horns to the forehead of the figure instead of tusks. I asked, "Has an elephant got horns?" He replied, "Yes, silver what you stick out," pointing to the corner of his mouth and placing his pencil into the position of a tusk. Evidently he was confused by the jargon words representing horns and impulsively added them to the picture; but he finally succeeded in explaining his error by gestures, which gave a correct interpretation of his intention. He subsequently learnt to draw a fair picture of an elephant; but, when on a later occasion he omitted the tusks and I suggested that he had left out something, he replied "bonezinks" (bone things) adding "I've been up India."

Appreciation of pictures. He understood pictures perfectly although he had great difficulty in describing their content. Shown a picture of two Belgian gunners explaining the mechanism of a field-gun to a British Red Cross worker at the Front, he said, "It's the ladies...come on the Hospital...come to see how men work it." "What sort of men are they?" I asked and he replied, "Till France...the men come from France...the Francemen...She might come from England...lady." To my enquiry, "What are they showing her?" he answered, "A gun...a 75 isn't it?"

I then allowed him to read the legend beneath the picture and asked him to explain it; this he did in the following words, "It's a guns belongs to Belgium...She a hospital lady from England...comes from England ...The Belgians just telling what it's made of...the different names, the words and..."

In this case the disorder of language mainly affected syntax and rhythm. The production of single words and their use as names were not materially disturbed; but groups of words could not be combined into coherent and effective phrases. This converted both external and internal speech into jargon and, in turn, interfered with his power of reproducing exactly what he heard or read and diminished his capacity to carry out suggestions given in the course of conversation.

Example IV. (Case No. 2.)

Captain C., an able young Staff Officer attached to the Indian Army, received a compound fracture of the skull from the kick of a horse on February 19th, 1918. At an operation performed shortly afterwards, the substance of the brain was found to have been reduced to pulp beneath the wound in the left parieto-occipital region. He was admitted to the Empire Hospital in September 1918, and the site of the injury was then represented by a well-healed, depressed, pulsating scar.

From the time when he first came under my care up to the most recent examination, his disorder of language remained the same in kind, although it diminished greatly in severity. I shall therefore attempt to weave my observations into a coherent account, so as to bring out the essential nature of his disabilities.

Articulated speech. Most of the words in ordinary conversation, in so far as this was possible, were well pronounced and intonation was normal. But, when he was unable to evoke a name or some nominal expression, he would try various combinations of sound more or less related to the word he was seeking. Thus, shown a match-box, he said "mat, mats, match"; blue was called "ber-loo," orange "or-ridge." This seemed to be due to difficulty in finding the adequate symbol rather than to lack of purely verbal aptitude. For he was able to give long and reasonable explanations of his inability to discover the right names; for instance, in order to show that he recognised black, he said, "I remember that now, because people who are dead...the other people who are not dead, they usually have this colour." Wanting to explain how he would walk from the hospital to the War Office he said, "I have no streets in London; no names at all. Suppose I was going from the Army and Navy (Stores) just round here, that's what it's called, I should then say some place to a hospital about a quarter of a mile away. I remember the hospital is on the left on the way to the War Office about half way"; he ended this conversation as follows, "You see, it's like this; with me it's all in bits. I have to jump like this, like a man, who jumps from one thing to the next. I can see them, but I can't express. Really it is that I haven't enough names."

He did not talk jargon and the syntax of his phrases was not affected, except in so far as he was perpetually at a loss for names; this frequently necessitated the recasting of a sentence before it could be brought to a conclusion.

12—2

He showed a tendency to employ ready made phrases and slang, which came more easily to him than orthodox expressions, although this was not his habit before he was injured. He would say, "I made a priceless blob" (error in tact); "The question of going to St Ives is a good egg" (a good idea). He was particularly fond of "putting heavy guns onto it," whenever he intended to imply that much effort had been used.

Asked to repeat single words or simple phrases he could usually do so correctly even if the same words might be badly pronounced in spontaneous speech. But at first he had difficulty in repeating exactly the names of colours said to him and, although the words of the man, cat and dog tests were perfectly enunciated, the content of the sentence was frequently incorrect. This was not due to defective word-formation, but to want of appreciation of verbal significance.

Understanding of spoken words. He had considerable difficulty in grasping the full meaning of what was said to him in ordinary conversation. When he had somewhat recovered, he explained his condition as follows: "I understand pretty well now what anybody says, unless it's anything that's rather...that's what I can't say...rather tricky, rather heavier...I can't quite get what I want to say. Everything I say is very little, like a child. I can't express what I want to say." One day, after having tea with me, he made the following comment on a fellow guest, "I like that young man; he's clever. I notice that clever people say everything in a few words so that I can understand. Stupid people take a lot of words and I can't remember what they have said; it confuses me."

He could not grasp the exact meaning of "to" and "past," "high" and "low," "up" and "down," "back" and "front," "right" and "left," when contrasted with one another. Asked, "Would you like to stop in or go out?" he would reply, "Either," in order to hide his want of complete comprehension. But if the question was put in a direct and not in an alternative form, "Do you want to stop in?" he would answer, "No"; "Do you want to go out?" "Yes," showing that he had definitely made up his mind to one course of action, but was puzzled by the two suggestions in one sentence.

At first he was extremely slow in choosing common objects to oral commands and the colour tests were so badly carried out that he might have been supposed to be colour-blind. But this was excluded by the rapidity and certainty with which he matched colours, when no words were employed. The defect was one of names and their significance; his gross errors were due to want of nominal recognition. Throughout his choice of colours to oral command remained slow, though at the last examination they were selected with two mistakes only. But his hand hovered in the air, whilst he pondered the meaning of the order, and then pounced on the object or colour named by me; he did not go straight for it, as when he had to find the duplicate to something seen or felt.

In spite of his inability to comprehend or evoke the exact names of the colours he was able to show by the use of similes that he recognised them correctly. For instance, when he could not remember the name for red, he said, "It's what the Staff...the same colour I had here," pointing to the lapel of his coat.

After a series of observations, in which by the use of such descriptive expressions he showed that he recognised the various colours, I carried out the experiment in another way in order to test his appreciation of the nominal value of these phrases. The colours were laid on the table as usual. I then said, "The dead," and he chose black; "What the Staff wear," red; "What is on your arm," blue and so on throughout the whole gamut. His difficulty lay in recognising the meaning of the words black, red, blue, etc., although he could choose each colour correctly if the order was given in some appropriate descriptive phrase.

If an oral command necessitated a more complex choice, as with the hand, eye and ear tests, his response was extremely bad and he made many errors. In the same way he failed to set the hands of the clock correctly, when I gave the order by word of mouth.

Throughout his attempts to carry out oral commands, he made movements of his lips without uttering a sound; he was evidently repeating the words to himself silently.

On one occasion during the coin-bowl tests he attempted to explain his difficulties as follows: "It is an extraordinary thing, with some of them I do it without thinking; then, if I think too much and say to myself 'third into fourth,' I don't know what it means. Now, if I say, 'the first into the fourth,' I pick up this (the first coin) and then I have to think what is 'fourth.' If I do it myself, I can do it as quickly as you like; but you tell me to do it and I have to think what it means, even if I say it to myself."

Reading. He could not read a newspaper to himself or appreciate the contents of a letter. Even after his powers had improved greatly, he found considerable difficulty in narrating what he had gathered from silent perusal of a set of printed paragraphs. After poring for ten minutes over a few lines about partridge shooting and motor cars fitted with

Dunlop tyres[1] he said, "It takes me an awful long time. In the early summer there are lots of young partridges...I think it is...That's as far as I've got."

Asked to read to himself three lines of print descriptive of a famous prize fight, he returned the paper with the following words, "Carpentier met Beckett in the Holborn...say...so...Sadium, I used to know it, and Carpentier being the champion now...who is...oh no...who met Beckett...now the champion of England...knocked...er...knocked ...er...Beckett out in seventy-four seconds...with a right...with right hook to the jaw."

But, when I said, "Can you see the fight?" an extraordinary change came over his behaviour; "Now I think about the fight I see the picture of Carpentier. I see Beckett falling...I see the Ref...Ref...what you call it...Referee...The last thing I can picture is Carpentier standing like this, with both hands like this." He sprang from his bed and assumed an attitude with both hands on his hips looking down towards the ground, in the position of Carpentier in the photographs of the termination of the fight. The change in manner from the puzzled aspect of a man slowly recalling what he had read to the brisk, vivid, smiling person describing what he saw was remarkable.

He chose correctly from a number of common objects the one indicated on a printed card; but, when it was a question of colours, he frequently made mistakes. He improved greatly in both these tests, although to the end his answers remained slow and hesitating.

He explained this delay as follows: "It's the interpreting words into pictures; when you give me KNIFE (printed card) I can't see the picture in my brain. All these things (passing his hand over the objects on the table) have no names at all until I really read K N I F E, and say 'knife' to myself; then I can say (indicate) what it is." I showed him the card bearing the word KEY and he replied, "I'm not quite sure of that; I was not certain if it was a key or a knife. I have to spell it K E Y, and I say 'key' and look down on the table and then that's the key" (pointing to it). "I still puzzle what K E Y means; if I see that (pointing to the key on the table) then I don't have to worry, I know K E Y is that...is a key."

I then handed him two cards one of which bore the word MATCHES and the other WATCH. He pointed to the match-box on the table and holding up the other card said, "Nothing here"; this was correct. Asked, "What is the difference?" he replied, "They are both written

[1] Vol. II, p. 34.

(printed); this one is here (pointing to the matches), the other there is nothing. I focus this one (matches) because it is here (pointing to the box on the table). I can't focus this (watch) because it is not so clear." He then moved his eyes round my room as if seeking something and added, "When I look at that big one (my consulting room clock) that helps me. I want to interpret the reading 'watch' into a picture or into that (pointing to the clock) watch. If I think of a watch and don't have to read it I think of a picture of my own watch. If you say it to me, I see it at once; if you show it to me like that (printed) I have to think, I don't get the picture easily." He added, "Suppose you had shown me 'looking glass' written like this (printed), I should have had to think a long time. But if I looked up and saw that looking glass (pointing to the one on the wall) I should have known it at once." Evidently he was helped to understand the printed card by seeing the object to which it referred in front of him; to imagine it and give a meaning to the name on the card was a distinctly harder task[1].

When the printed command necessitated a more complex choice, his response remained extremely bad throughout. At first he was completely unable to carry out this form of the hand, eye and ear tests; even during the last series of observations, although he made no mistakes, his lips moved as he read the card repeatedly in silence. "What worries me," he said, "is the name of eye and ear; they are very similar. It is the names that bother me."

From the first he could set the hands of the clock if the time was given in printed figures, although he failed to do so correctly to an order in printed words. For instance he succeeded with "6.50," though with "10 minutes to 7" he set 7.10; in the same way with the coin-bowl tests he had no difficulty, when the printed order was given as "1st into 3rd," etc.; but, with "First penny into third bowl," his actions became slow and uncertain. He said, "I see where the trouble is. I can't get its name. You see the first is like writing in numbers; with the other I have to read it."

Single words were read aloud badly and he was greatly hindered in comprehending their meaning, if he tried to spell them out letter by letter; this confused him and he usually ended by making a guess at their significance. Yet he read the alphabet correctly, though somewhat slowly, and readily recalled the sound of the letters; but he could not appreciate their meaning as constructive elements in a word. Thus, he frequently succeeded in spelling out correctly all the letters of a simple phrase, though he failed completely to produce the words; given, "The

[1] Cf. Lotmar [96], p. 223 et seq.

cat and the man," he deciphered it letter by letter, but at the end said, "The cat, I know that's the dog (pointing to cat). No, I cannot tell you any more."

As his powers improved, he was able to read aloud more or less correctly such paragraphs as that on partridge shooting and cars with Dunlop tyres; but, whenever he failed to produce the exact verbal equivalent, that word puzzled him and frequently spoilt his comprehension of the whole sentence. Apart, however, from this cause of misunderstanding, he usually gave a very confused account of what he had just read aloud; many of the phrases he had reproduced accurately evidently failed to communicate their full meaning.

When, however, he was told in print to make a simple choice between different objects or colours laid before him, reading the order aloud was of distinct assistance. Thus, at a time when he was responding badly to printed commands read silently, he made a perfect series of answers to the colour tests on reading the names aloud. A similar result occurred even with the more complicated hand, eye and ear tests.

Writing. He wrote his usual signature, consisting of his name, rank and regiment with perfect ease and rapidity; but he was completely unable to add his address. At first he could not write a letter or a sentence of any length, although he amused himself by making lists of words, especially those which came into his head spontaneously. Of these the following may serve as characteristic examples: "Post offest" (Post Office), "The King One" (The King's Own Regiment), "Arbes" (Arabs), "Masptmeran" (Mesopotamia).

By repeated practice he recovered to a considerable extent his power of writing spontaneously. But he remained to the end extremely slow and inaccurate; he was accustomed, when composing a letter, to put it aside for correction and then to recopy it. He wrote me a long and vivid account of how one of his fellow patients at the hospital came by his spinal injuries; the train of thought was consecutive, but the errors in spelling went far beyond simple mistakes in orthography. Thus he wrote "smached it into Tinder by mashen gun fire" and ended, "and that is how the officer in question became a spin case (spine case), three or four times badly wounded and paraliesed."[1]

Even after he had read the story of the Carpentier-Beckett fight, first silently and then aloud, he wrote "Carpanter the Hevey Champion of [Phrance] France met Beckett the English Hevey waite at the Holborn [Sadeon] Stadium on Thursesday the 4th Dec after 74 minutes fight

[1] Vol. II, p. 33.

[with] Carpomter [nockered] knocked out Beckett with a right hand nunch in the [gor] jaw." The words in square brackets are those he wrote and then erased.

The days of the week and the names of common objects and colours were extremely badly written, even those which he could pronounce with some approximation to accuracy. He failed to write down movements made by me and reflected in the glass, although he imitated them without hesitation.

Dictation did not help his writing materially. His name and address were so badly reproduced that they were unrecognisable and many of the days of the week bore little relation to the words said to him beyond the initial letter, which was uniformly correct. On the other hand, the monosyllabic words of the man, cat and dog tests were well written, but the content of the phrase did not always correspond to the pair of nouns dictated. Even when he was permitted to say the words aloud after me, he wrote them badly although he spoke them correctly.

From the first he was able to copy printed words in capital letters, although his power of transferring them into cursive handwriting was faulty. Sometimes he combined the one form of lettering with the other, producing a mixed script. Long after he could copy such simple phrases as those of the man, cat and dog tests in excellent handwriting, he still showed a tendency to make mistakes in the particular combination placed before him. His disability did not consist simply in forming the words, but he also failed to recognise the verbal meaning of the copy and so fell into errors of appreciation.

Appreciation of pictures. His comprehension of pictures was remarkably good, and he not only noticed the various details, but recognised their full significance. Pictorial jokes he saw easily, though he was frequently puzzled by the legend.

He liked to have everything that was said to him illustrated, as much as possible, in a drawing or a diagram. Thus, when his sister was teaching him music, she told him that the scale consisted of three tones, a half tone, two tones and another half tone. This puzzled him completely; she played the scale and he still failed to grasp it. But as soon as she drew a diagram, where each tone was represented by a horizontal line, each half tone by a short vertical one, he understood and from that time never forgot it.

But in spite of this ready appreciation of pictures, pictorial commands, such as those of the hand, eye and ear tests, were badly executed throughout; and yet they could be carried out with perfect ease, if reflected in the glass. For, when the picture was held in his hand, he was compelled to formulate the command in some form of internal language, whilst to obey the mirrored order was, as he said, "just copying."

Drawing. He could make an excellent drawing of a complicated object, such as a spirit lamp, placed on the table in front of him and later reproduced it almost exactly from memory. He amused himself, when in hospital, by making pictures of animals he had shot in Cashmir; on one occasion, when trying to describe the difficulties of transport in the East, he drew spontaneously a spirited picture of a camel. When, however, he was told to draw an elephant he produced an absurd figure without trunk, tusks or ears. He was extremely troubled about the trunk and the tail, saying, "Oh! that certainly comes from there (pointing to the tail and then to the mouth); this I know he generally takes from there (pointing to the rump) and brings round to there (the mouth) to eat with; with that on there he can generally eat." Thus, his inability to find the correct names led to a general confusion with regard to the nature of the tail and the trunk. When, however, I drew the rough outline of an elephant and asked him to point to the various parts as I named them, he did so accurately and without hesitation; the name once given to him was immediately attached to the appropriate part of the body.

Numbers. From the first he could count correctly and with perfect enunciation, though he had difficulty in manipulating numbers as direct symbols. Told to pick out five objects, he did so by counting them in the usual way; but, asked to add five to any written number, he made five dots on the paper and counted them up starting from the given numeral. This he did with all numbers up to ten; above this a number, e.g. eighteen, had no meaning for him unless he had reached it by counting.

This corresponds with another experience, which throws light on the nature of his disability. Suppose he were told that something had happened on Thursday March the 12th, it conveyed nothing to him until he had repeated to himself, "Monday, Tuesday, Wednesday, Thursday," and then, "January, February, March," finally counting up to twelve. Telling him the day or the month did not convey to him at once the part of the week or of the year in which it fell. He could reach the meaning by enumeration of a sequence, but not as an act of immediate apprehension.

This was also evident, when he attempted to tell me how many of one coin corresponded to another of higher value, both laid on the table before him; his tendency was to give the requisite additional number rather than their direct relation. Thus, with a penny and a shilling he said "Eleven," and with the former and a two-shilling piece he actually carried this process so far as to answer, "Twenty-three."

This tendency to reach the value of a numerical symbol by counting greatly reduced his capacity to carry out simple arithmetical exercises. He was aware of the nature of the process involved in addition and subtraction, though his method of action was clumsy. When about to add 8 and 6, he did not take these numbers as entities, but counted up to eight and then on for another six, saying finally, "Fourteen." This was a difficult task and required several attempts before he reached the correct answer; with 3 and 6 on the other hand he easily counted up to nine. By this cumbrous method he frequently failed to arrive at an accurate result, especially if he had to carry over a digit from one column to the next.

He could write the numerals in figures as a consecutive series; but as soon as he attempted to put them on paper in verbal form he made the most curious mistakes. For instance seven, eight, nine and ten became "nenn," "nert," "new," "ten"; yet, as he wrote each numeral, he whispered or said aloud its name with perfect accuracy.

Some of the most instructive observations were made with the *clock tests*. At first he was unable to tell the hour set for him on a clock, although he had a definite appreciation of the time of day and was punctual for his appointments. Even when he failed to name the hour, or did so incorrectly, he was able to explain, "It's when you eat," or, "That's when we went there," and was always right.

Commands given orally or printed in the usual nomenclature were badly executed; but from the first he could set the clock if the order was given in printed figures. For under these conditions he rapidly placed the short hand on the number of the hour named on the card and then swung the long hand round to the position corresponding to the minutes. In the same way, asked to choose a printed card corresponding to the time set on the clock face, he gave perfect answers, when the legend on the card was in numbers, but failed badly if it was in the ordinary nomenclature. Evidently 1.55 conveyed a clear idea to his mind, which was not the case with 5 minutes to 2. At first he was unable to write down the time even in figures; but later, as he became able to tell the time accurately, his power of transposing it into written words returned, although he still had difficulty in setting the hands to oral and printed commands. He regained his capacity to name the time in spoken or written words before he was able to set the clock with certainty and celerity to oral or printed commands expressed in the ordinary nomenclature.

Orientation and relation to one another of objects in space. He had no difficulty in finding his way about the hospital and showed by his actions that he knew the position of his room. When, however, we walked from my house to the hospital he made frequent mistakes, even after he had made the journey on foot several times. He would take the wrong turning and look round puzzled; what he saw did not correspond to what he expected and he retraced his steps slowly. At certain salient points he described correctly some incident he had seen as he passed that morning. After several mistakes he turned into the street which led to the hospital, looked up and said, "That's it." Asked how he knew, he replied, "There you see that...where the Padre is (pointing to the spire of a church); that's near the hospital." He then walked along rapidly, took the right turning to the entrance and ran upstairs to his room without hesitation.

Throughout he found difficulty in comprehending right and left; and yet the following conversation shows that he still possessed a conception of this aspect of space, although he could not use these abstract terms. As we were walking along the street he said, "I've been so long out of the Old Country that I don't know which way cars come. If I were riding in one up the street I should be riding there." He swung round to place himself into the position of a moving vehicle and tapped the left-hand curb with his stick. Then he added, "But that's not there," waving his stick to signify a foreign country.

During my explanation, which preceded the hand, eye and ear tests, he complained that he did not know his right hand from his left. But, on this occasion, he obtained the knowledge he wanted by throwing himself into the correct boxing attitude with the left hand in front; at the same time he said, "I know if I were going to fight I'd go like this." Then he exclaimed, "Now I know, this is the right, this is the one with which I used to do this," making the movements of writing.

From the time when he first came under my care, there was no doubt that he recognised the spacial relation to one another of various pieces of furniture in some familiar room. If I drew a four-sided figure on paper to represent the ground-plan, he could point to the position of the various tables, chairs, cupboards, windows, etc., correctly. As soon, however, as he was asked to produce a ground-plan of the room, he failed entirely; he drew a number of objects in elevation, evidently guided by the images of his visual memory, but could not transpose them onto a plan.

When he was asked to point to an object, corresponding to one he had just seen or held in his hand out of sight, he did so with great rapidity and certainty; during these tests, I noticed that he did not pass his hand along the series on the table in front of him, but pointed straight to the object he wanted. So certain was he of its position, that I repeated the experiment without removing the screen. He still indicated the place of the thing he was seeking in spite of the fact that it was covered from his sight; and yet he was unable to express correctly in words the serial order in which the objects lay, though he could name them correctly. He said, "If you hold it up I see it at once. The fact of thinking too much ...I can't say what I want to say." Evidently when the act was one of those he could perform easily, he not only selected the true duplicate of what he had seen or felt, but knew its position in space. If, however, he was compelled to formulate its relation to the other objects of the series, he was unable to do so.

Games. From the first he was able to play chess well and taught his sister the game. He was extremely clever at draughts, "fox and geese" and all games that did not demand the expression or comprehension of names. Once he had found the solution of a puzzle he never forgot it and could solve the problem time after time.

In conclusion, this patient may be said to have lost the power of recognising verbal significance and of applying names to objects. The structure of words and phrases was not materially affected except in as far as he was deprived of their use and comprehension as specific indicators. This disturbed some acts of speaking, reading and writing, whilst others were left more or less intact. Even imitation of certain movements was defective, provided verbal formulation was a necessary link in the process. He had no difficulty with numbers in sequence, but he could not use them easily as abstract symbols, for instance in relating the value of two coins to one another or in simple arithmetical exercises.

Example V. (Case No. 10.)

Lieutenant R. M. was wounded accidentally by the premature explosion of a hand grenade on March 17th, 1916. There were two small wounds in the left parietal region; at the operation performed next day, the dura mater was found to have been perforated and a few minute fragments of bone were removed from the substance of the brain.

When, a month later, he was admitted to the Empire Hospital under my care, the wound had healed. But throughout a period of seven years, during which this patient was under my observation, his intellectual difficulties remained in principle unchanged. His power of performing the serial tests and his general aptitudes improved materially.

Where originally he made many gross errors, he later carried out the task slowly and with hesitation; but the nature of his disorder was fundamentally the same, though much less severe. I shall therefore give a combined description of this condition under the same headings as I have done in the previous examples. But in this case no such description can convey a complete impression, unless we bear in mind that all the actions of the patient, in as far as they necessitated symbolic formulation, showed weakness of intention and lack of complete comprehension of the significance of commands.

Articulated speech. He had no difficulty in finding words to express his ordinary needs; they were correctly enunciated and all his phrases were perfectly formed and spaced. But in general conversation he paused repeatedly like a man confused, who had lost the thread of what he wanted to say.

He could repeat anything said to him, provided the sentence did not contain several possible alternatives. Any mistake he might make depended on faulty comprehension or memory and not on want of verbal capacity to reproduce what he had heard.

He named a set of geometrical figures and the usual colour series correctly and was able to evoke the names he required for common use. At first he had some difficulty in telling the time; his answers were characterised by a curious inaccuracy rather than by positive misconception.

Understanding of spoken words. From the first he could carry out oral commands expressed in a single word. It was the remote or ultimate meaning of a phrase that puzzled him, rather than the verbal significance of its constituent elements. Thus, he made many errors in setting the hands of a clock, when the order was given by word of mouth; this was still more evident with the more complex hand, eye and ear tests. In spite of greatly improved powers, these defects persisted, mainly in the form of slowness and hesitation.

Reading. The manner in which he executed orders given in print was almost exactly comparable with his response to oral commands. Single words did not puzzle him, but a more difficult task, such as the hand, eye and ear tests, troubled him greatly and was carried out slowly and with hesitation. This occurred even when my movements were reflected in the mirror; for he could not grasp the general conception that this was pure imitation. He tried to argue the matter out with himself silently and consequently became confused.

He showed profound inability to grasp the full significance of what he read silently; he would start briskly to tell the story, but lost the thread and his narration tailed away aimlessly.

He read aloud correctly and with perfect enunciation; this undoubtedly helped him somewhat to carry out printed commands more easily than he would have done otherwise.

Writing. He wrote with extreme rapidity as if in fear of forgetting what he intended to express. Letters were badly formed, words wrongly spelt and his handwriting gave the impression of extreme negligence.

At first he employed a common sign for several dissimilar letters. This gradually passed away; but although he could say spontaneously, repeat correctly and read aloud the alphabet in perfect order, he continued to have difficulty in writing the letters. This was manifest, whether he wrote them spontaneously or to dictation and even when he copied capitals in cursive handwriting. On one occasion he said, "I found some difficulty. I always have difficulty with a k; I always write h; then I know it is different. I can't get started somehow with an r; the same with the t...I wasn't sure until I came to put the stroke and then I found I was right. I had to risk it." The following account, which he wrote spontaneously, is a good example of the manner in which he expressed his ideas in writing. "Shall now try to tell you of a very Difficul tast you set me, that is trying to write the Letters of the alphabet. This test is one which I always felt would be Difficut. he trouble is mostly in beginning the Letters i.e. actual Letters of the alphabet while I can write straight on beginnin a new letter or sentence troubles me. This may not be intellegable to you, but if I may, I shall try to explain my somewhat rambling..." He then ceased and appended his signature, as if he had come to a natural end. He had no difficulty in reading this letter when written; he appreciated where he had gone wrong and corrected some of the mistakes.

Although he could read aloud from print or from pictures all the combinations of the man, cat and dog tests, he had difficulty in writing them down spontaneously or to dictation; he even failed to copy them accurately from the printed cards. In the same way, during the earlier stages, he was unable to write the names of the geometrical shapes; those of the colours were correct, though the words were badly spelt. He could not put down on paper the time shown on a clock; but this passed away as his power of telling the time improved.

Numbers, etc. He could count perfectly, but was unable to carry out simple arithmetical operations. He complained, "I seem to get tangled up in the process." Later on he said, speaking of the six sums he had been set to solve, "I found difficulty in them all. I found the subtraction more difficult than the addition. When there was a carry, it seemed to be more difficult. What I feel about it is, if I were to begin my education, like a boy at school, I shouldn't know where to begin. In those sums you gave me I did the addition almost involuntarily, I think the result of former practice. The subtraction...the simplest one I did in the same more or less involuntary way...but the more difficult I had to think what subtraction really meant." This was the more remarkable as he had been an accountant in civil life, accustomed to handle complex masses of figures.

He could name any coin or piece of paper money correctly, but found considerable difficulty in expressing the relative value of any two of them placed on the table in front of him. At first he made many mistakes; later on, however, his difficulty was manifested mainly in the slowness and hesitation of his answers.

On making a purchase he was unable to calculate the amount of change he should receive. At one time he was accustomed, when buying tobacco, to place a two-shilling piece on the counter and expected to receive two ounces, together with threepence in change; and yet he could not tell me the cost of one ounce of tobacco. Suppose he gave a ten-shilling note in payment, he asked the tobacconist to give him the change in florins; if he received it in shillings he "was lost." When he wanted to buy a box of matches in addition, he waited until the first transaction was over and then took a penny from his pocket to pay for the matches.

Significance of pictures. Shown a picture and asked to describe what he saw, he went over it in detail, usually beginning at one side and working across to the other; but as a rule he failed to appreciate its complete significance.

In consequence of this difficulty in recognising the full meaning of pictures, most jokes in graphic form were incomprehensible. Suppose, however, that the humour consisted solely in the details of the drawing, it might be appreciated; but any demand for coordination between its various parts or with the text beneath it, met with little response. On the other hand he was sometimes surprisingly quick in seeing the point of a picture, if it depended on details, especially when each one bore its explanatory label.

Drawing. At first he could not draw at all, either from the model or to oral command. Five years after the injury he was able to make a feeble drawing of a simple glass jug, placed before him as a model. Ten minutes later, on attempting to draw it from memory, he reproduced his first drawing exactly and was evidently repeating from memory his previous motor acts. Asked to draw an elephant, the result bore no relation to any known animal and ultimately he became completely confused. He then said, "I'll draw you a bee-skep" and produced a rude but accurate representation of the sort of hive he was using for his bees, together with the stand and the metal cover to keep off the rain.

Visual images. There can be little doubt that in normal life he possessed strong visual imagery. But since his injury he has had difficulty in evoking these images to command and holding them for voluntary use.

A few days after I had tested his power of drawing, he volunteered the following remarks: "I thought of what you asked me to do, drawing the glass...I was trying to see the glass bottle; the picture seemed to evade me. I knew it was a bottle, and I could describe the shape of it, and I remember making a drawing of it, and I could describe the drawing. But, when it came to seeing it as a picture, I was more or less nonplussed. I often seem to have got the picture, but it seemed to evade me."

On the other hand he could evoke at will a visual image of his wife's photograph and could see a bee alighting at the mouth of the hive, laden with yellow pollen. But in both cases the pictures were recalled spontaneously and not to command. "The more I try to make them come," he said, "the more difficult it is to get in touch with them, as one might say."

Orientation and the relation to one another of objects in space. With his eyes closed he had no difficulty in pointing to the position of the various objects in the room where we were working. When he was asked to say how some one of them stood in relation to another, e.g. the fireplace to the door, he entirely failed to do so; allowed, however, to say, "The fire is there and the door is there," he pointed to their position with complete accuracy. He knew exactly where they were and was certain that he could see them "in his mind"; but he could not express their relative position to one another.

Asked to draw a plan of some familiar room, he habitually failed; he could not translate what he saw into this diagrammatic form.

But, when the examination was carried out in the following manner, he was able to execute this task, impossible under other conditions. I took him into another room, closed his eyes and told him to point, as I named them, to the various objects in the one we had just left; this he did perfectly. His eyes were then opened and I put before him an outline plan on which he indicated with his finger the position of the various pieces of furniture. Then I asked him to draw a plan of the familiar room; this he was now able to do, at any rate as far as its main features were concerned. After he had been made to indicate on a blank plan the position of the various objects, he was able to retain it in his memory and to reproduce it on paper without difficulty.

He was completely unable to find his way alone. He never took his bearings and, if he was going to a place for a second time, did not recognise landmarks, or appreciate that he was passing over the same ground again.

He was puzzled which way to turn and, if he took the opposite side of the road, became confused not knowing in which direction to walk. Given the number of a turning to the right or left he could never find it correctly; but told to take the "next on this side" he was able to do so. Left and right puzzled him greatly; he tried to work them out by thinking which was the left half of his body and frequently brought out an incorrect answer.

Appreciation of the ultimate meaning of things perceived. His lack of power to grasp the full meaning of a question, order, or series of formulated perceptions led to perpetual confusion in his daily dealings with others. For instance on a sunny spring morning, before we began work, I said, "I hope you don't feel it cold; shall I put the window up?" He answered, "Yes"; but, as soon as I began to raise it, he called out, "No, no." Then he explained, "When you said, 'have the window up,' I thought you meant open...more air. You want to put the window like that (waving his hand upwards) and I thought no, no, more air, that's what I want."

Starting from errors of this kind, he was perpetually liable to arrive at mistaken conclusions. Seeing a young lady on a station platform, who was an old acquaintance, he denied that she was married, in spite of his brother's statement to the contrary; this was based on the absence of a wedding ring from what he supposed to be her left hand, but was in reality her right.

He was incapable of grasping the full consequences of "summertime." He knew it had something to do with the Daylight Saving Act and was able to explain that it was intended to give more daylight during working hours; but could not formulate with certainty what happened to the clocks when it came into force, or when we returned in the autumn to normal time.

His difficulty in appreciating ultimate meaning came out clearly, when he was given a chosen passage and was asked to reproduce what he understood in speech and in writing. He remembered all the salient details, but was puzzled by the suggestion at the end that the wedding cake was emblematic of the state of marriage. After he had read it several times to himself and aloud, and had written it spontaneously and to dictation, he still remained in a state of confusion. But, when I asked, "What is an emblem?" he answered at once, "Oh! an emblem is a... well...the Cenotaph might be taken as an emblem of sacrifice and adhesion to a great principle." The word "emblem" was not only correctly understood, but its meaning was illustrated by an apposite example. When, however, a series of detailed characters appertaining to a wedding cake were said to be "emblematic" of the marriage state, he was unable to complete the mental synthesis necessary for complete comprehension.

Appreciation of the general intention or aim of an action to be performed. This lack of complete recognition of the goal at which he was aiming made most games impossible. After I had beaten him easily at a simplified form of draughts, he complained, "The chief bother was trying to follow the consequence of the next move. I couldn't foresee what would happen."

He was never skilled at billiards, but since his injury could not play at all. "A straight shot," he said, "with two balls is not so bad, but the third ball confuses me. I seem to think of the three functions at the same time and get muddled." I therefore tried the following experiment. A basket was placed at the end of the room and he threw into it balls of paper even more accurately than I could; but, when I placed a screen in front of it, his shots became extremely bad and he said, "When I could see the basket I could follow the line of vision; when it was covered I didn't feel so confident it was in the same place...I'd seen the basket before you put the screen there; I knew you hadn't changed the position, but in some odd way I didn't feel perfectly confident in my own mind that it was in that position."

This disability greatly hindered the due performance of his daily work. When making frames for his bee-hives, he could thread the wire from side to side consecutively, but was unable to pass it from corner to corner; for this necessitated a fresh starting-point. He made the four portions of a bee-hive under the guidance of the instructor, but was unable to fit them together.

I placed before him all the breakfast utensils requisite for one person and asked him to set the table. He quickly placed the cup, the saucer and the plate correctly. Then he became confused, laid the knife across the plate and removed it, set the spoon to the right of the plate and took it away again; finally after much hesitation he placed the fork to the left, the knife to the right and the spoon above the plate. He explained his difficulty as follows: "There was something missing, something unusual. I got the knife and the fork, I couldn't find...let us say the bacon and eggs. Then the spoon puzzled me; I wasn't quite sure why it was there. If I was laying my own breakfast-table I should know because I always take porridge. If I saw the spoon I should look for the bowl for the milk and so on; but there seemed nothing like that, so I thought the best way out of the difficulty was to place the spoon in a position in which it might be convenient for any purpose."

In this example of the disordered use of language the patient could evoke both words and names for voluntary use. He appreciated their meaning and that of the isolated details of a picture. Syntax and grammatical construction were not primarily affected. But he could not comprehend and reproduce correctly the total or ultimate meaning of what he heard or read, and failed to appreciate the full intention of an act he was about to perform, either to command or on his own initiative.

CHAPTER III

THE NATURE OF THE DISTURBANCES OF FUNCTION IN APHASIA AND KINDRED DISORDERS OF SPEECH

§1. THEY CANNOT BE CLASSIFIED AS AFFECTIONS OF SPEAKING, READING OR WRITING

HAD it not been for the trend of scientific thought at the time when the facts of aphasia were discovered, no one would have imagined that a lesion of the brain could affect exclusively such complex modes of behaviour as speaking, reading and writing. But it was assumed that man had been endowed at his creation with certain "faculties," situated in different parts of his brain and these it was thought were disturbed by the cerebral injury.

This theory seemed to receive support from the fragmentary and insufficient examination of the earlier observers. The patient was said to be able to read or write, although he could not speak. Sometimes, on the other hand, he could speak but could not write. As observations accumulated and the first novelty of the discovery wore off, it became obvious that pure instances of "aphasia," "alexia" or "agraphia" must be extremely rare, and most patients were said to show a "mixed affection" of speech.

From 1866 onwards Jackson opposed such conceptions, and laid stress on the importance of recognising that there was no "faculty of language." In the same way he denied the existence of a "faculty of memory" apart from things remembered. But although the doctrine of human faculties may have passed out of fashion, the ideas upon which it was based are still enshrined in the terms "aphasia," "alexia" and "agraphia." Many still hold that it is of value to record solely that a man has been deprived of power to speak, to read or to write, without specifying exactly the conditions under which these acts are disturbed.

"Speechless" patients are not of necessity "wordless"; for they can swear or even ejaculate appropriate exclamations. A man usually speechless may at times produce a complete phrase. Thus No. 21 could reply "yes" and "no" correctly, but could not repeat these words at will; asked to say "yes," he answered "No, I can't" and, told to repeat "no," he usually shook his head, but once replied, "No, I don't know how to do it." He could at times use the expression "Thank you" appropriately

and when puzzled would say, "Can't get it; I know what it is, I try."
Once, when excited by the request to draw an elephant, he said "Yes,
I've been all over; seen lots! I've got some on my what you call it,"
alluding to figures on his sideboard at home. Words were not at his
disposal for voluntary use, but they existed for comprehension and could
be called up under emotional stress. Voluntary power was diminished
with retention of the capacity to evoke the same action in a more automatic manner.

Even if the power of forming words is still preserved the patient may
be unable to use them to denominate objects or to express his meaning.
Thus No. 2 was unable to name colours and might have been thought
to be colour-blind; and yet he could indicate perfectly the difference
between them in words, if he was allowed to use metaphorical expressions, such as, "What they do for the dead," or even "dead," instead
of "black."

We are face to face with exactly the same difficulties when we attempt
to record the power of appreciating spoken words. What, for example, is
the condition of a man who cannot draw a "square," when asked to do
so, but, told to draw a "block of wood" at once draws a perfect square?

Moreover, in attempting to discover if the patient can read, we not
uncommonly find that he can choose a familiar object without fail if
the name is presented to him in print, although he is unable to carry out
a simple command to touch some part of his body with one or other
hand. He can no longer execute the printed order because of its greater
complexity.

The majority of those who are said to be suffering from "agraphia"
can write their names and are able occasionally to add the address. One
patient under my care wrote his name followed by the full address of
his home; yet he failed to write that of his mother with whom he lived.
The written words could be evoked, when they applied to himself and
were more nearly automatic, but not in connection with another person.

Jackson pointed out the close association between speaking and writing,
insisting on their coincident variation. He thought of internal speech
as words that had not passed over the vocal organs, and he used writing
as a means of testing its condition. Now internal speech in this sense
plays an essential part in many other acts besides speaking and writing.
When a patient sitting opposite me, attempts to imitate movements of
my right or left hand brought into contact with eye or ear, some degree
of internal verbalisation occurs as a phase of the normal act. No sound
need be uttered; but the words "right" and "left," "eye" and "ear,"

or some more inclusive expression such as "opposite" or "the same," are essential to correct imitation of this kind. But similar movements made by the examiner and reflected in a mirror can be copied with ease, because this is in most cases an act of matching, no symbol intervening between the command and its execution.

For the same reason patients may experience considerable difficulty in carrying out these tests, when the order is placed before them in the form of a picture; although if it is reflected in a mirror, the movements are imitated correctly, no internal verbalisation now being necessary.

Obviously therefore we have no right to be satisfied with the statement that the patient is unable to speak, read or write. It is our business to discover the conditions under which he can or cannot perform these acts. As soon as we examine the clinical phenomenon from this point of view, we find that no one of them is affected alone by any unilateral lesion of the cerebrum; a disturbance of one aspect of speech is invariably associated with some other disorder in the use of language or allied functions.

§ 2. THE "MOTOR" ASPECT OF THESE DISORDERS OF LANGUAGE IS NOT DUE TO A PURE "ANARTHRIA"

In 1906, Pierre Marie broke away from the orthodox views of aphasia and propounded the theory, that the "motor" aspect of disorders of speech was due to "anarthria," a high-grade disturbance of articulation. On the other hand he held that the "aphasic" aspect was nothing more than a manifestation of diminished general intelligence. "Il n'y a rien d'aphasique," he says, " dans le trouble *moteur* de l'anarthrique. L'anarthrique comprend, lit, écrit. Sa pensée est intacte, et l'expression en est possible par tout autre moyen que la parole, le langage intérieur n'étant pas altéré."

He laid down that the aphasia of Broca was not a clinical entity but a "syndrome," composed of two distinct troubles, "anarthria" and "aphasia," of which the former consisted solely in want of mastery over verbal articulation. On the other hand, the latter was the sensory aphasia of Wernicke, characterised by troubles of internal language, which showed themselves directly in alterations of speech, reading and writing.

This statement had the advantage of clearing the ground of older preconceptions, but unfortunately substituted a theory which does not agree with the results of more extensive clinical observation. Marie contends that the "anarthric" patient, in his sense of the term, or the "motor" aphasic, as it was the custom to call him, understands what is said to him, reads and writes; his powers of thought are intact, he can express himself by every other means except words, and internal speech is unaffected. Now it is true that such patients may be able to read and write; but the statement of Marie and his followers implies that these acts can be executed perfectly, and that emissive speech is alone disturbed as a consequence of the cerebral lesion. Closer observation shows that this is not strictly correct.

Amongst my military patients were three who would have been classified as uncomplicated examples of "motor" aphasia; they could read and write, and exhibited no defect of general intelligence. Further investigation, however, showed that other acts were affected besides those of emissive speech and this was borne out in each case by the statements of the patient himself. Thus No. 17, who talked slowly and was frequently at a loss for a word, said that at first he did not dispose of a more than "twenty word vocabulary." Often when he had to alter the form of a sentence, because he could not find the word he required, he substituted some more picturesque expression, such as "dig it up" for "remember." He had difficulty in recalling the right adjective and described a person as "strong-willed" and "strong-headed," when he wanted to say "head-strong." He was liable to become confused by the sound of verbal symbols; thus, when saying the alphabet aloud, he stumbled over R and explained that he wanted to say A because he was thinking of "are." These are no mere articulatory defects, even in the highest meaning of the term, but demonstrate some interference with the power of verbalisation, internal as well as external.

He could understand what he read aloud or to himself, if he went slowly, and he executed even complex printed commands. But he confessed that he could not read a book with ease or pleasure; for, although he understood each isolated sentence, he was obliged to go back, when he reached the middle of the paragraph, and to start again from the preceding full stop. He had forgotten or missed several of the words.

Asked to read a few lines from a book to himself and to write down shortly what he remembered, he did so slowly and with great effort. Moreover, his errors were exactly of the same order as those evident in vocal speech. He explained that, although he could write, he did so with difficulty; he was forced to spell every word even the little ones. He forgot the order of the letters and wondered, when writing to "Holt and Co." his bankers, whether the l came before the t or vice versa. Prepositions troubled him; he had to say "of" and then was compelled to debate in his mind was it "to" or "from" or "of." Shown a set of geometrical figures he named them correctly, his pronunciation alone being defective. He was then asked to write down their names without speaking and, although he never failed to designate their shape correctly, he wrote "pymared" and "pymerad" instead of pyramid; these mistakes corresponded closely to those he made in pronunciation. It is obvious that, like most normal persons, he said the words to himself silently before writing them down and, since the power of verbal formation was defective, written and spoken words showed faults of the same kind.

Even stronger evidence that "motor" aphasia is something more than an uncomplicated disturbance of emissive speech appears when the alphabet is used as a test. Although a patient has recovered considerable power of speaking, reading and writing, he may still find difficulty in saying or writing the letters in due sequence; and yet he can read them aloud, repeat them and copy them correctly. In such circumstances, he will almost certainly be unable to put together with normal facility the twenty-six block letters to form an alphabet. Something more than external articulation is at fault; that form of internal speech, necessary for writing the letters or for placing them in order, has obviously suffered, and indeed most persons, when asked to think of the alphabet, say the letters to themselves silently.

In the same way, if the patient is asked to execute some complex movement shown on a picture held in his hand, he is liable to make mistakes, or at any rate carries out the order slowly and with hesitation. He is compelled to translate the pictorial commands into words, though no words are uttered. But as soon as the picture is reflected in a mirror the act becomes one of pure imitation; no silent verbalisation is necessary and the movements are executed with ease and rapidity.

Of all my patients with "motor" aphasia No. 19 came nearest to being a case of "anarthria" in Marie's sense of the term. He showed almost complete loss of word-formation with no disturbance of appreciation of verbal meaning. He understood what he heard or read and executed oral or printed commands correctly. Moreover, he recognised names; for he selected without fail a card bearing the appropriate designation of an object or colour shown to him.

In so far articulated speech alone would appear to have suffered. But further examination showed that writing was grossly affected. He could not even write the alphabet spontaneously and failed to arrange the block letters in due order. He could count in spite of his lack of words but was unable to solve simple problems in arithmetic. Internal speech was undoubtedly affected in addition to external verbalisation.

All these facts and many more which will be brought forward in the course of this work show how little the "motor" disorders of speech can be explained as due to an uncomplicated "anarthria."

§3. THESE DISORDERS OF LANGUAGE CANNOT BE CLASSIFIED AS "MOTOR" OR "SENSORY"

General opinion refused to limit the conception of "motor" aphasia to a high-grade disturbance of articulated speech and to gather together all the manifestations of the "sensory" form under defects of general intelligence. Most observers gave a wider interpretation to the term "motor," making it include all executive processes, internal as well as external, associated with the acts of speaking and writing. On the other hand "sensory" aphasia, or amnesia, was divided into "visual" and "auditory."

This view was clearly formulated by Collier[1] in the discussion which followed my Hughlings Jackson lecture in 1920. He spoke as follows: "Whatever conception we may have of the localisation of function in the cortical speech region, we are bound to admit the existence of afferent paths to the speech region upon the auditory side and upon the visual side, and efferent paths therefrom by which speech is usually exteriorised, both spoken and written; and in these paths there is surely strict anatomical and physiological separation." A lesion, situated in such a position that it severed more or less completely one or other of these separable paths, would produce (1) failure of acceptance of speech, on the visual side word-blindness, on the auditory, word-deafness; or (2) failure of exteriorisation of speech, resulting in motor aphasia and agraphia. Purves-Stewart[2], who took up a slightly different standpoint, divided the clinical manifestations into "psycho-motor" and "psycho-sensory," adding that the first was "verbal apraxia," the second "verbal agnosia."

Most recent observers have adopted some general hypothesis of this kind, which is capable of explaining many of the clinical facts and falls in readily with the conceptions current in neurology. For from the periphery to the cortex all acts can be classed as motor or sensory, and, since sight and hearing play so important a part in the use of language, it is natural to suppose that on the afferent side defects of speech can be classed as visual or auditory.

Underlying this argument is the prevalent fallacy that, when a highly complex process breaks up, its component elements are betrayed by the

---

[1] [44], p. 415.   [2] [44], p. 424.

loss of function or negative effect. But we cannot even analyse normal speech strictly in terms of motion or sensation; most acts depend on both these factors for perfect execution. For the use of language is based on integrated functions, standing higher in the neural hierarchy than motion or sensation, and, when it is disturbed, the clinical manifestations appear in terms of these complex psychical processes; they cannot be classed under any physiological categories, motor or sensory, nor even under such headings as visual and auditory.

No. 21 was an example of severe "motor" aphasia in the wider sense of the term. All articulated speech was impossible, except for a few words uttered under the influence of emotion, and even these he was unable to repeat at will. Want of words prevented him from naming any single object or colour, although he was obviously conscious of its correct designation, for he could select without fail a card bearing its name in print. All power of writing spontaneously was abolished; even his name was given imperfectly and he was completely unable to reproduce the letters of the alphabet. He could neither speak nor write and in so far might have been classed as a case of "aphasia of expression."

On the receptive side, he undoubtedly understood what was said to him, choosing common objects or colours correctly to oral commands. In a similar way, on the visual side, he was able to point to an object named in print and, during the man, cat and dog tests, he selected that card which bore the names of the two figures shown to him in the form of pictures. Evidently he was not suffering from auditory or visual "agnosia."

But this simplified version of his condition gives an absolutely false impression of the nature of his disabilities. For, although he could not write a single letter spontaneously, he succeeded fairly well in reproducing the alphabet from dictation; his "agraphia" was certainly not due to a general "verbal apraxia." He understood what was said to him and could make a simple choice in response to words said by me; yet he was unable to place a certain coin into the right bowl, or bring his hand into contact with eye or ear, to oral commands. The increased complexity of verbal formulation had made these acts impossible. In the same way, although he could read the names on a card and make an accurate choice of objects or colours, he was unable to carry out other printed commands.

Further observation showed that he had lost the capacity to perform acts not usually comprised under the use of language, but profoundly dependent on the power of internal verbalisation. He was unable to imitate movements, which were made by me when we sat face to face or were represented on a picture held in his hand; yet these same actions were perfectly executed, when they were reflected in a mirror. These phenomena are entirely inexplicable on any theory of "motor" and "sensory" aphasia, "apraxia" and "agnosia," or similar analytical conceptions; but they fall into place at once if we assume that the main defect consisted in loss of power to evoke verbal symbols at will and to formulate them with a view to action.

None of the conventional theories can explain the clinical manifestations even of so straightforward a case as No. 20. Removal of an extra-cerebral tumour of non-malignant character from a region well in front of the fissure of Rolando was followed by flaccid hemiplegia and so-called "motor" aphasia. At no time was there any disturbance of sensation; vision and hearing remained intact. All forms of articulated speech and writing were grossly affected, but objects could be chosen correctly, when the names were said by me or presented to her in print. But closer observation showed that the "receptive" aspect of her use of language had not in reality escaped; for she had difficulty in setting the hands of a clock and could not carry out the hand, eye and ear tests either to oral or printed commands. Moreover, she was unable to imitate these complex movements if we sat face to face, although she did so perfectly when they were reflected in a mirror.

This is an excellent example of the difference between my point of view and that usually adopted by other observers; for, so far as the physical signs were concerned, this patient suffered from a loss of motor power with complete integrity of sensation. But, from the point of view of speech, the loss of function consisted of inability to employ words for the purposes of any action beyond the simplest choice.

The more completely such cases are examined the less do they conform to the current views of the nature of aphasia and the less easy is it to explain the clinical manifestations. If this is true with "motor" defects of speech, the difficulties become multiplied indefinitely in the so-called "sensory" forms. This is evident in the account of the subject given by von Monakow in his voluminous monograph on cerebral localisation[1]; for whilst his account of "motor" aphasia corresponds fairly closely with the actual results of clinical examination, that given of "sensory" aphasia or amnesia is, as he is compelled to confess, indefinite and confused.

The fourth example I chose in Chapter II, to illustrate the various defects of speech due to a unilateral lesion of the brain (No. 2), would

[1] [107].

probably be classed by most observers as predominantly a "visual amnesia" accompanied by hemianopsia. The posterior situation of the injury would be adduced in support of this view. But, when we attempt to reduce the clinical manifestations to these terms, they become completely incoherent and confused. For the patient could talk, offering long and reasonable explanations of his difficulties, and yet executive speech was affected, judged by the deformation of many of the words he employed. He was unable to name colours, but described them accurately if he was allowed to employ metaphorical expressions, such as "what they do for the dead," or even "the dead," in place of "black." He could not choose common objects to oral commands; with colours he also failed to make a perfect selection, unless I asked him to do so in a metaphorical phrase in place of the proper name. Obviously this was due to defective appreciation of verbal meaning and not to any loss of "auditory" appreciation. His power of understanding what was said to him depended on the way in which the words were presented. Asked if he would like to stop in or go out, he replied in an indeterminate manner; but to the question, "Do you want to stop in?" he answered "No," "Do you want to go out?" "Yes," showing that he had definitely made up his mind and was only puzzled by the two alternatives in one sentence. In the same way he was confused between "right" and "left," "to" and "past" the hour, "up" and "down," "high" and "low."

Exactly similar contradictions occurred, when he attempted to read or carry out printed commands. He could select common objects correctly, but failed to execute the more complex hand, eye and ear tests. He set the hands of a clock if the order was printed in railway time (e.g. 3.40), but not to ordinary nomenclature (20 minutes to 4). He made an excellent drawing from a model and reproduced it later from memory; but he was entirely unable to draw an elephant to command, though he was perfectly familiar with these animals from his service in India. None of these defects can be explained by any form of "visual amnesia" or "agnosia"; they depend on lack of power to appreciate and reproduce nominal and other symbols.

If there were any validity in the views usually held with regard to the nature of "sensory" amnesia, they should be capable of explaining such a case as my third example in Chapter II (No. 15). For the bullet traversed the temporal lobe from before backwards and made its exit just behind the left ear. His speech was that agrammatical jargon, which has so often been associated with lesions in this situation.

This should have destroyed the higher forms of auditory appreciation;

yet he recognised the names of common objects or colours and even carried out slowly but correctly the complex hand, eye and ear tests. Asked to perform these tasks to printed commands, his behaviour was identical; there was not that difference of response between the auditory and visual modes of presentation that might have been expected according to the current doctrine. Moreover, if he read a short paragraph to himself, he reproduced its contents equally badly in speech and in writing, showing that internal speech also suffered from defects of balance and rhythm. This distinctly diminished his capacity to comprehend what was said to him in ordinary conversation; for he could not retain and repeat to himself the exact contents of what he had heard. This was no "auditory agnosia," but inability to manipulate language in a coherent and grammatical form, accompanied by loss of balance in the production of words and phrases.

Many might consider that my fifth example, chosen to illustrate the various forms of aphasia, did not belong to this category at all, but was an instance of "ideational agnosia." Now "tactile," "visual" or "auditory agnosia" are comprehensible terms, for they signify that things touched, seen or heard are no longer fully appreciated intellectually. A patient with "auditory agnosia" hears sounds, but does not know their meaning and thus fails to understand words said to him. Similarly "visual agnosia" is betrayed by want of comprehension of written or printed symbols. But "ideational agnosia" can only signify that ideas are no longer recognised; the use of this term for a state, in which the patient fails to formulate and retain the general conception of what he intends to express in speech or writing, does not explain the condition. Moreover, since this abnormal condition leads to definite defects in the use of language, no account of these disorders of speech would be complete from which it was omitted.

The patient in question, No. 10, would talk fluently, read aloud perfectly and name correctly; but in conversation his sentences tended to die away, as if he had lost the thread of what he wanted to say. He chose common objects and colours to oral and printed commands, but made many errors in setting the clock and was grossly at fault with the hand, eye and ear tests. He wrote with extreme rapidity, as if afraid of forgetting what he was about to put down on paper, and the words were badly spelt. He had lost all power of carrying out simple arithmetical exercises and could not give the relative value of two coins or manage the simple monetary transactions of daily life. Such expressions as "summer-time" puzzled him; he was perfectly aware of the meaning of each word separately, but could not remember or argue out for himself in which direction the hands of the clock were altered. Drawing was impossible and he failed to construct the ground-plan of a familiar room, although he was able to indicate the actual position of each piece of furniture. He became confused, when he tried to lay the table for breakfast, to construct his bee-frames, or to put together the parts of a hive he was making. He threw a ball of paper into a basket placed at a distance better than I could, but he failed completely if a screen was placed so as to hide it from his sight; he had lost the objective of his aim and could not replace it in imagination.

This want of power to retain, or express as a proposition, the general intention or meaning of some form of behaviour, extended from the common acts of daily life to the logical processes of thought. Since these defects interfered with speaking, reading, writing and numerical calculations, they come under the heading of disorders of language; but they are entirely inexplicable on any theory, however extended, of separate loss of the "emissive" and "receptive," "motor" and "sensory" functions, which are supposed to accompany speech.

§4. THE ESSENTIAL NATURE OF THESE DISORDERS OF LANGUAGE

No conception we have so far considered is in harmony with the clinical manifestations of these disorders of language; for any satisfactory hypothesis must be capable of explaining why a patient succeeds in reading or writing under certain conditions, although he fails completely if the task is presented to him in a different manner.

Consider the condition of No. 21, who was almost completely speechless. He could just use "yes" or "no" correctly, but could not repeat them to order; yet under the influence of emotion he was able to produce a phrase of considerable length and use the expression "thank you" appropriately.

When I gave him a command by word of mouth he executed it extremely badly, failing in twelve out of fifteen attempts to place the coin named by me into the right bowl. With the hand, eye and ear tests his errors were just as gross; and yet he had no difficulty in pointing to any one of a set of objects, or in choosing the correct colour named to him orally. It was not comprehension of words that was lacking, but the power to use them in a certain manner.

The most remarkable incongruity was shown when he attempted to read. Given a printed command, such as to touch eye or ear with one

or other hand, he made no effort to carry out even the simplest movement. He shook his head saying, "I can't, I know what it is, I don't
know what it says." In the same way with the coin-bowl tests he was completely unable to execute an order printed in words or in numbers. But
in spite of his inability to carry out these printed commands requiring
some more or less complex choice, there was no doubt that he could read.
On seventeen out of eighteen consecutive occasions he was able to point
to an object named in print. He even carried out the following more
severe test on similar lines. The six printed cards of the man, cat and
dog tests were laid on the table in front of him; he was then shown
pictures of one pair of the series, for instance the man and the dog, and
picked out correctly ten times in succession the card which corresponded
to the combination he had seen. Once he chose a card with the inscription
"the cat and the man," but rejected it for one bearing "the man and the
cat," the order from left to right in which the figures had been presented
to him. Later in the same set of observations he again chose a card with
the right names in the reverse order, but immediately corrected his
mistake. Thus, he was not only accurate with regard to the verbal
significance of print, but also paid attention to the order in which the
words stood upon the card.

His signature was reduced to one word "Beadon" (Beaton) and he
was totally unable to write the alphabet, when asked to do so; but, if
it was dictated, seventeen of the letters were written perfectly and many
of the remainder were recognisable.

Most patients with aphasia imitated my actions extremely badly, when
we sat face to face, or if the order was given in the form of a picture;
when, however, these movements or their pictorial representations were
reflected in a mirror, they were usually performed without fail. For in the
first case the words "right" or "left," "eye" or "ear," or some similar
verbal symbol, must be silently interposed between the reception and
execution of the command; but, when reflected in the glass, the movements are in many instances purely imitative and no verbalisation is
necessary. It is an act of simple matching and such immediate recognition
presents no greater difficulty than the choice from amongst those on the
table of a familiar object laid before his sight or placed in his hand.

Ask him, however, to write down the movements he has seen in the
mirror and he will make as many mistakes as if he attempted to describe
them sitting face to face. The verbal formulation necessary for writing
has introduced the need for symbolic representation and in this way
has destroyed the intuitive nature of the act.

All patients suffering from these disorders of language can choose from amongst a set of common shapes and colours the one which corresponds to that which they have been shown. If a familiar object or geometrical figure be placed in his normal hand out of sight, the patient can indicate without hesitation the similar one from a group in front of him. He can in fact carry out any operation not demanding the use of verbal or other symbols. All forms of immediate recognition are possible; but in these cases of disordered language acts of symbolic formulation and expression are liable to be more or less seriously affected.

Words are the commonest and most obvious symbols used in thinking, and any action is liable to suffer, which demands for its perfect execution any form of verbalisation. A gesture which can be accurately imitated, when reflected in the glass, cannot be performed with certainty if patient and observer are seated face to face; for the attitude necessitates translation of the movement with some verbal formula before it can be carried out.

An act demanding for its correct execution any kind of proposition will certainly suffer, whilst the more closely it corresponds to matching the less will it be affected.

This conception almost exactly corresponds to the views put forward by Hughlings Jackson from 1868 onwards. He stated that the words disturbed in consequence of unilateral lesions of the brain were those employed in the "formation of propositions"; those which remain to the "speechless" patient are the same words used "non-propositionally," or in the lowliest form of proposition. Less severe destruction of speech disturbs the use of words in such a way, that the higher and more abstract the "proposition" the more likely is the patient to fail, not only in the emission of a correct verbal equivalent, but in the recognition within himself of the full value of the "proposition." As Jackson expounded this theory in paper after paper, it assumed a form which includes the greater number of the facts I have observed.

It is with the greatest reluctance, therefore, that I venture to change his nomenclature; for I believe that under the uncouth word "propositionising" is included what I understand by "symbolic formulation and expression." This Jackson contrasted habitually with what he called "lower forms" of speech and thought. But the question as to what constitutes a proposition is so disputable, that it is better to avoid a term which is liable to be misunderstood and to lead to controversy. Moreover, it is doubtful whether the term is strictly accurate, even in Jackson's sense and it certainly does not cover all the abnormalities observed in cases of aphasia and kindred disorders.

I would therefore suggest that the functions affected in such pathological conditions can be grouped under the descriptive phrase "symbolic formulation and expression." But I am anxious that this term should not be thought to define the limits of the disorder. I should have preferred to adopt some entirely neutral appellation and to indicate its meaning by enumerating one after the other the various activities found to be affected on clinical examination.

I have combined under the general heading of "symbolic formulation and expression," the disorders of language produced by a unilateral lesion of the brain, because in the majority of instances the gravest disturbance is shown in the use of such symbols as words and figures. But any form of mental behaviour is liable to suffer which demands perfect reproduction and use of any symbol between its initiation and fulfilment. I do not believe that it is possible to include within one categorical definition all those activities which experience shows to be affected; and yet from a physiological point of view they form a group of defects as definite as those of sensation.

§ 5. SYMBOLIC FORMULATION AND EXPRESSION

Most previous observers assumed that the perfect use of language in its various forms demanded certain activities of mind and body, and that these could be deduced by a priori reasoning on general grounds. These factors were supposed to form categorical groups, which were exposed by the disintegrating effect of disease, and thus, by examining the clinical manifestations, we could discover the synthetic elements out of which speech was composed. Some observers adopted as units the acts of speaking, reading and writing; others divided the phenomena into "motor" and "sensory," "emissive" and "receptive," whilst many were content with the purely descriptive terms of "apraxia" and "agnosia," which have no more explanatory value than the word "aphasia" itself.

Analysis of the facts of clinical observation have led me to fundamentally different conclusions; for, when a complex mode of behaviour, such as the use of language, is disturbed by structural disease, the loss of function is manifested in terms of the process itself and does not reveal the elements out of which it has been built up. Moreover, the various mental activities, interrupted during acts of symbolic formulation and expression, can frequently be exercised in a normal manner during some other form of behaviour. Thus the patient may have profound difficulty in manipulating visual images at will for the purposes of verbal expression, although he can employ them with ease in other modes of thinking. It is not images as such that are disturbed, but images used in a certain manner directed towards a definite end.

By symbolic formulation and expression I understand a mode of behaviour, in which some verbal or other symbol plays a part between the initiation and execution of the act. This comprises many procedures, not usually included under the heading of the use of language, and the functions to be placed within this category must be determined empirically; no definition can be framed to cover all forms of action which may be disturbed at one time or another according to the nature and severity of the case. If clinical experience shows that some particular aspect of behaviour is affected in association with these speech defects, it must be included, although it is not logically implied, in the purely descriptive term "symbolic formulation and expression."

Since, then, it is impossible to define the exact limits of this group of functions, I shall attempt to enumerate shortly the various acts, which may be thrown into disorder, when a unilateral lesion of the brain disturbs the use of language.

It is not the "general intellectual capacity" which is primarily affected, but the mechanism by which certain aspects of mental activity are brought into play. Behaviour suffers in a specific manner; an action can be carried out in one way, but not in another. In so far as these processes are necessary for the perfect exercise of mental aptitudes, "general intelligence" undoubtedly suffers. For a man who, in the course of general conversation, is unable to express his thoughts, or comprehend the full significance of words and phrases, cannot move freely in the general field of ideas. If in addition he cannot manipulate numbers with ease, or find his way from one place to another, he will certainly appear to be more stupid than his fellows. Moreover, it must not be forgotten that the intellectual life of civilised man is so greatly dependent on speaking, reading and writing, that any restriction of these powers throws him back upon himself; he shuns company and cannot occupy himself with the newspaper or social intercourse. This inevitably leads to a diminished field of thought and many aphasics gradually deteriorate in mental capacity. Yet closer observation shows that this "want of intelligence" is based primarily on some distinctive defect in a definite form of behaviour.

The more nearly the task approximates to a simple act of matching, the less does it suffer in those forms of defective speech on which this work is founded. All my patients could choose some familiar object, colour or geometrical figure, which corresponded to the one shown to them.

14-2

For in such tests the sensory pattern aroused by visual stimulation is matched with that produced by some one of the forms or colours on the table. No symbolic formulation intervenes of necessity between perception and the act of choice.

In the same way if one of the geometrical shapes or implements of daily use is placed in the normal hand out of sight, the patient can select its duplicate from amongst those on the table in front of him. Here tactile sensations evoke a perception, which has obvious similarity with the visual impressions produced by some object within his sight.

But any act of mental expression, which demands symbolic formulation, tends to be defective and the higher its propositional value the greater difficulty will it present. Thus a patient may execute a command to hold up his hand, although he is unable to carry out an order to touch with it his eye or his ear. The addition of the second factor has rendered it too difficult; the larger the number of possible alternatives presented by the task, the more certainly will the desired action be defective. By this means it is possible to grade the patient's disability. He is first required to carry out a series of movements such as "lift your hand," "shut your eyes," etc., which name one part of the body only. Then the right or left hand is specified and the task is gradually increased in severity, until at last it is brought up to the multiple alternatives of the full hand, eye and ear tests. Somewhere on this ascending scale of difficulty the aphasic will break down, and this gives a rough indication of the degree to which this particular form of behaviour is affected.

Any modification of the task, which lessens the necessity for symbolic representation, will render its performance easier. Thus, a patient who finds extreme difficulty in imitating gestures accurately, sitting face to face, makes no mistake when they are reflected in a mirror; for this is in most cases an act of direct imitation. But if, instead of reproducing the movements he sees in the mirror, he is asked to write them down on paper, he falls into the grossest errors, because he is now compelled to express them in verbal symbols. Acts which can be imitated with ease cannot be formally expressed.

Many patients cannot find words sufficient for current speech or the accurate designation of objects; yet they can choose correctly both to oral and printed commands. For the verbal formula is presented to them ready made and comprehension of its meaning is an easier process in such cases than the act of evoking it at will. Once the word has been presented to the patient it calls up a response, which corresponds to the name of some object before him; but naming is impossible, because he cannot reproduce the adequate verbal symbol to demand.

The more abstract the symbol the greater difficulty does it present in cases where the use of language is defective. The words "knife," "penny," "match-box," are direct verbal symbols, appropriated exclusively to these objects by long familiar use. The names for colours on the other hand are more abstract; from the materials before us, consisting of paper, cloth or silk of different shape and texture we abstract one quality which we call its colour. Thus many aphasics, who can designate correctly objects of daily use, fail when they attempt to find the names for colours.

On this principle we can explain the behaviour of No. 2, who, though unable to name colours, described them appropriately if he was allowed to employ a simile or metaphorical phrase. For example, when he failed to recall the name for "black," he described it as, "What you do for the dead"; this he shortened to "dead" and could employ the single word to designate the colour because of its metaphorical significance, although he was unable to evoke the more abstract term "black."

It is a well-known fact that many aphasic patients, who are unable to write spontaneously, can copy printed matter in capital letters; in most cases this requires little more thought than imitative drawing. But to copy print in cursive handwriting is an act of transliteration demanding a certain degree of symbolic formulation. It is not surprising, therefore, that this form of behaviour is frequently disturbed, although it suffers less than spontaneous writing.

Sometimes it is possible to grade the extent of the patient's disability by means of these tests. He may be completely unable to write spontaneously, but does so, though imperfectly, to dictation and can copy with comparative ease. For the last demands a relatively slight amount of symbolic formulation and expression, whilst to write spontaneously requires exercise of these powers to a high degree. But in some instances, especially if verbalisation is mainly affected, copying from print may be gravely disturbed; like most normal persons, the patient glances at the words to be copied and then says them over to himself, as can be seen from the soundless movements of his lips. Copying from print becomes in fact a form of self-dictation and suffers from the same defects as if the words were dictated by the observer. In other forms of aphasia, however, copying is the least affected of all forms of writing.

The alphabet forms one of the most valuable means of investigating these defects in the use of language, provided the tests are carried out systematically. It is remarkable how many aphasics are unable to say the letters, or to write them in correct sequence, although they can repeat and write them to dictation. Under such conditions the patient not infrequently fails to construct an alphabet out of the twenty-six block letters; for he is unable to formulate them in due order.

It is comparatively easy to count and to say the days of the week, or the months of the year, in sequence, provided it is possible to form the necessary words; long familiarity has made such tasks almost automatic. But to recognise immediately the significance of any single number, day, or month demands a higher power of symbolic recognition. Thus, a patient who can count correctly and say the days of the week or the months may be unable to comprehend the meaning of a definite date such as "Thursday, March the twelfth." He is obliged to reach an understanding by recapitulating each series up to the word he is seeking to comprehend, just as he adds $6 + 3$ by counting 6, 7, 8, 9.

The clock tests reveal a similar difference in the ease with which an order can be obeyed according to the nomenclature employed. A patient may be able to set the hands correctly at "3.40," but not when he is told to place them at "20 minutes to 4." For in the first instance he moves the short hand to 3, and then swings round the other consecutively up to 40 minutes; in the latter he sets the hour hand at 4 and then stops puzzled, doubtful of the meaning of the words "20 minutes to."

These tests also show the existence of symbolic meanings that are not expressed in words or numbers. The short and long hands of the clock have acquired a significance, which converts each of them into a direct symbol, and they are confused or used wrongly in many forms of aphasia. Moreover, we are in the habit of dividing up the space between any two numbers on the clock face into portions of an hour. Told to set "half-past one," we not only bring the long hand opposite to the figure 6, but we bisect the space between 1 and 2, and place the hour hand in this position. The interval between the two figures marking the hours has in itself a symbolic value. In many cases of aphasia this is affected, and the patient no longer sets the hour hand at a point proportionate to the position of the minute hand; he places the former opposite the figure 1, whilst the latter indicates 6. Or, more confusing still, when told to set "a quarter to six," he may place the short hand at 6 and the long hand opposite 9, so that it is impossible to discover without questioning him whether he intended to set 6.45 or 5.45. Not only the hands of the clock, but their relative position on the face have acquired a symbolic value which is disturbed in many cases of aphasia.

Recognition of the passage of time and of its intervals is not strictly affected. A patient may be unable to tell the hour set for him on the clock, although he has a definite appreciation of the time of day and is punctual for his appointments. Even though he fails to name the hour, he may describe it correctly as "when you eat" or "when we went there."

In the same way sense impressions can be appreciated and recalled, but the aphasic may find difficulty in expressing the relation between them. Thus, when tested with the compass points, he may be unable to answer in speech or writing whether he has been touched by two or one, although he possesses the necessary words to do so; and yet we can prove that his sensibility is not affected. For, if the figures 1 and 2 are written on a sheet of paper, he may by pointing be able to indicate correctly whether the contact was double or single. When this test is carried out in the ordinary manner, he is compelled to formulate his sensory impressions and express their relation in suitable words. But by the second method the processes of thought required are simpler; he has only to match the impression produced by his afferent impulses with one of the two verbal patterns in front of him.

To the functions of the superior cerebral centres we owe predominantly our capacity to appreciate the various qualities and relations of external objects. By the time man developed speech, he already possessed the power of discrimination to a high degree, and definite symbols, such as words and numbers, were invented to register these differences.

When we are shown a coin and are allowed to handle it, we receive certain sensory impressions; these we abstract from it and speak of them as its objective characters. It is hard, brown, cold, round of a certain size and is commonly called a "penny." But, in addition to these sensory attributes, it has other relations such as its position in space with regard to its surroundings. Place a set of familiar objects or colours on the table and ask the patient to point to the duplicate of one he has just seen; he not only chooses correctly, but after a time his finger will move at once towards the position of the object he wishes to indicate, even though the whole set is still screened from his sight. But as soon as he is asked to formulate the order in which they lie on the table, that is their serial relation to one another, he may fail completely.

In the same way a patient with his eyes closed may be able to point to the position of various objects in some familiar room with regard to himself, although he cannot formulate their relation to one another. He can say "The window is there, the fire-place there," but is unable to express the situation of the one with regard to the other. This makes it impossible to draw a ground-plan, which demands somewhat complicated acts of symbolic formulation.

But such an object as a coin has a still further relation to others of the same order, namely its monetary value. If two coins are placed on the table, many aphasics are unable to state how many of the one would be required to correspond with the other; given a sixpence and a two-shilling piece, they fail to reply that four of the one "go into" the other. Yet from a number of pieces of money they can build up a pile on the one hand, which exactly corresponds in value to the two shillings on the other. It is not appreciation of monetary value that is at fault in such cases, but the power to express the relation of one coin to another. In the same way No. 10 remembered that, when buying tobacco he placed two shillings on the counter and received two ounces and three-pence in change; but he was unable to say how much it cost. He could register the facts of the purchase correctly, although he could not relate them to one another and draw the obvious deduction.

Another form of activity, which is more particularly disturbed in a certain group of speech defects, is what may be called the ultimate intention of the symbol. Some patients have no clear or certain conception of the goal of an action they are asked to perform. This is profoundly evident in all that concerns words and figures; but it is not the individual words in their primary sense which are affected. No. 10 understood the meaning of "summer" and "time"; he was well aware that with the advent of "summer-time" the clocks were changed, but he was entirely unable to say whether the hands were put forward or back, and tried in vain to work out the problem. Such patients cannot add or subtract with certainty; they have lost their knowledge of the processes of arithmetic, but not of the direct significance of figures.

This failure to formulate the intention or ultimate goal of a desired action leads to loss of capacity to perform tasks not directly associated with words and figures. Thus, when No. 10 was threading a quadrilateral frame for his bee-hives, he could carry out the operation if the action consisted in bringing the wire across from one side to another, and then back again through neighbouring holes; but, as soon as he attempted to go from corner to corner, he failed entirely. He could carry out a strictly consecutive action, but found difficulty when he was compelled by the discontinuity of the task to formulate his intention. Such patients cannot collect the various objects they require for shaving and may fail to lay the table correctly for breakfast. All such games as billiards and cards become impossible, because of the difficulty in formulating beforehand the aim or goal of some particular act.

I have attempted to describe shortly the various actions which may suffer when "symbolic formulation and expression" are affected. It is impossible to find any single term to include all these disorders of behaviour, which extend on the one hand from mechanical aptitudes to exercises in formal logic on the other. I therefore chose an empirical designation to indicate that the defects produced by the lesion are manifested most often and most profoundly in the use of words, numbers and other analogous symbols.

CHAPTER IV

DIVERSE CLINICAL MANIFESTATIONS ASSUMED BY
THESE DEFECTS OF SYMBOLIC FORMULATION
AND EXPRESSION

IN the previous chapter I have suggested that the various defects of
speech produced by a unilateral lesion of the brain might be classed
together as disorders of symbolic formulation and expression, an
empirical group of functions more or less necessary for the proper use
of language. All these forms of psychical activity are rarely disturbed
uniformly in any one instance and sometimes one set of tests, sometimes
another, yields the more abnormal results. This leads clinically to the
appearance of diverse "types" of aphasia, each of which represents
some particular form of functional derangement.

Disorders of language of this kind cannot be classified as isolated
affections of speaking, reading and writing; for these acts are more or
less disturbed whatever the primary nature of the defect. Nor can they
be attributed directly to destruction of auditory and visual images or
to any other analogous processes, which belong to a relatively low order
in the psychical hierarchy. Each clinical variety represents some partial
affection of symbolic formulation and expression; the form it assumes
depends upon the particular modes of behaviour which are disturbed
or remain intact.

Sensation, as I have shown elsewhere, may be affected in an exactly
analogous manner in consequence of destruction of certain parts of the
brain. Injury to the so-called "sensory" cortex disturbs the orderly
course of those physiological processes, which underlie the discriminative
aspects of sensibility. But a local lesion of relatively small extent and
slight severity may disturb some forms whilst others remain intact. Even
if the immediate results of the injury are sufficiently grave to affect all
these discriminative functions, some will certainly be restored before the
others during the progress of recovery and thus lead to various manifestations of disordered sensibility.

Such clinical phenomena do not express the elements out of which
sensation is composed, but reveal the various ways in which this complex
psychical act can be disturbed by organic brain injury. The results are
expressed in sensory terms; one aspect of sensation is affected whilst

another remains unchanged. Closer examination of these disorders, however they may arise, shows that they cannot be classified as isolated or combined affections of touch, pain, heat or cold. They tend on the contrary to fall into the following three groups. Sometimes the spacial aspects of sensation are alone disturbed; at others the sole defect is found in appropriate response to graduated stimuli or, lastly, in the power of appreciating relative differences in size, shape and weight.

But it is important to remember that the form assumed by the clinical manifestations also depends on the severity of the disturbance of function and not only on the specific nature of the sensory loss. Suppose for instance that spacial discrimination is alone affected by an organic lesion of the cortex. The means we employ for investigating this particular aspect of sensibility are threefold; we estimate the recognition of passive movement and posture, the appreciation of two compass points and the power of localising the site of the stimulated spot. All these methods depend for their exact performance on the integrity of spacial discrimination; but they can be graded as tests in three, two and one dimensional space, and are not of the same order of difficulty. The easiest task is to localise the position of the stimulated spot whilst the most difficult consists in recognising the exact direction in which some part of the body has been moved passively; between these two lies appreciation of the compass points. Now a more difficult task is affected sooner and more severely than one which is simpler of execution; the three tests therefore tend to suffer to a different degree, but always in the same order. A cortical lesion, which disturbs spacial discrimination, affects first and to a preponderating degree appreciation of posture and passive movement, whilst the power of localisation is disturbed last and least.

Thus the clinical picture may vary from two fundamentally different causes. Firstly, the loss of function may fall into diverse specific groups and each case will then illustrate a different "type" of sensory affection. Or, in the second place, the same aspect of sensibility may be disturbed in two patients and yet the amount of the loss be so different that many tests, which yield abnormal results in the one, are carried out perfectly in the other.

Aphasia and allied disorders of language follow the same principles. If the disturbance of function is comparatively slight, it may be so partial that certain acts of symbolic formulation and expression can be carried out perfectly, whilst others are gravely affected. A severe lesion in appropriate parts of the brain may destroy all orderly speech to such an extent that the patient retains the use of a few words only and cannot read or write consecutively; but, if the structural changes do not progress, some power will certainly return and the various tests will not be uniformly affected.

In each case we must determine which acts have suffered and to what extent they are affected; by comparing the results obtained in a series of suitably selected patients we can then determine the empirical groups of aphasia and kindred disorders of speech produced by an organic cerebral lesion.

The majority of observers have fallen into the error of supposing that these clinical manifestations could be classed categorically as defects of speaking, reading and writing. On the contrary all the acts suffer more or less according to the severity of the loss of function; for the degree to which they are affected depends more on the gravity of the disturbance than on its specific character. Two persons may possess very different powers of speaking, reading and writing, although their defects of language belong to the same category. In a similar way an individual patient may regain the capacity to carry out one or more of these acts and yet remain a typical example of the same form of aphasia. Time may profoundly change the extent of the loss of function, as indicated by a series of language tests, without changing the essential nature of the defects. Lastly, we must remember that a more difficult task is affected earlier and more severely than one of a lower order, although both depend for their performance on the same aspect of symbolic formulation and expression.

Provided we bear these principles in mind we are justified in recognising the existence of certain classes of aphasia. For the clinical manifestations are so obviously different according as the loss falls mainly on one or other group of the functions necessary for language in its widest sense, that some formal differentiation or grouping of the phenomena is necessary.

This I shall now attempt to carry out. The various defects discovered by clinical observation can be arranged under four headings, to each of which I have given a name indicating the verbal or grammatical errors by which it is characterised. These designations are empirical; they have no value as definitions and must not be employed to limit the extent of that loss of function to which they are assigned. Each group includes disorders of wider extent than those comprised under the name by which it is known.

§1. VERBAL DEFECTS

Any disturbance of this aspect of symbolic thinking and expression is revealed primarily by defective word-formation. The patient is unable to find the words he requires for ordinary conversation; in the severest cases he may be reduced to "yes" and "no," together with a few expressions, which he employs automatically or solely under the influence of emotion. So grave a disorder of articulated speech is always accompanied by some loss of power in writing and want of verbal memory for the content of sentences read silently.

One of the advantages derived from observations on patients with gun-shot wounds of the head is the tendency they show to recover. However severe may have been the original affection of language, it disappears, to a greater or less extent, provided the wound heals satisfactorily. During this process some functions are restored before the others; but all the various aspects of symbolic formulation and expression rarely return completely to their normal fluency and perfection. By noting the tests which are most severely disturbed and those which to the end yield an abnormal response, we can grade in order of severity the various aptitudes which are affected, when verbalisation is at fault, and so obtain an insight into the essential nature of this disorder of symbolic formulation and expression.

Of the six traumatic cases which fell into this group, four patients came under my observation in the severe stage with gross loss of speech, reading and writing. Two showed the characteristic defects in a much slighter form and had already regained a considerable vocabulary; it is these which throw most light on the essential nature of this affection of symbolic formulation and expression. For I was not only able to carry out an elaborate series of observations, but could obtain from these patients themselves some account of the difficulties they experienced in performing the tasks that were set them. Fortunately both No. 4 and No. 17 were highly intelligent officers, who were able to give introspective information of the greatest value.

However fluent they may ultimately become, these patients always find difficulty in pronunciation. Words of more than one syllable tend to be slurred and shortened. No. 4 complained that he had difficulty with "tenical terms" (technical terms). "Yesterday," he said, "I had diff-ulty in remembering what you do with a skull...tri...tre...trephine." "I'm confine (confined) to the words I've got back." No. 6 spoke of "the claration of war by the Ollies" (declaration of war by the Allies). Moreover, especially in rapid conversation, words were dropped out in the struggle to convey the desired meaning; but there was none of that omission of the syntactical parts of speech which in other forms of aphasia leads to a "telegraphic style" of utterance.

Even after they had regained a considerable vocabulary, these patients tended to lapse into errors due to defective word-formation. Utterance was slow, in short groups of words or syllables each of which was separated by a pause, and speech had a staccato rhythm. All the normal component elements were present; syntax was not fundamentally affected, but the patient was frequently compelled by want of a word to go back and reconstruct the sentence on a different plan.

But it must not be supposed that the loss of function in such cases was purely articulatory. Any process of thought, which demanded fluent verbalisation, was affected, even though the patient remained silent and made no obvious movement of his articulatory apparatus. Silent word-formation was profoundly disturbed and showed the same sort of defects as external speech.

No. 17 complained, "At first I don't think I had more than a twenty word vocabulary." "I want to say a word, but it is at the back of my mind, I can't dig it up. I sometimes have to alter a whole sentence because I have difficulty in finding the word." He frequently substituted a more metaphorical expression for the usual and more direct word, as for example "dig it up" for "remember."

Some noun or adjective which forms a significant factor in the narrative may be forgotten unexpectedly, even though it has just been uttered by the observer or read by the patient silently. No. 17 said, "A few days ago I said a person was 'strong-willed' and 'strong-headed' and I knew it was not what I wanted to say; and about half a day afterwards I said 'you wanted to say headstrong.'" He gave a remarkably accurate rendering of a passage he had read to himself, but failed at the end to find the word "contrivances"; "but I never found we were much in pocket by her...her...thrift...or her...I want another word, but I can't get it." Six months later he recalled that the word he was seeking was "economy."

A characteristic feature in severe cases is an inability to repeat words, which can be uttered under the influence of some appropriate occasion or emotion. Patients who can say "yes" or "no" in answer to a question, may be unable to repeat these words to command. Occasionally they utter sounds, which give some indication of the word they are struggling to reproduce; but more commonly they shake the head silently or express their inability by some such phrase as "Don't know."

As recovery proceeds, the power of repetition rapidly returns. In the less severe stages of the disorder, words are articulated better when repeated than when spontaneously enunciated, although their formation shows the same kind of faults. These patients suffer from a defective power of verbalisation; they cannot produce with certainty the word they require, either for external or internal speech. They usually appreciate the significance of words presented to them and can therefore execute both oral and printed commands; but they are liable to become confused in general conversation or if an order is given too rapidly. No. 4 said, "Some words, when I listen to them, I can't collect (recollect) the meaning. Nurse said something about your coming this morning; but she said it too quickly, I couldn't collect it; she had to say it again." But one of the earliest functions to return is the power of carrying out oral commands; for with all such tests the words are given by the observer and the patient is required to exercise his power of internal word-formation to a slight degree only.

All these patients could name objects correctly provided they possessed sufficient mastery of articulated speech. The sounds emitted might be extremely defective, but they bore some obvious relation to the usual nomenclature. Even when the patient did not possess sufficient articulatory power for this purpose, he could pick out correctly the card which bore the name of an object or colour he had seen[1].

Lack of free and fluent internal verbalisation is liable to interfere with the power of silent reading. No. 17 said, "I can't read a book to myself because I'm bothered when I say the words. I can get the meaning of a sentence, if it is an isolated sentence, but I can't get all the words. I can get the middle of a paragraph. I have to go back and start from the preceding full-stop again." This does not materially interfere with the execution of printed commands, provided they are conveyed in one word; but if they demand choice between several alternatives, the patient may fail because he cannot retain in his mind exactly the terms of the order. This is liable to occur in the severer cases with the hand, eye and ear tests, although the patient is greatly helped to make a correct choice by the existence of the words on the paper before him; when in doubt, he can look back to them for guidance as often as is necessary.

Reading aloud usually conveys the meaning better than if the patient reads to himself; for the sound of the words, though badly pronounced, reinforces his understanding of the significance of the paragraph as a whole.

[1] No. 19, Vol. II, p. 285.

Writing shows defects analogous to those of articulated speech; but they tend to be overlooked, especially in the slighter forms of aphasia, because they consist mainly of faults in spelling and word-formation. When No. 17 was asked to read a short printed passage silently and to write what he had learnt from it, he wrote slowly and with great effort. He then said in explanation, "I always have to spell out every word, even the little ones. I have to say 'of'; I know it is a preposition, but then I have to think, is it 'to,' 'from' or 'of'? Prepositions are always a bother to me." "It's not the long words that stop me. When I am puzzled over a word like 'help,' I have difficulty in knowing whether the l, or the p, comes last. My bankers are Holt and Co.; at first I had difficulty in knowing whether the l, or the t, came last. Now I've written to them so often I've learnt it." "My spelling of Latin derivatives is better than that of other words."

"I can't spell. I think I can write if I have tried on the blotting paper. I have difficulty in writing the words, because I speak the thing out when I write it." As a matter of fact he did not utter the words aloud; but he evidently referred to that distinct internal verbalisation, which so commonly accompanies writing in normal persons. "When I write a letter hurriedly," he continued, "I hurry on and leave out lots of 'to's' and 'at's' and words. The easiest way for me to correct is to get somebody to read aloud and I say, Wait a minute, I want to put in an 'of' or a 'to.'" "I'm teachable. If I spell a word wrong, my wife tells me; I get it right. When I wrote to my bank man-ger (manager) I always spelt 'man' and 'ger.' She told me that; now I get it right." Here his pronunciation of manager coincided exactly with the way in which he had been in the habit of writing the word. "It's no use my trying to spell out the words, when I'm blocked with a word. But if I can visualise it, I'm all right; visualise the word as it is written."

The form assumed by written words corresponds in a remarkable way with the errors of external verbalisation. In the speechless stage these patients write with extreme difficulty and may be reduced to their signature only. No. 19 could write his name and the address of his previous home in the country; but he failed to complete that of the house in which his wife had lived for a year, although it was the place to which he returned every time he left the hospital on leave. As these patients improve in speech, the power of writing increases, but to the last it tends to show defects analogous to those still evident in pronunciation.

Asked to write the names of common objects or of colours, without saying them aloud or under his breath, the patient produces words which are recognisable and correspond to the proper nomenclature. Even though he may be unable to complete them, as is usually the case in the severer forms of this disorder, he can not uncommonly write one or more letters, which sufficiently indicate that he is familiar with the name of the object. With slighter degrees of verbal defect, spelling or the written structure of the word may be alone affected and writing reproduces exactly the faults of pronunciation. Thus, in the case of No. 17, pyramid became "pymerad," scissors "sissiors" and ovoid "oboid" throughout a series of observations.

Writing to dictation is slow and words may be omitted. No. 4 said, "I can't carry many words at a time. If you give me a phrase containing four words, I can do three and then have to get you to dictate further, or read it again." An extremely easy task, such as writing down the various combinations of the man, cat and dog tests to dictation, presents no serious difficulty in the slighter cases; one word is not substituted for another, nor is the order reversed, common faults in other forms of aphasia.

On reading over what he has written to dictation, the patient notices many of the errors and omissions and attempts to correct them more or less successfully.

If he is able to write at all, he can translate simple pictures into written words correctly. The actual names of any two pictures of the man, cat and dog tests may be indicated accurately and in proper order, although the rest of the phrase is omitted and the formation of the words defective.

The power of copying printed matter in cursive handwriting is not lost except in the severest cases. It is restored early in the course of recovery and is always carried out more easily than spontaneous writing. But although the final transcript may be accurate, the patient usually writes slowly, frequently referring to the print in front of him, as though he found difficulty in retaining the words he is copying.

The most striking evidence of a disturbance of internal speech is given by the hand, eye and ear tests. Most of these patients found considerable difficulty in imitating my movements correctly, when we were face to face. At first sight it might seem as if this had nothing whatever to do with speech. But analysis of our own experience under similar conditions, shows that such imitative movements depend for their perfect performance on internal verbalisation. Although we may not enunciate to ourselves "eye" or "ear" we undoubtedly tend to say "right" and "left" or some equivalent verbal formula; this is fully borne out by the patient's own statements.

When, however, he is told to imitate my actions reflected in a mirror, he is able to carry out the test perfectly without hesitation. For under such conditions the movements can be performed without the necessity for any form of verbalisation; they are the result of direct imitation or matching, and no verbal symbol intervenes between the reception of the command in gesture and its execution.

If the patient is then asked to write down my actions seen in the glass, he again falls into error. Writing necessitates the interpolation of words into what would have been a non-verbal intuitive act; this spoils the response to a test, that could otherwise have been carried out perfectly. No. 4 explained his slowness and occasional mistakes as follows: "I say to myself 'left hand'; then I have to say to myself 'left ear or eye.' When I've said it, when I've decided, I can write it quite easily."

An exactly similar result is obtained when the order is given pictorially. A set of cards are prepared, each bearing a representation of the essential factors in one of the test-movements; these are handed to the patient one by one and he is asked to obey them without speaking. If he holds the card in his hand, looking on it as he would at a picture, the records contain many mistakes, just as with face to face imitation. No. 17 said, "It's like translating a foreign language, that I know but not very well. It's like translating from French into English."

But when the figure on the card is reflected in the mirror, imitative movements are carried out perfectly and without hesitation. For no verbal activity intervenes between the visual reception of the order and its performance.

The truth of this general explanation is supported by the remarks of those patients who were able to carry out the hand, eye and ear tests with unusual accuracy. Alluding to imitation of my movements, when face to face, and to the execution of pictorial commands, No. 17 said, "It doesn't make much difference to me except the first time or two. I think, if you use that hand (pointing to my left), I shall have to use this (holding up his left) and then I am ready. As soon as I have learnt my lesson, I can go easily; I never say it to myself; I know. I have rehearsed it whilst you are getting ready and I don't say it. Before I commence I say 'if he does it with that hand (my right), it is this hand' (his right). I've done a lot of signalling." The records he gave were unusually good to both forms of the test.

No. 19, a severe but stable example of this form of aphasia, gave at first a set of answers on face to face imitation, which were slow and contained several faults. Similar defects were present in his response to pictorial commands. But after practice in the hospital, he learnt to do these tests without mistakes. This he explained as follows: he thrust one hand forwards and drew the other backwards at the same time; then he made similar movements in the opposite direction to indicate that his actions and mine should be conversely related. As soon as he had firmly acquired this idea, his responses became excellent, although they never attained the rapidity of the same movements imitated from reflections in the mirror. Any formula or concept, which reduces the amount of internal verbalisation, materially improves the accuracy of the response.

The alphabet forms an extremely instructive test in the more severe forms of this disorder of language. No. 19, asked to say the letters in order, made a few meaningless sounds and gave up the attempt. He read them aloud so badly that the majority were unrecognisable. Told to repeat each letter after me, A B C were reproduced correctly together with E F I O U V and Y; the others were very badly pronounced, although it was usually possible to trace some resemblance to their proper sound. When he attempted to write the alphabet spontaneously, he succeeded up to F, but in spite of repeated attempts could not carry the series further. To dictation, however, he wrote them without material mistakes. He was given the separate letters of the alphabet on cardboard and asked to arrange them in order; but, after reaching G successfully, he gave up altogether. I then said them aloud to him, one by one, and he tried to select each letter from the heap on the table; he succeeded somewhat better than before, but the alphabet he put together contained many faults.

This striking experiment shows that his disability was more than a defect of articulation, even in its widest sense. For he was not only unable to say or to repeat the alphabet, but he could not arrange the cardboard letters in their proper order.

As capacity to employ the verbal aspect of language increases, the patient regains the power of saying and writing the letters spontaneously and he can then arrange them in due sequence; but, to the last, pronunciation tends to be somewhat defective.

The verbal aspect of numerals is affected in exactly the same manner apart from their significance. Thus, in the early days after the injury, the patient may be unable to count, because he has not those verbal symbols, which are numbers. As recovery proceeds, this is replaced by various troubles with compound numbers and inability to carry a long list of figures in the memory. Thus No. 17 said, "When I first began to look at reference books like the Army List, I couldn't say it was 982, when I looked the page up; but if I didn't try to say it, I could look up the page without difficulty. When I tried to say it, I would say different numbers and then I would muddle myself and have to look it up again. Silent thought was easy, but vocal thought was muddling."

He played an excellent game of bridge, but complained, "When I am scoring in a game, I say 28, when I mean 41. But this makes no difference to my score. I count 41, though I may say 28. I do the sum right but get the figures I say wrong." Addition and subtraction sums were solved correctly and he checked his own bank-book.

No. 4, however, found some difficulty in carrying over a number, when adding or subtracting, although the actual calculations were correctly performed. He had worked in a bank before the war, and was accustomed to add up long columns of figures in his head; this he now found difficult because he could not retain the numbers sufficiently long in his memory. Such loss of power to verbalise numerals with ease may lead to actual faults in simple arithmetic, if the disturbance is severe or the patient has been poorly educated (No. 6).

When the loss of word-formation is extremely grave, counting may be affected in a most instructive way. If the patient can utter the simpler numerals, he uses them to arrive at the desired result by some roundabout method. Thus No. 19 could enunciate all the numbers, except seven, up to ten; then he continued, "one one" (eleven), "one two," etc., ending the decade with "one and nine." He counted on in this way until he came to "six and nine" (sixty-nine), when he exclaimed, "Ah! you've got me." I suggested "seven"; he replied, "I know, that's what I want—sed" and continued to count "sed one" (seventy-one), "sed two," etc. A hundred and two became "one no and two." Now it is obvious that his conception of each numeral and of its place in the series, when counting, must have been intact. But, instead of using the customary nomenclature, he could only employ the method of expression we habitually use when asking for a telephone number. He could not say "a hundred and two" and so substituted the more direct translation of the figures, "one, oh, two" (or "one no and two"). In this case the images which were thus reproduced were almost certainly visual, for he could write the numbers perfectly in the usual manner.

None of these patients failed to name coins correctly, if they could find the requisite words; however badly pronounced, the sound bore some relation to the actual name. They could always indicate the relative value of two coins placed in front of them, even if they were obliged to do it in dumb show on their fingers.

Drawing is not affected and the outline of a simple model can be reproduced from memory. Told to draw an elephant the result is recognisable and exhibits all the salient points of the beast. These patients have no difficulty in drawing a plan of some room with which they are familiar; this is a true ground-plan and does not show that tendency to lapse into details of elevation, so common in other disordered forms of symbolic formulation and expression. They can find their way with ease and certainty, and describe a journey from one place to another without error or confusion, provided they have sufficient words at their disposal.

They can look at pictures with pleasure and understanding, appreciate jokes expressed pictorially or in print, and are capable of playing games at an early stage of recovery. No. 4 found "jigsaw" puzzles very "re-edji-kate-ive" (re-educative).

One of the most striking faculties possessed by this group of patients is the power of recognising their errors. They struggle to correct their defective articulation and utter one sound after another corresponding more or less with the word they are seeking. In the same way they go over what they have written correcting many of the mistakes and omissions. Moreover, they remember, and can correct at some subsequent period, their failure to recall some salient expression, whether in speech or writing. Innumerable examples might be collected of this power of appreciating whether some verbal act has been rightly or wrongly performed. It is one of the most characteristic features among the manifestations of this form of aphasia.

This variety of aphasia consists mainly in a defective power of forming words, whether for external or internal use. Articulated speech is limited to a profound degree and, in the severer stages, the patient may be unable to repeat even the few words at his command. He cannot evoke the verbal symbols he requires, although he understands the meaning of single words and can carry out an oral command, provided it is not too complex. Even if he is unable to designate a single external object, he knows its name; for he can pick out without fail a card on which the correct word is printed. In the same way he can indicate on his fingers numbers which he cannot pronounce. It is the structural formulation and expression of words that is mainly defective; comprehension of their meaning is relatively intact, except in the most severe cases.

§2. SYNTACTICAL DEFECTS

This form of disturbance of language can be distinguished by the fact that the patient talks jargon. In other varieties of aphasia he may not be able to evoke the word he desires to use and, in his efforts to find it, gives vent to sounds that do not correspond to any recognisable language symbols. If he is of a lively temperament he tries again and again to correct his faulty nomenclature and may fly to metaphorical expressions in order to circumvent his want of ability to express his meaning; but this cannot be described as true jargon.

On the other hand with a syntactical disorder of language the patient talks with great rapidity, when once started. Individual words may be recognisable, but the grammatical structure of the phrase is liable to be badly affected. He talks fluently in short jerky sentences, slurring or omitting many of the junction words. Even when they are present, it is difficult to hear the articles, conjunctions and other components necessary to a perfectly formed sentence. Asked what he had done since his admission into the London Hospital, No. 15 said, "To here, only washing, cups and plates. That's about all you've got to do here." "Have you played no games?" I enquired, and he replied, "Played games, yes, played one, daytime, garden."

One day, during a set of observations, No. 14 suddenly exclaimed, "Funny thing, this worse, that sort of thing," and seizing his note-book wrote "as, at." I asked, "You mean conjunctions and prepositions?" and he replied, "Yes, that sort of thing."

Not only are the rhythmic movements of the phrase affected, but the internal balance of its constituent elements is disturbed. The patient cannot "touch off" the words so as to produce an accurately coherent sentence and the articulatory rhythm of polysyllables tends to be disordered.

Moreover, his extreme rapidity of utterance leads to indistinct enunciation even of smaller words. Labials and dentals are slurred and past becomes "pass" or black "back." When a patient of this kind mispronounces a word, he does not as a rule go back and try again; he dashes on in the hope that he will be understood. If checked and asked to repeat what he had said, and especially if told to speak slowly, he usually becomes confused or angry. The more he is pinned down to some word that is incomprehensible to his hearer, the more confused he grows and the worse becomes his speech. Finally he may refuse to speak altogether.

Such difficulties may occur even when he attempts to formulate silently what he intends to say. No. 13 is employed in an Insurance Office; if, as he walks along the passage to his chief's room, he attempts to repeat to himself the message he was bidden to deliver, he cannot make himself understood. But, when he "thinks nothing about it," he can make his meaning plain.

In the slighter forms of this defect words and names may be intelligible, especially if the subject of the conversation is known. Thus when No. 15 was given quinine, as one of the tests for the sense of taste, he said, "Rotten to drink it. Something medicine or that. Make you drop of water after it, so to take out of your mouth." On a later occasion, wanting to explain to me how he came to develop an inguinal hernia he said, "I got that rupture, after left hospital, when dark, no lights, when air-ships came over. Couldn't see, smashed the wall, the house like, smashed into wall, couldn't see. Had a pain, saw doctor, pushed it up. If it should come up, press it up and use what you call 'em. When it do go up, pain inside."

Sometimes speech closely resembles baby language; for example, asked what his right hand felt like, No. 13 said, "Tiff-rent from uffer 'um...kā tell ooh, know zis 'un seems strong," and he complained that a tactile stimulus "tittles." Occasionally his answers would have been incomprehensible without a knowledge of the context; I pointed to a white scar on his scalp and he answered, "Aevus ah a baby" (Naevus as a baby). Thus, he was able to find the name and form the essential part of the word rapidly and with certainty, although it would have conveyed no meaning to anyone unfamiliar with the origin of the scar.

But occasionally this patient became completely unintelligible; describing to me a picture of a tramway car with a woman at the wheel and a male conductor he said, "Here's lay, here handle, the man condukr, on the nines, shot seats on it, zee passengers, two man, lady" (Here is the lady; she's at the handle; the man conductor; on the lines; it's got seats on it; three passengers, two men and a lady). He then read the legend at the top of this picture as "Mins bixet o-er man" (woman's victory over man).

No. 14 was a more severe example of syntactical defects. His voluntary utterances consisted of a flood of jargon, containing occasional good and apposite phrases; but the sounds usually seemed to bear little direct relation to the form of words he wished to employ. He could say "yes" and "no" correctly and answered "come in" to a knock at the door. He was extremely intelligent in the way in which he used the few words at his voluntary disposal to explain a map, a book or a picture. He accompanied his lively and significant gestures by "there, there," "down there," "up there" and other indicative expressions. He used words or short phrases, but could not amplify them or repeat them at will.

The power of naming an object, in sounds that are comprehensible to a listener, varies with the severity of the affection. Thus No. 13 evoked single names perfectly to indicate common objects; but when attempting to name colours he "jargoned" orange, green and violet, although in every instance the sound bore a correct nominal significance. No. 15 was somewhat unstable in his nomenclature, using "blacking," "pencil" and "black lead" indiscriminately for pencil. He found difficulty with the words orange, violet ("volley") and to some extent with green; but the truly monosyllabic colours were named correctly.

With No. 14 the sounds, though emitted volubly, seemed to bear no relation to the customary name of the object; thus, matches became "Sten-min-ness." He then seized a pencil and wrote "match," proving that he knew the name. Shown a penny he shook his head, said "No," but wrote the name correctly; in some instances, however, he could neither say it intelligibly nor write it at all. Here the jargoning had become so severe as to destroy all power of producing names at will.

Comprehension of the meaning of words is always in excess of their use as names or in conversation. These patients can choose common objects or colours without fail to oral commands in the form of a single word, although No. 14, who was the most severely affected, found some difficulty with geometrical shapes. If, however, the order was given as a spoken phrase, it might not be understood correctly; the complex commands of the hand, eye and ear tests were frequently misapprehended and the clock was badly set in two out of the three cases of this disorder.

In daily intercourse these patients suffer from inability to recall with certainty what they have been told. Not only is phrasal utterance defective, but phrasal memory is also transitory. This leads to uncertainty in carrying out commands given in the course of current speech and also, in the severer instances, makes consecutive conversation difficult and imperfect. No. 15, when asked to repeat one by one three simple statements, did so with almost complete accuracy; but he failed to say all three phrases in direct sequence, complaining, "I can't think." His father stated that it was impossible to employ him in the business, because he could not comprehend exactly what he was told to do.

Time after time, in general conversation, No. 14 failed to understand what was said. He was reading an account in French of Napoleon's Russian campaign and wanted to tell me how closely the dates coincided with the retreat of the Russians, which was then taking place (September 1915). He took the book in his hand, pointed to the words "15 Septembre" saying, "Now, just the same, there, yes, over there." I answered, "Yes, that was also a beautiful summer and the snow came early." He replied, "Yes, oh! did it, oh! yes." He showed so much interest in the similarity of the two events, that I asked him when Napoleon first had difficulty with the snow; but he turned the pages of the book aimlessly. I then questioned him as to the date on which Napoleon first reached Moscow (September 14, 1812), the starting-point of our conversation; but he shook his head and could not answer. Spontaneous thought was rapid and correct, though the power of comprehension and symbolic expression in answer to questions was evidently defective.

Reading to themselves was a favourite recreation with these patients and, although they showed remarkable powers of understanding what they read, the meaning was evidently hampered by the disorderly structure of the phrases of internal speech. No. 15 confessed, "Don't always know what they mean going to talk to."

No. 14 followed all the movements at the Front on large scale military maps and enjoyed demonstrating to me the changes reported day by day in the newspapers. But he was quite unable to follow up a conversation suggested by what he had read to himself.

In all cases printed commands were well executed. Common objects and colours were chosen correctly and the clock was accurately set. No. 15 alone, a man of comparatively defective education, failed to carry out the hand, eye and ear tests to orders given in print. It is noticeable how much more easily these patients can carry out printed than oral commands.

But, as soon as an attempt is made to read aloud, all the troubles of articulated speech become evident in a severe form. The simple monosyllabic phrases of the man, cat and dog tests can be pronounced correctly, although they are not infrequently shortened by the omission of one or both of the pronouns. The printed names of common objects or of colours, read aloud, correspond fairly closely to the same words uttered spontaneously; but an ordinary sentence from a newspaper may become completely incomprehensible without a knowledge of the text.

This leads to the curious anomaly that a patient may be able to write a fairly coherent letter, although he cannot reproduce a word of it aloud (No. 14). The clue to this observation is given by cases where the loss of speech was less severe. Thus No. 13 composed an excellent letter; but, when he attempted to read it aloud, the words were so badly articulated and the phrasing so faulty, that the whole became incomprehensible. Had his voluntary speech been as badly affected as that of No. 14, he would not have been able to read it aloud at all.

A printed order, read aloud as complete jargon, may be executed perfectly; No. 14 made all the movements of the hand, eye and ear tests without a mistake, although as he read them aloud they seemed to be incomprehensible nonsense.

But, in the course of general reading, this tendency to jargon greatly hampers comprehension of matter read aloud and the patient tends to invest the words with an incorrect meaning. Thus No. 15 read aloud from the heading of a newspaper, "Mr Lloyd George says red take, take must go," instead of "red tape." Asked what this meant he said, "Mr Lloyd George says...Act beer something." The substitution of "red take" for "red tape" evidently confused him and, on attempting to reproduce the meaning, he substituted legislation about beer, much discussed at the time.

The power of writing suffers on the whole less than external speech, because the defect is essentially one of balance or rhythmic utterance. Thus No. 14 made unintelligible sounds when asked to name a set of common objects on the table before him; but, in eleven out of eighteen serial attempts, he wrote their names correctly. When they were placed in his normal hand out of sight, he gave up all attempts to indicate them orally, although he succeeded in writing their names in fifteen instances. Single words were so much more easily written than spoken, that this patient always carried about paper and a pencil to help him out of his conversational difficulties.

In the course of the man, cat and dog tests, the patient is shown two of these pictures in combination and asked to write down what he has seen in the form of a simple phrase with which he is already familiar from previous observations. As a rule he omits the articles and sometimes the conjunction, shortening the whole to "man, cat," etc.; and yet the actual content is correct. But No. 13 exhibited a curious tendency to reverse the order, reading from right to left, so that, when shown the man and the cat, he wrote "cat, man." This was not fortuitous, for it was a prominent feature, when he said the words aloud, and it is another example of that uncertainty in phrasing so characteristic of this disorder of language.

After the period of neural shock has passed away, it is always possible to obtain some recognisable signature and usually the address can be correctly written. Even No. 14 wrote his name and appended that of one of his estates in the country, shortened so that it resembled a telegraphic address.

Any variation, which renders this habitual act less automatic, is liable to prevent its performance. Thus, No. 15 wrote his name and address perfectly, but could not write that of his mother in whose house he lived; the unfamiliar beginning interrupted what would otherwise have been an almost intuitive action.

Except in the severest stage of such a defect in language, the patient can compose a letter and such spontaneous writing is carried out much better than might have been expected from the character of external speech. Even No. 14 left to himself wrote, "I am going to London seeing a Doctor. In the night the darkness is very funny. The weather is good for the corn and not now spoiled." But he could not read a word he had written and when I asked him what it contained, he answered "I can't, I know, I suppose in time, not now, funny thing why." No. 13, who was much less severely affected, wrote a perfectly coherent and well-spelt letter, but jargoned badly on attempting to read it aloud.

The power to write from dictation shows all grades of disturbance from almost complete loss in No. 14 to a difficulty with consecutive phrases, but not with isolated words or sentences. Thus No. 13 succeeded perfectly in writing the man, cat and dog series to dictation but failed badly with a passage chosen by himself from the newspaper.

All these patients could copy correctly, and transcribed print into cursive handwriting without hesitation.

The nature of this disorder of language can be demonstrated by setting the patient a task which combines tests for speech, reading and writing, together with the comprehension of words and pictures. No. 13 chose a picture from the daily paper showing a box for the receipt of flowers for wounded soldiers, placed on the platform of a railway station. Underneath was the legend, "This box has been placed on the platform at Snaresbrook Station as a receptacle for flowers for the wounded. Many of the passengers contribute nosegays daily from their gardens, and these are forwarded without delay to the Bethnal Green Infirmary." As a Londoner in an East End Hospital this interested him greatly.

Asked to put down on paper what he had gathered from his reading and from the picture, he wrote, "At Sanbrook station they have large box which are collicting flowers for the wounded soldiers, and they are sending to the Belnah Green Hospital." I dictated the printed description with the following result: "This box has been placed on the platform a smatbrook station as sesful for the wounded many of the passengers

contic nonsgay from there garndens and these without delay to the
Belnelth Green imfirary"; but he was able to copy the printed sentences
in perfect handwriting without a fault or omission. Given the paper and
asked to read it aloud, he produced the following jargon: "Zis box had
been place on the plakform at Senbrook Station as a...for flowers for
the wounded...Many ob le pasn-gers contribute nosezays from their
gardens and these are for-boarded without delay to Besnal Green In-
ternary." When his attention was directed to the picture, he pointed
out all the various significant objects without hesitation, giving them
recognisable names. "Box. Flowers for wounded soldiers. On the back,
plakform, Senfbrook. Ladies see, putting flowers into box."

He evidently understood the significance, both of the printed legend
and of the picture, but he could not reproduce his conception in coherent
words or in writing, although he could copy correctly.

The same picture with its printed legend was shown to No. 15 with
strikingly similar results. But when, after reading the printed paragraph
silently, he put down on paper what he had understood, he happened
to write in error that the flowers were "for sail." This misled him throughout all the subsequent tests, so that finally he pointed out in the picture
the two ladies "buying flowers" and said the station-master was "selling
'em."[1]

Except at a very severe stage of this disorder of speech, the patient
can count freely and shows none of that hesitation in finding the correct
word, obvious in some other forms of aphasia. The numerical order is
accurate and the name, given to each number, corresponds recognisably
to its proper designation, although it may be badly pronounced.

Here again we find that variable nomenclature so common a feature
of this group of cases. Thus, No. 13 counted between twenty and thirty
as follows: "Twenty, henty-one, henty-two, henty-free, tenty-four,
penty-fi, twenty-six, twenty-seven, twenty-eight, penty-nine." Thirty
was sometimes pronounced correctly, at others it became "sirty."

The power of carrying out simple addition and subtraction varies
according to the normal capacity of the patient. For instance, Major X
(No. 14), the most severely affected of the three war-cases, found no
difficulty with arithmetical operations, checked his bank-book and could
act correctly on the financial questions put to him by his banker and
steward. He could make out a cheque, if the action was performed
spontaneously; but, when told to fill it in for a certain sum, he was liable

---

[1] For the results of alphabet tests, see No. 13, Vol. II, p. 202 and p. 210.

to insert numbers in the place of words, although the actual amount was correct. On the other hand No. 13, though intelligent in ordinary life, failed to solve any of the subtraction sums; he confessed that he was "No good arithmetic at all; I no good at all that at tool" (school). But No. 15, who was a soldier in the regular army, answered all these simple tests correctly.

All these patients recognised the relative value of any two coins placed on the table and none of them experienced any difficulty with change.

The clock tests proved unusually interesting because, according to the results they yielded, the three patients could be arranged in consonance with the known severity of the disorder. The hands of the clock were set correctly both in imitation and to printed commands. To oral commands, No. 14 made several gross mistakes, No. 15 was doubtful and hesitated, but his errors were less grave, whilst No. 13 carried out the task perfectly. On attempting to tell the time No. 14 failed in every instance; No. 15 made two errors only in substance, but adopted an extraordinary nomenclature; No. 13 was slow, although he named the time correctly. Asked to write down the time shown on a clock set by me, the results were identical and No. 15 showed the same extraordinary nomenclature as when he told the time aloud. At one time he wrote "45 to 9," at another "20 past 11"; he called 8.10 "2 past 8," because the long hand, pointing to ten minutes past the hour, stood opposite the figure 2. This is another example of that instability in the use of language, so common in these cases[1].

Drawing from a model, or from memory of the same object shortly after it had been removed from sight, was not affected; in fact No. 15 produced a remarkably successful picture of a spirit-lamp and said, "I was a good drawder, drawer, at school." But, when he was asked to draw an elephant, which he had seen during his service in India, the outline of the body somewhat resembled this animal, devoid of trunk or tusks. He proceeded to fill in the mouth, saying the word aloud; then he said "Highons," "Irons" (horns) and immediately added horns to the drawing. After we had discussed the parts he had omitted, I pointed to the horns on the head of this figure and asked, "Has an elephant got horns?" He replied, "Yes, silver, what you stick out" (pointing to the corner of his mouth and placing his pencil into the position of a tusk). "What are they made of?" "Kind of a white bone one, what grows in the mouth, on the roof, on the edge of the mouth." Evidently he was

---

[1] Cf. also Major X (No. 14), Vol. II, p. 224.

confused by the jargon words representing horns, and impulsively added them to the figure; but he was finally able to explain his error by gestures and gave a correct interpretation of his intention.

None of these patients had any difficulty in finding their way or in pointing out from memory the position of the principal objects in the ward.

They enjoyed games and both the privates played dominoes well.

No. 14 was musical and played me Chopin, Op. 20, Largo, very slowly, reading the notes and giving the change of key correctly. The right hand was clumsy owing to the cerebral injury; but he succeeded in bringing his fingers on to the right notes of the chord, and if he was wrong immediately corrected his error. Keeping his eyes on the music, he recognised by ear when he had struck a false note, and that it did not correspond with the text of the music. He played to me other pieces of Chopin, correcting the faults due to the clumsiness of his right hand; but the slow pace of the Largo was in his favour, whilst the complexities of the change in key showed how clearly musical notation conveyed to him its intended meaning.

All the members of this group recognised that their utterances were inadequate to express what they wanted to say. Once started, they usually poured out a torrent of speech in the hope that it would be understood. Recognising that their words were incomprehensible, partly from the puzzled looks of the auditor and also from their own perceptions, they blushed, grew confused or angry and did not care to try again to express that particular thought.

Moreover, they no longer possessed the power of reproducing to themselves exactly a series of words or phrases heard, read or formulated from pictures, so necessary for the complete voluntary use of language. Inaccuracies of this kind led to confusion of thought and were frequently followed by some perverted explanation of the original text.

Single words could be evoked with comparative ease and articulated speech tended to consist of short isolated verbal groups. Internal speech was also affected in the same way though to a less degree. This was shown by the fact that these patients could often write what they could not utter intelligibly; for instance No. 14 helped himself out of his conversational difficulties by writing single words in a note-book which he carried about with him.

In spite of these hindrances to thought and frequent misunderstandings, general intelligence may remain on a surprisingly high level. The following incident in the life of No. 14, whilst under my care, shows how accurate may be the processes of perception and thought even with a severe syntactical disturbance. He was walking in Kew Gardens with the medical officer in charge of the hospital, when he pointed out a new variety of heath. The doctor said "Scotch," to which the patient replied, "No, no, you and me." It was a rare Irish heath, and both the patient and his companion were Irishmen.

During one of our sittings he touched the depressed part of the wound and then wrote "Forest branche." As I failed entirely to understand his meaning, he made me fetch from the cupboard in his room a book on forestry; he turned the pages until he came to a picture of a wood with undergrowth to which he pointed, saying "branch," at the same time touching his head. By this means he was able to make me understand his fear that, when walking through a coppice, the branches might injure his wound. He was at once satisfied when I told him we would cover it with an aluminium shield.

On another occasion he succeeded in communicating to a friend, who was visiting him in hospital, a piece of information not generally known. The visitor asked, "Who told you that?" and as the answer he received was incomprehensible jargon, he suggested, "Was it the Admiralty?" "No, no," was the reply. "Was it the War Office?" The patient repeated, "No, no," and seizing a pencil wrote "Lansdowne." This greatly puzzled the friend until he remembered that the Marquis of Lansdowne had once been the Head of the Foreign Office; he therefore enquired, "Was it the Foreign Office?" "Yes, yes," replied the patient, who had employed the familiar name of a previous Foreign Minister to represent the department over which he no longer presided.

This disorder of symbolic formulation and expression consists essentially in lack of that perfect balance and rhythm necessary to make the sounds uttered by the speaker easily comprehensible to his auditor. The phrase may be faulty and even single words are badly pronounced, although their nominal use and meaning remain intact. All those smaller words, such as articles and conjunctions, which bind together the more significant parts of the sentence, tend to be slurred or dropped. Speech becomes a series of disconnected categorical statements.

The internal use of language also suffers, though to a less degree. All these patients experienced difficulty in formulating to themselves some statement they were desirous of making, and in retaining it exactly for future use. The basic idea was precise, unless it had been confused by verbal mispronunciation, either external or internal. Single words conveyed their correct meaning and oral commands were well executed, except when they demanded the exact recall of a spoken phrase. In the course of ordinary conversation this frequently led to confusion in the mind of the patient and rendered him unable to carry on a subject, even if started by himself.

These defects in the use of language are not due to imperfect auditory images. They are manifestations of a disturbance in the rhythmic aspects of symbolic formulation and expression. Not only is the articulatory balance of words or word-groups affected, but the structural form of the phrase is disordered from want of those verbal elements which help to knit it together. For this reason I have spoken of these defects as syn-tactical, rather than as agrammatism, because they go deeper than grammar and affect the very basis of one aspect of the formation and use of language.

§3. NOMINAL DEFECTS

In this disorder of symbolic formulation and expression, we are not dealing with a difficulty in shaping words or phrases, but with a dis-turbance of their nominal significance. A name is a pattern which, if appropriately chosen, fits an external object or state of things around us. When a set of geometrical figures are ranged before me and a cone is placed in my hand out of sight, I know that it resembles one of the objects on the table, and this in spite of a diversity in size or material. A pattern has been produced as the result of the sensation from my hand, which agrees essentially with what I see. If, however, I give the object a name and call it a cone, I evoke a symbol, which indicates that pattern. In the same way, when I give the time as "five minutes to eight," I not only utter a series of words, but name a position on the clock, which differs fundamentally in significance from "five minutes past eight"; the two are as diverse as a cone and a pyramid distinguished by touch.

During the first few weeks the patient may be almost dumb with little or no spontaneous speech, unable to read or to write even his signature. Should he be suffering from a disorder of the nominal aspect of symbolic thought and expression in an uncomplicated form, some power of speaking returns rapidly. His enunciation becomes normal, except when he is in doubt for a word, or is seeking a correct appellation. Like an un-practised public speaker, who cannot find the expression he requires, he goes back to the beginning and tries to convey his meaning by changing the form of the phrase. So far as he can find words they are enunciated correctly and united into coherent phrases. There is none of that profound disturbance of pronunciation which runs through all the utterances of the verbal aphasic; nor are the sentences jerky and ill balanced, as with syntactical defects of language.

These patients can frequently give long explanations of the difficulty they experience in finding the right form of words. Thus, when I asked No. 7 if he could remember any of the songs he used to sing, he replied, "I've always tried...to see if I could think of them...but I've never been able to think of any of them...I used to think of them...before I went over (waving his hand to show he meant over the top)...I used to say them...but now...since (putting his hand to his wound)...since that...I can't even think." And yet at this time he could not name one of the common objects presented to him, nor repeat the words after me. When No. 2 was unable to find a suitable designation for black, he said, "I remember that now, because people who are dead...the other people who are not dead, they usually have this colour."

He also showed a tendency to employ ready made phrases and slang which came to him more easily than orthodox expressions, although this was not his habit before he was injured. He would say, "I made a priceless blob" (a mistake in tact); "The question of going to St Ives is a good egg" (a good idea). He was particularly fond of "putting heavy guns on to it," whenever he intended to imply that much effort had been used.

This disorder of language depends essentially on inability to designate an object in words and to appreciate verbal meaning. Names cannot be evoked readily for voluntary use, and they do not lead to a perfect and immediate response when presented in the form of oral or printed commands. To consider the manifestations of this form of aphasia under the headings of speech, reading and writing is misleading. I shall therefore describe first of all the results obtained by serial tests with common objects and colours which clearly reveal these general defects in appreciating verbal significance.

No. 7, who was the most severely affected of this group, could not name one of the common objects and was almost equally bad with colours. When they were placed before him he failed in every instance to write down their names correctly, although he could copy them from print in capital letters. If they were said or presented to him on printed cards, he occasionally chose correctly, but made many mistakes and experienced great difficulty in selection.

When first No. 2 came under my care he showed a less severe disturbance and has since steadily improved. It was therefore possible to estimate the relative value of these tests as indications of the intensity of the affection. In his first state he could pick out common objects with much hesitation to oral and to printed commands; but he made many mistakes with colours. When he attempted to name either common objects or colours, he failed grossly both in speech and in writing. Much improvement occurred and he then had little or no hesitation in selecting the object or colour presented to him orally or in print. Naming was still difficult, but correct; the words he wrote were badly spelt, but bore a recognisable relation to the name he was seeking.

Thus in this form of aphasia evocation of the correct name for use in speech or writing is most severely affected; next in order comes, as a rule, comprehension of single words in print, whilst oral commands are executed somewhat more easily. But this depends to some degree on the state of the patient's education and general intelligence.

Although it is impossible to name an object with any certainty, he may be able to do so by using some metaphorical designation instead of a single word. For example, during the tests with colours, No. 2 made such gross mistakes that he might have been thought to be colour-blind; for white was called "green," black "red," and green "blue." Exactly the same kind of error occurred when he chose a colour from its printed name on a card; on this occasion he even chose white for black, and black for green. More or less similar mistakes were made by all the patients of this group, and No. 22 was sent to me as an example of aphasia with colour-blindness. But not one of them had the slightest difficulty in choosing, from amongst the colours on the table, that which matched the one I had shown him.

From these observations we might be tempted to think that they had lost this knowledge of the nature of colour, that they were in fact "mind-blind." But No. 2, in his attempts to explain to me his difficulty in reading the printed cards, began to point to my white coat, to his khaki tie, the blue band on his arm which he wore as a wounded officer, and the green of the trees outside his window. Instead of the names of the colours, he was therefore encouraged to use a set of similitudes; black was "what you do for the dead," red "what the Staff wear," or, pointing to the lapel of his tunic, "where the Staff have it"; blue was "my arm," green "what is out there" (pointing to the trees), white was "what you wear" (a white coat), yellow "this one" (holding his tie). Twelve times he was shown cards bearing the name of one of these colours and in every instance he gave the right answer.

I then reversed the procedure, saying to him "the dead" and he chose a black piece of silk from a set of colours on the table in front of him; for "what is on your arm," he selected blue, "what the Staff wear" red, "what is out there" green, "like your tie," which he was not allowed to look at, led to his choosing yellow. For violet we had agreed on a lamp-shade that stood by his bed; this had been removed from the room before these observations began, but to the words, "like a lamp-shade," he chose violet. Throughout fourteen consecutive tests he made no mistakes. This demonstrates that his sense of colour was acute; it was names he lacked and they were imperfectly understood, when presented orally or in print.

No. 22 had been a house painter; when he found it impossible to name the colours, he described to me correctly how he would mix his paints in order to make them. For orange he said, "It's easy enough to make it if I'd the stuff; a bit of red, a bit of yellow and a bit of white lead." In the same way to designate violet, "It's made with black, red and a bit of blue; white lead would be the prevailing thing and stain it afterwards."

These observations, made with the help of familiar objects and colours, show that this disorder in the use of language depends, not only on inability to evoke names, but on want of capacity to fit a word, presented orally or in print, to its appropriate object. Capt. C. (No. 2) threw much light on this difficulty. When a command was given orally, his hand hovered in the air whilst he pondered over my words. He said, "I can do it, but it takes some seconds to get my brain straight." This delay for consideration was an equally striking feature with printed commands, and he volunteered the following explanation. "It's the interpreting words into pictures; when you give me KNIFE (printed card) I can't see the picture in my brain. All these things (passing his hand over the objects on the table) have no names at all until I really read K N I F E, and say 'knife' to myself." I showed him the card bearing the word KEY and he replied, "I'm not quite sure of that; I was not certain if it was a key or a knife. I have to spell it K E Y, and I say 'key' and look down on the table and then that's the key (pointing to it). I still puzzle what K E Y means; if I see that (pointing to the key on the table) then I don't have to worry, I know K E Y is that....is a key."

I then handed him two cards, one bearing the word MATCHES, the other WATCH; the first of these objects was amongst those on the table, whilst the other was not. He pointed to the match-box and holding up the latter card said "nothing here." Asked for the difference, he replied, "They are both written (printed); this one is here (pointing to the matches), the other there is nothing. I focus this one (matches) because it is here. I can't focus this (the watch card) so well because it is not so clear." He then moved his eyes round my room, as if seeking something, and added, "When I look at that big one (my consulting room clock) that helps me. I want to interpret the reading 'watch' into a picture (image) or into that watch (pointing to the clock). If I think of a watch and don't have to read it, I see a picture of my own watch. If you say it to me I see it at once, the picture is alright; if you show it me like that (printed) I have to think, I don't get the picture easily." Later on he added, "Suppose you had shown me 'looking glass,' written like that (printed), I should have had to think a long time. But if I looked up and saw that looking glass (pointing to the one on the wall), I should have known it at once."

Even though single words may yield a sufficiently accurate meaning to lead to correct choice from amongst a limited number of objects on the table, more complex commands, given orally or in print, are badly executed. The response required is more elaborate; the task is on a higher grade of difficulty and the words fail to communicate their full significance.

When the command is presented in the form of a phrase, complete verbal comprehension depends definitely on the complexity of the intellectual problem. Thus No. 7 could carry out such simple orders as "Shut your eyes," "Touch your nose," etc., given orally, but failed grossly with the more complicated hand, eye and ear tests.

The following remarks made by Capt. C. (No. 2), after a series of observations with the coin-bowl tests, show that this fact may be familiar to an intelligent patient. Throughout his hesitating attempts to carry out oral commands to place a certain coin into a definite bowl, he made movements of his lips without uttering a sound; he was evidently repeating the order to himself silently. He then said, "It is an extraordinary thing. With some of them I do it without thinking; then, if I think too much and say to myself 'third into fourth,' I don't know what it means ...If I do it myself I can do it as quickly as you like; but you tell me to do it and I have to think what it means, even if I say it to myself. I think the whole thing is it gives me one more...what do you call it... if you do two or three things together...factus, factor...do you call it factor, when I get two or three things together?"

This want of complete verbal comprehension is liable to lead to difficulties in ordinary intercourse. No. 2 said, "I notice that clever people say everything in a few words, so that I understand. Stupid people take a lot of words and I can't remember what they have said;

it confuses me." He added, "I understand pretty well now what any-body says, unless it's anything that's rather...rather tricky, rather heavier."

But he had difficulty in grasping the exact meaning of "to" and "past," "up" and "down," "high" and "low," "back" and "front," when contrasted with one another. Asked, "Would you like to stop in or go out?" he would reply, "either," in order to hide his want of exact comprehension. But if the question was put directly, "Do you want to stop in?" he would answer, "No"; "Do you want to go out?" "Yes," showing that he had definitely made up his mind to one course of action, but was puzzled by the two alternatives in the same sentence.

In severe forms of this disorder repetition, even of single words, is difficult or impossible. No. 7 was unable to repeat the names of common objects and colours with certainty, although the sound he uttered bore a distinct relation to that of the word said by me; in some instances it approximated sufficiently closely to be reckoned a correct response. For example key became "kay," pencil "pintil," matches "mats"; twice in this series penny was pronounced correctly. Asked to repeat scissors, he said "sis—I can't open far enough," pointing to his jaw.

The power of repetition is one of the earliest activities to be restored. But, even after he had recovered to a considerable extent, Capt. C. (No. 2) found difficulty in repeating the simple phrases of the man, cat and dog tests; twice in a series of twelve observations he failed to reproduce the correct combination, although the words of the phrase were accurately pronounced. No. 23 was almost completely successful, but stumbled in the middle of the series; he said in explanation, "Anything like that I can pick up quick. I can't hold it. I can say things after people quicker than I can say them myself, but I can't hold them."

All these patients tend to move the lips silently without uttering a sound, when attempting to repeat a phrase, especially if in doubt. Still more is this the case should it contain an order of some complexity. Silent repetition also suffers in nominal aphasia, because the patient has difficulty in retaining in his memory the word of the proper meaning; he becomes confused owing to the incorrect words he repeats to himself.

Except in the earlier stages, these patients can read to themselves, but with great slowness and uncertainty. They are particularly liable to grave misunderstandings, due to defective appreciation of the significance of the words they are reading. No. 2 was asked to read to himself the following account of a famous prize-fight, a few days after its occurrence. "Carpentier, the French champion, met Beckett, heavy-weight champion of England on Thursday, December 4th, at the Holborn Stadium. Beckett was knocked out in 74 seconds by a right hand hook to the jaw." At the end of six minutes he returned the paper and started to tell me what he had read in the following words. "Carpentier met Beckett in the Holborn...say...so...Sadium, I used to know it, and Carpentier being the champion now...who is...oh no...who met Beckett...now the champion in England...knocked...er...knocked...er...Beckett out in 74 seconds...with a right...with a right hook to the jaw." He then added, "I wasn't thinking so much of the fight...but what I had been reading...I saw the picture of 74...seconds...saw what I had read."

I then asked, "Can you see the fight?" and an extraordinary change came over his narration. "Now I think about the fight, I see the picture of Carpentier. I see Beckett falling...I see the Ref...Ref...what you call it...Referee...The last thing I can picture is Carpentier standing like this with both hands like this." He sprang from his bed and assumed an attitude, with both hands on his hips, looking down towards the ground, exactly that of Carpentier in the photographs of the termination of the fight. The change in manner from the puzzled aspect of a man, slowly recalling what he had read, to the brisk, vivid, smiling person, describing what he saw, was remarkable.

If what they are given to read silently is in the form of a command, this want of appreciation becomes still more apparent; for not only must the patient understand the printed matter, but he is compelled to formulate the meaning to himself, before he can carry out the order that lies behind it.

No. 7 was given a series of cards, one by one, each of which contained a simple order such as "Shut your eyes," "Touch your nose," etc. He was told to read it to himself and to "do what it says." This presented great difficulties; sometimes, when told to shut his eyes, he brought his hand to his eye, or, asked to give his hand, he touched the left with the right. Once only in eight attempts did he carry out such orders correctly.

Reading aloud seems to add to the difficulty and is no aid to understanding the import of the printed matter, as with some other forms of aphasia. The patient tries to spell out the words and becomes confused, because he is uncertain of the nominal value of the different letters of which they are composed. At a time when No. 2 could say the whole alphabet and read or write it without mistakes, he was unable to read aloud the simple words of the man, cat and dog tests. Occasionally he succeeded in spelling out all the letters correctly, and yet he could not deduce from them the verbal content of the phrase. Once, after naming correctly in sequence all the letters of "the man and the cat," he suggested that it was "the dog and the cat," and added "it might be anything." This is a fair sample of the way in which all these patients tended to read aloud a combination of simple words not containing a command. Offered the short phrases in print, they attempted to decipher them letter by letter and became confused owing to lack of power to combine the printed characters into a verbal symbol, which bears the correct meaning[1].

When, however, pictures of the man, the cat and the dog are shown in pairs, in place of the printed words, they can be named accurately and without hesitation in all but the severest cases[2]. Evidently these patients still possess the power of evoking simple words in response to pictures. But as soon as they were made to carry a command, as in the hand, eye and ear tests, the action demanded is as badly carried out as if the order had been given in print. The necessity for formulating the significance of the pictures gives them a high nominal value.

As might be expected, the power of writing spontaneously is gravely reduced. No. 7, the most severely affected of this group, wrote his surname with difficulty and could not complete his somewhat unusual Christian name, or that of the town in which he lived. Capt. C. reproduced his usual signature with the name of his regiment, but was unable to add his address.

None of them could write a coherent letter or a sentence of any length. But Capt. C. amused himself by making lists of words which came into his head spontaneously; of these the following may serve as examples, "Post offest" (Post Office), "Arbes" (Arabs), "Turskes" (Turks). By repeated practice he recovered to a considerable extent his power of writing spontaneously. But he was extremely slow and inaccurate; he was accustomed, when composing a letter, to put it aside for correction and then to recopy it. With much labour he wrote for me spontaneously the vivid account, given on p. 33, Vol. II, of the adventures of a fellow patient, a young naval officer. All the facts were correctly reproduced, but the composition was poor and the spelling incredibly bad for a highly educated Staff Officer.

All these patients were able to write the simple words of the man, cat and dog tests in response to pictures. Even No. 7 could reproduce these combinations correctly although he failed to write the name of a single colour shown to him. Not uncommonly, however, the content of

---

[1] No. 23 made a good record so long as he did not attempt to spell out the words.

[2] No. 7 hesitated over the verbal form but the content was correct throughout.

the phrase is inaccurate; one noun is substituted for another and there is a tendency to spell "Dog" "God," a common mistake of childhood.

When the words to be written are a description of some movement made by the observer, as in the hand, eye and ear tests, the results are usually unsatisfactory. They show the same sort of mistakes that mar direct imitation; but, in addition, one of the factors may be omitted or "eye" may be mistaken for "ear."

Once the stage of shock has passed away words can be copied in capitals, letter by letter. If the disturbance of speech is very severe, patients belonging to this group may be unable to translate print into handwriting; but so great a limitation of power is uncommon, except in the earlier stages or where education has been defective. Usually they can transcribe printed words or short phrases into cursive script. This contains many faults; capitals are interspersed meaninglessly, the spelling is defective in spite of the copy, and the same kind of mistakes occur, as when the patient attempts to name an object placed in front of him.

One of the most instructive facts, illustrated by this disorder of language, is the close association between the power to write to dictation and to copy print in cursive script. Both show the same sort of errors; when one is defective the other also suffers and during recovery both are restored together. Evidently, during the act of turning print into handwriting, the patient is dictating to himself, whereas to reproduce the printed characters is an act of simple imitation.

The nature of the difficulties, which obstruct the perfect use of language in nominal aphasia, can be revealed by setting the patient some task that tests systematically his various powers of speech, reading and writing. The simplest of these is the alphabet, which also serves as a useful measure of the severity of the disturbance. Thus, No. 7 could not say the letters in sequence spontaneously; he repeated them slowly and with difficulty; but read them aloud correctly. He could not write them down in order without prompting and, when they were dictated, he wrote very slowly, his lips moving silently throughout. He copied the alphabet in printed characters, but could not transcribe it into cursive script. Thus, the more he was compelled to evoke the significant value of the letters, as when speaking or writing them spontaneously, the harder became the task. On the other hand he could repeat or copy them in capitals without difficulty; these acts were closer to pure imitation. It was not the verbal form of the letters that was at fault, but their symbolic associations and meaning.

With slighter affections of this order the alphabet may be said spontaneously, perfectly repeated, and read aloud slowly. It can also be written, but capital letters are interspersed amongst the cursive script. In this state the patient experiences no difficulty in copying all the letters in his normal handwriting. Finally, even the power of spontaneous writing is restored although capitals tend to appear in an otherwise correctly written alphabet.

Even more valuable information can be obtained with the help of a printed paragraph, provided the patient can write at all. I gave Capt. C. (No. 2) the lines headed "Partridge Shooting"; "Birds are fairly plentiful this year thanks to a warm late May and June. It is a pleasure to see the old hands gathering round again and, as before the war the cars bringing the guns were fitted with Dunlop tyres, so the cars of to-day are similarly equipped."

After he had pored over these paragraphs for ten minutes, I asked him, "What have you read?" He answered, "It takes me an awful time. In the early summer there are lots of young partridges...I think it is... That's as far as I've got."

He then read the whole aloud slowly but correctly, ending as follows, "so the cars of to-day are simul...sinerly...simuly...ecuped, whatever that means...yes, equipped."

I asked him to tell me what it was about, and he replied, "It has been a good warm May and June, from which the young pheasants are... are...I should say in thousands. The rest is about Dunlop tyres. I don't quite see the joke...quite what it is about. I suppose because people... No, I don't see why they should have Dunlops at all."

On dictating these sentences to him, he wrote them slowly; all the words were reproduced, but with incredible faults in spelling. The difficulty he experienced was to translate what I said into written symbols.

I then asked him to put down for me on paper a short account of what he had just written to dictation, with the following result: "There are a lot of young Phesionts this year at June and May and as there are are many Dunlop cars running out for shooting." He then ceased, protesting, "As a matter of fact this is quite wrong, because it is not the time to shoot partridges."

He could, however, copy these paragraphs slowly and accurately in cursive handwriting, correcting any errors he may have made.

Here the power of translating knowledge gained from silent reading into articulated or written speech suffered most severely. Writing to dictation was also badly affected, because it necessitates translation of auditory impressions into written symbols of similar meaning; but copying, even in cursive handwriting, could be carried out correctly. He failed to comprehend accurately the significance of the earlier phrases about the plentiful supply of young birds in May and June; this confused him, because he recognised that these were not the months for shooting. He also tended to substitute pheasants for partridges. It was not words he lacked, but the power of selecting the one which bore the exact meaning he required. It is interesting to notice how closely orthography is associated with such accurate verbal selection; this might have been anticipated from analogous observations carried out with the alphabet.

In the case of No. 22 the tests were arranged somewhat differently[1]. He had been a house painter, but loved music; in the summer he used to play in an orchestra at a sea-side watering place and possessed a double bass, of which he was very proud. I combined these details of his life into a series of printed sentences and, when he had perused them silently, he was requested to tell me what he had understood. This he was unable to do; after three attempts he handed the paper back to me saying, "I can't get at that somehow." He read it aloud with considerable difficulty, spelling many of the words, but again failed to reproduce its meaning when asked to do so. I then read the sentences aloud to him and he could still give no coherent account of what they contained. But as soon as I asked him to tell me his story in his own way, without thinking of the words he had read or heard, he gave all the details mentioned in the printed paragraphs; in some instances he employed the identical words, embodied in the account, which he had previously been unable to reproduce.

The nature of this disturbance of symbolic formulation and expression comes out particularly clearly with the clock tests. There was not the slightest difficulty in setting one clock in direct imitation of the other; the short hand was even moved into a position proportionate to the number of minutes shown by the long hand. But none of these patients could tell the time or write it correctly; they could not find the adequate spoken or written symbols[2]. They set the clock badly to oral commands, or when the order was given in the form of printed words; this was evidence of defective appreciation of verbal significance. But the response might be perfect, if each card bore the hour in so-called "railway time" instead of in the ordinary nomenclature. Given such a number as 4.45,

---

[1] Vol. ii, p. 334.
[2] No. 23 is an exception because he had been specially taught to tell the time.

the patient first places the hour hand at 4 and then sweeps the other one round to a position he associates with 45 minutes. But, if he is asked to set "a quarter to five," the temptation is to set the one hand at 5 whilst the other hovers uncertainly between "a quarter past" and "a quarter to." This difference does not, however, apply when the patient attempts to tell the time; it is equally difficult for him to find the designation "four forty-five" as "a quarter to five."

Throughout these tests there is a profound tendency to confuse "to" and "past." Moreover, the number of the hour has an overwhelming attraction; for example, when setting twenty minutes to six, the long hand may be rightly placed, but the hour hand points to six. Not infrequently the symbolic significance of the two hands is mistaken and the long one set to the hour. The character of these errors sometimes makes it extremely difficult to record exactly the nature of the response.

All this does not signify that the patient is ignorant of the time of day. No. 2 said, "That is when you eat," or "when we were there," of some particular event and was always right, although he could not mention the time in either case. He was punctual for his appointments and never missed a train, provided the time was written down for him in figures. Moreover, when shown the test clock set at some definite hour he could select without a moment's hesitation a card, on which the corresponding time was printed in figures. It is not knowledge of time that these patients lack, but the symbolic means of expressing, even to themselves, what they know; they also find difficulty in understanding the nominal significance of words, spoken or printed, in which they are told how to set the clock.

The power of saying the numbers in sequence may be disturbed in the more severe cases (No. 7), but is rapidly recovered. No. 2 had no difficulty in counting correctly with perfect enunciation, when he first came under my care. But he could not employ any particular number directly and with certainty in simple arithmetical operations. He could pick out five things, when told to do so; but asked to add five to any number, he would count on his fingers or place five dots on the paper. When about to add 8 and 6, he did not take these numbers as entities; he counted up to eight and then on for another six, saying finally, "fourteen."

He confessed that numbers puzzled him; if "eighteen" was said, the meaning did not come to him until he had counted it up. This difference between the ease with which a number can be appreciated in series and as an isolated word, is familiar to us all in a foreign language; many, who can rattle off French numerals, experience a moment's hesitation when told that the price is "quatre-vingt-douze francs." Moreover, some educated persons habitually count during addition, instead of employing the numbers as direct denominators.

No. 2 experienced a similar difficulty when he was told that an event had happened on some definite date such as "Thursday, March the twelfth." Telling him the day of the week or of the month conveyed nothing to him until he had repeated to himself, "Monday, Tuesday, Wednesday, Thursday," and then "January, February, March," finally counting up to twelve. The date did not convey to him at once the part of the week or of the year in which it fell.

All these patients failed to carry out simple arithmetical exercises. They could add such numbers as 356 to 231 on paper, but they tended to fail, whenever it was necessary to carry over a number from one column to the next. No. 7 wrote down the sum of each pair of figures separately as follows: $\frac{3}{8}$ $\frac{4}{6}$ $\frac{5}{8}$ and, when subtracting, took the lowest number from $\overline{11}$ $\overline{10}$ $\overline{12}$ the highest, whether it was in the upper or lower line of the sum.

As might have been expected, there was considerable difficulty in finding the usual names for coins, although it was obvious that they were still recognised correctly. Thus, a sixpence was called "half a shilling," two-and-six was "two and a half," a ten-shilling note was "half a pound"; and yet many coins were given their usual names and there was no evidence that any one of them was mistaken for another of different value.

But, when the patient was asked to express in words the relative value of two coins, such as a sixpence and a shilling, laid in front of him, he became confused; he tended to add them, saying, "one and a half"; with a penny and a sixpence Capt. C. said "seven." When, however, the question was put in the form, "How many of that (sixpence) would you have to give me for that (a shilling)?" he answered "Two; one more of that (pointing to the sixpence) to get one of that (the shilling)." Then he suddenly burst out, "One more sixpence to get a shilling." Through-out this series of tests he could never name the relative value directly of any two pieces of money; and yet by these indirect means it was possible to show that he had understood perfectly. No. 7 experienced exactly the same difficulty in formulating the relationship, but was able to pile up a heap of coins on the one side, which exactly equalled the larger one in value. Given a shilling, he collected together a sixpence, a threepenny bit and three coppers; a two-shilling piece was placed before him and he chose from the money on the table a sixpence, a threepenny bit, a shilling and quickly added three coppers. Yet when asked, "How many of this (sixpence) go into that (two-shilling piece)?" he said, "Two...two... two shillun," and with one shilling and a two-shilling piece replied, "Three shillun." Behind this difficulty in expression lay a correct comprehension of the relative value of the coins to one another. This is borne out by the fact that these patients have no difficulty in manipulating change.

Nearly two years after the injury Capt. C. (No. 2) was able to fill up a cheque spontaneously; but he could not be certain that the written words and figures corresponded with one another. He drew a cheque in my presence for eighty-five pounds, ten shillings and sixpence, but filled in the figures as £80. 10. 6. He noticed this discrepancy and succeeded finally in making the correction; but the cheque would not have passed the bank.

All these patients could draw from a model and, after its removal, reproduced the drawing from memory. But when No. 2 and No. 7 were asked to draw an elephant, the result bore no relation to that animal; it was without trunk, tusks or ears. This was the more remarkable as Capt. C. (No. 2) used to amuse himself by drawing pictures of the animals he had shot in Cashmir; on one occasion, when talking about means of transport in the East, he drew spontaneously a spirited rough picture of a camel, to supply the name he was unable to evoke. Visual images were not destroyed, but they could not be called up with certainty to command. No. 22, who had played in the band at a circus, and was familiar with elephants, failed altogether when told to draw one of these animals. He asked, "That's the gentleman with the long...yes quite so, with the long trunk," and added, "No, I can't think, I can't call it, sir" (recall). But he drew from memory a jug shown to him and described the colours of the pattern upon it.

This difficulty in formulating visual images to command is particularly evident, when the patient is asked to draw a rough ground-plan of some place he knows well. Sitting in my work-room, No. 7 was asked to put down on paper the relative position of the objects in the ward he could see from his bed; he failed completely. But, when I drew an oblong on the paper, saying, "That is your bed" and asked him to point to the situation of the various things he could remember, he was astonishingly accurate. For instance, he pointed to the left saying, "There's only my bed," and to the right, "There's a bed; no one there now"; he then indicated the head of the bed and touched the wall of the examining room to signify that here was a wall. All these details and many others were correct, but he could not transfer them to paper. Captain C. (No. 2) started to draw a plan but filled it in with details in elevation. He could copy his images but could not translate them into a symbolic formula.

When I applied the same test to No. 22, who had been a house painter and decorator, he fully understood what I required, saying, "Do you want a floor plan?" But he could only draw in elevation, and relinquished the attempt with the words, "No, no, I know what you mean, but I can't get at it."

Orientation is unaffected and such patients have no difficulty in finding their way, provided they are not asked how they intend to go from one place to another. After he had made the journey several times on foot I accompanied Capt. C. from my house to the Empire Hospital, allowing him to be my guide. If he took the wrong turning, he looked round puzzled; what he saw did not correspond to what he expected and he retraced his steps slowly. After several mistakes he turned into the street which led to the hospital, and said, "That's it." I asked how he knew and he replied, "There, you see that?...where the Padre is (pointing to the spire of a church); that's near the hospital." He then walked along rapidly, took the right turning to the hospital, which he recognised at once, and ran up to his room without hesitation.

In spite of the fact that he could always find his way he was unable to describe how to walk from one place to another. This he explained to me as follows, "I have no streets in London; no names at all. Supposing I was going from the Army and Navy, that's what it's called, just round here (the Army and Navy Stores), I should then say some place to a hospital about a quarter of a mile away. I remember the hospital is on the left on the way to the War Office, about half way. I believe it's the Abbey. No, it's near the Abbey on the way to the War Office." He added, "I saw the hospital"; I put as a question, "The Abbey?" and he replied as follows: "It's here, but then it's gone again and I have to feel for it again. The only thing I can remember of it is the opening, the big opening, where everybody goes in. I can get that" (moving his hand in the form of a large arch). Since it was obvious that he had described Westminster Hospital and Westminster Abbey, which are close to one another, I asked, "Have the Hospital and the Abbey anything to do with one another?" He answered, "Nothing except my focus, the place of them; the distance, that is all. I should say how far the Hospital is to the Abbey in re...in re...that's where I go wrong. I want to say in re- something (relation). There are just little bits in expressing what

I want to say; little bits in which I have to turn my brain another way to get what I want to say, whereas a year or two ago I should have said it without thinking. You see, it's like this; with me it's all in bits. I have to jump like this," marking a thick line with his pencil between two points. "Like a man who jumps from one thing to the next. I can see them, but I can't express. Really it is that I haven't enough names. I've got practically no names."

It is evident from this conversation that he was able to recall visual images of objects on his way from the Empire Hospital in Westminster to the War Office in Whitehall. First of all he saw the Army and Navy Stores and then Westminster Hospital on his left, with the great door of Westminster Abbey on the right; but want of names prevented him from connecting the two except in position, and he was compelled to jump from one image to another without the connecting links of symbolic formulation.

In the same way he retained a conception of right and left, in spite of his inability to express the idea in abstract terms, or to carry out commands, which necessitated choice between them. As we were walking along the street, he said, "I've been so long out of the Old Country that I don't know which way cars come. If I was riding in one up the street, I should be riding there," indicating the left-hand side of the road and tapping the left curb with his stick. Then he added, "But that's not it, there," waving his hand to indicate a foreign country.

Pictures apparently conveyed their full meaning so long as they did not imply a command to carry out some action. Thus No. 2 saw all the points in a Bairnsfather picture of "Old Bill" boxing with Hindenburg, but carried out pictorial orders badly. Jokes presented in the form of pictures are appreciated with considerable difficulty if they demand a verbal formula for their comprehension; but, so long as the humour is inherent in the drawing itself, it is recognised with ease.

No. 2 liked to have everything that was said to him illustrated in a drawing or diagram. Thus, when his sister was teaching him music, she told him that the octave consisted of three tones, a half tone, two tones and another half tone. This puzzled him completely; she played the scale and he still failed to grasp it. But as soon as she drew a diagram, where each horizontal line represented a tone and each short vertical one a half tone, he understood and from that moment never forgot it.

All power of understanding musical notation is destroyed by these symbolic defects. No. 22, who had always played the cornet and the double bass from notes, lost all capacity to play either instrument. On the other hand No. 7, though a professional singer, had never read music easily and, when under my care, was completely unable to do so. But he sang by ear in perfect time and tune without words. No. 23 could correct his friends when they played the violin or piano, though he could not read the notes.

These patients enjoyed games and could play dominoes and draughts. Capt. C. was above the normal average at chess, but could no longer play bridge; "The names of the cards bother me," he said. "It's just names; I used to play a good game of bridge."

In spite of these disabilities general intelligence may remain on a remarkably high level. Many of these patients succeeded in communicating to me introspective observations of the greatest value. I need scarcely draw further attention to the many luminous remarks of Capt. C., which have been already detailed in this section. No. 22 was a charming companion when his mind was turned on to reminiscences of his past life as a musician (cf. his account of the Empress of Austria and her private circus). No. 23 could not rise above the position of a farm-hand, because of his difficulty in expressing himself and transmitting orders to those under him; but his employer reported that he was a most intelligent worker on the farm and far above the average standard. He was extremely good at any job connected with machinery; he could take a bicycle to pieces and put it together again perfectly.

He complained, however, that "When I think of anything, everything seems to be rolling along; I can't hold it...I can see what it is. I seem to see it myself, but I can't put it properly into words like you ought to. I can see what it is myself like. My mind won't stop at one thing. They keep on rolling. Myself, I imagine, when you're talking, you're only thinking of what you're talking about. When I'm talking to anybody it seems a lot of things keep going by." "If I go and feed the sheep, things keep passing in my mind. I do it, but whilst I'm doing it things keep coming into my head, I can't hold it whilst I'm talking about it." "If I do it wrong first time (in the farm work) I can see what I done wrong. I know what I want to say; I seem to get half there and then I forget. I get muddled."

These defects of speech consist essentially of loss of power to employ names together with want of comprehension of the nominal value of words and other symbols. Although the patient has plenty of words at his command, he may be unable to designate familiar objects; yet he can describe their use or composition, either directly or in some apt metaphorical phrase, and he can repeat anything said to him provided it is simple and easy to understand. Asked to point to an object named by the observer, he is unable to do so, or makes his choice slowly and with effort.

He reads and writes with extreme difficulty. He can usually count and say the alphabet, but suffers from defective appreciation of the meaning of single numbers or letters.

Drawing from a model is easily performed; but when the patient is asked to draw some definite figure from imagination, the result is unsatisfactory. He is unable to produce a ground-plan of a familiar room, but has no general loss of orientation and can find his way unaided.

§ 4. SEMANTIC DEFECTS

I have described the various changes in speaking, reading and writing, which occur with what have been called verbal, syntactical and nominal affectations of symbolic formulation and expression. One other form of disorder emerges from analysis of the clinical phenomena due to unilateral lesions of the brain. This may be called "semantic,"[1] because it is comprehension of the significance of words and phrases as a whole which is primarily disturbed.

These patients tend to talk rapidly as if afraid of forgetting what they wanted to say; at times this actually occurs and the conversation tails away aimlessly. They suffer from no difficulty in pronunciation and, although the sentences may be somewhat short and jerky, syntax and intonation remain undisturbed. Pure verbal repetition is in no way affected. They can name common objects and indicate without fail the one that has been mentioned orally or in print. Sometimes, though colours are named correctly, the patient may confuse red and orange, orange and yellow, violet and blue, especially when choosing to oral commands; this does not occur except in the severer cases.

We can only understand the peculiar nature of this disorder of symbolic formulation if we bear in mind that the fault is essentially a want of recognition of relative significance and intention. Everything tends to be appreciated in detail, but the general significance is lacking. This is evident, when the patient is given a picture and told to say what he sees

---

[1] From σημαίνειν, to signify. This term was used by Bréal in his well-known *Essai de Sémantique*, a study in the science of the ultimate meaning of words. Since I am dealing here mainly with a loss of power to comprehend the full significance of words and phrases together with a want of capacity to employ such modes of expression as a whole, I have not hesitated to adopt this term, which has already become part of the English language.

in it. He looks at it like a child, pointing out one thing after another, and not uncommonly misses some important feature; asked what the picture means, he may be entirely at a loss and either gives up altogether or invents some preposterous explanation.

I showed Dr P. (No. 24), who was an ardent student of politics, a cartoon of Mr Lloyd George playing the harp from the same score as M. Briand, who held in his hand a French horn. After contemplating this picture for some time he said, "It's the Welsh Prime Minister with the Celtic instrument and the other man has a musical instrument, a blowing instrument. He's a foreigner probably; whether he's a French editor I don't know." I then uncovered the legend beneath the picture, which ran, "The world's premier duettists," and he replied, "I don't understand it; it doesn't help me."

No. 18 was shown a series of drawings of a man in evening dress, who, arriving late at the theatre, inadvertently stripped himself to his shirt-sleeves to the horror of the surrounding spectators. He said he understood it and proceeded to explain it as follows: "It's about a man who goes into a theatre late. He gets in everybody's way when he's taking his coat off and he disturbs them, when he's seated. I couldn't say exactly what was making them so excited. After looking a long time I saw it was him laughing." This explanation satisfied him completely until I said, "Don't you see he has taken off both coats; he is in his shirt sleeves?" He then looked at the picture again and replied, "I can see it now; I thought it was because he was laughing so loud."

This want of power to combine details into a coherent whole is peculiarly evident, when comprehension of a printed legend is necessary for the complete understanding of a picture. No. 5, who was a gardener from the country, chose from the paper the picture of a man riding a cow over which stood the description, "Mayor's Curious Steed." He said, "That's a man riding on a colt. No it isn't, sir, it looks more like a cow...or a young cow...no, it isn't...heifer, sir." After he had read the legend I asked, "Who is the man?" and he replied, "A farmer, sir. No, Major...no, the Mayor curse sted...the Mayor curious stid. It's something you don't see every day, that stid; something very uncommon that animal. It's in a horse's place instead of where it is. I should think myself they are going to show that animal; it's uncommon, that stid, more so to see a man riding on it...You don't often see a man riding on a stid." When I asked, "What is a stid?" he replied, "It's something the same family as a cow."

In consequence of this difficulty in appreciating the full significance either of pictures or of print most examples of pictorial humour are in-comprehensible. Supposing the joke consists solely in the details it may be understood, but any demand for coordination between various parts of the drawing and the meaning of the text beneath it meets with little or no response.

On one occasion I showed Miss S. (No. 25) a picture from *Punch* in which a country gentleman says to a tramp, "It's about time you chaps started to do something; hard work never killed anybody." The mendi-cant replies, "You are mistaken, sir, I lost three wives through it." She said, "There's no joke in it; he lost three wives, but I don't know what by." About ten minutes later she exclaimed, "Oh! now I see it. It was the wives who were killed by work." She laughed heartily and added, "That's very characteristic; when once I've seen it I wonder how I have been so silly not to have seen it at once."

When these patients read to themselves a story or consecutive passage, they are liable to miss the general sense and to omit words or phrases essential to the argument. This tendency becomes evident if they are asked to give a coherent account of what they have just read silently. For instance, I gave No. 18 a short series of simple sentences bearing on the much discussed question of the advantages of "summer-time." He took the paper in his hand, read it through carefully and started to tell me what he had understood; in this he succeeded fairly well until it became necessary to remember that the clock was put forward, when he gave up. Asked what happened to the clocks in summer-time he recog-nised that they were altered an hour, but did not know in which direction and complained, "It's always a puzzle; I've given up thinking about it." But later in the conversation he assumed that summer-time was an hour *later*, showing his inherent confusion with regard to the ultimate meaning of what he had read.

The tendency becomes particularly obvious when they are asked to write an account of what they have just read to themselves. For instance, I handed No. 5 his own story in print, "My name is Charles H. and I live at Laurel Cottage, Pilley. Before I joined the army I worked for Miss D. for nearly two years. I worked in the garden and looked after the pony. He was a forest pony, bay, with a dark mane and tail." This he read to himself and then wrote, "I was worked for Miss D. and looked after a pony and trap," adding, "That's all I remember." He was then asked to read it aloud, which he did perfectly and without hesitation; but all he could communicate in writing was as follows: "I worked for Miss D. and I looked after a pony and trap and helped in the garden."

This loss of capacity was not based on any defect in the power of writing, for he copied his own story perfectly in cursive handwriting and was able to write a coherent letter to his relatives, mentioning the friends who had visited him by name. Symbols could be utilised better for spontaneous thought than for an intellectual effort made to command.

This is not due to want of education, for Dr P. (No. 24) showed exactly the same disability in an even more pronounced degree. I gave him the following sentences to read silently to himself: " But my country now is Italy where I have a residence for life and literally may sit under my own vine and my own fig tree. I have some thousands of the one and some scores of the other with myrtles, pomegranates, oranges, lemons and mimosas in great quantity. I intend to make a garden not very unlike yours. In a few days, whenever the weather will allow it, I have four mimosas ready to place in front of my house and a friend who is coming to plant them." Asked to put down on paper what he had gathered he wrote, " I have Italy as my country and mimosa, 4 bushes," and then ceased. The printed paragraph was again placed in his hand and he read it through silently and deliberately. He then said, " I know Italy. I have an interest in Italy. You know it...and mimosas and pomegranates. I forget the rest." He read the whole aloud without material mistakes, but doubted in the middle if it made sense. I then asked what it was about, and he replied, " Well, the country is Italy. You have this mimosa and these shrubs. You intend to make a garden not very unlike...You have four mimosa and a friend...I have to take the ideas as they come. I think it is a difficult subject; it is involved. It wants concentration of thought. That's what I can't do." To my dictation he wrote, " But my country now is Italy where I have a residence for life and literaly six under my own vine and own vig tree. I have some 1000 of the one and scores of the other with Myrtles, Ponegranates, Oranges, Lemons and Mimosas in great quantity. In a few days when even the weather will allow it I have 4 mimosas ready to place in front of my house and a friend who is coming to plant them." But although he copied the whole paragraph without a mistake, he was unable to recapitulate the contents of the sentences he had so often read and written; he said, " I've a general idea of it. It's Italy. You have these mimosas, pomegranates and so on...and, er, you make a home in Italy for life. I don't remember anything else." Finally, he added, " I'm wonderfully clear minded in some respects. I know, but I can't keep it in my mind. I've no constraint of thought and, if I attempt it, I get worried. I've no sequence of ideas; involved sentences are inapplicable."

We can only understand the nature of these difficulties, if we bear in mind that they are due essentially to want of power to combine mentally into a single act a series of relevant details. This has usually been spoken of as an "amnesia"; but it is an affection of the same functional order as the other forms of aphasia, which I have already described. The difference lies in the fact that semantic defects are manifested mainly in want of ability to appreciate and retain the ultimate significance or intention of words and phrases combined in normal sequence.

In severe cases this may even lead to hesitation and defects in writing the letters of the alphabet. No. 10 used the same symbol "Ϩ" for D F O R T and V and wrote with great rapidity, saying, "I had to risk it." Both No. 18 and No. 25 were puzzled by the shape of the letters. But all the patients of this group could say the alphabet spontaneously and repeat it letter by letter, although they showed a tendency to "go full tilt" as if afraid of forgetting what they were about to say.

At first, as in the case of No. 10, the patient may find it impossible to write the name of an object, although he has no other difficulty in nomenclature. Five months later each name was correctly given, but he wrote at a tremendous pace as if in a desperate hurry. The words were carelessly written; cylinder became "cilande" or "cylander," ovoid "ovoad" and cube was shortened to "cub." This excessive rapidity was also evident during the man, cat and dog tests, when he wrote from dictation or from pictures. He said, "I write very hurriedly so as to keep track of it." But, if he was given a printed card and asked to copy it, he wrote with greater deliberation and his handwriting improved considerably. The character of the script and the orthography depends on the ease or difficulty of the task; thus No. 25 copied printed matter in excellent handwriting, but any attempt to use it for the expression of general ideas led to profound deterioration. She explained that, "So long as I take in the sense at a glance I can put it down from sheer habit." Her spelling suffered in the same way; the harder the task the worse it became until the faults reached a degree unknown in an educated person.

A simple letter written spontaneously to friends or relatives may be coherent and reasonable; and yet these patients complain that they "cannot pull it together," or are uncertain whether it is wrongly written or not. But an attempt to put on to paper spontaneously more complex thoughts and ideas may lead to difficulty and confusion in severe degrees of this affection. When I asked Dr P. (No. 24) to write down the gist of his political conceptions he produced the following sentences: "Why are National Colonies dissastified (dissatisfied)? India Eagptian (Egyptian)

Crpress (Cyprus) all dissastified and hating the English. Where as the free Colonies are loial (loyal). the natives of Egypt say the (they) know the govt is good but they admit they hate us. and would rather be under a bad govt such as the Turk. This appears to be due to gealousey (jealousy) and due to the educated man he as he believes looked down upon and the contempt of olor" (due to the educated man, who as he believes, is looked down upon and contempt of colour).

The nature of this disorder of symbolic formulation and the defective general recognition of the aim of some act to be performed are clearly revealed by the clock tests. In no other form was there the least difficulty in setting the hands of one clock in strict conformity with those of another; but patients belonging to this group tended to carry out this manoeuvre slowly, with hesitation, and might even become confused by what is little more than an act of matching. They were puzzled by the significance of the hands and failed to understand exactly what they were expected to do. As a rule they could tell the time correctly and this task was performed more easily than any other of this series of tests. But, when asked to set the clock in response to either oral or printed commands, the errors were extremely gross. The long and short hands were confused, "to" and "past" were mistaken and even the hour was wrongly indicated in some instances. Since the patient could tell the time correctly this inability to set the clock to order must have been due to want of appreciation of spoken and written commands or to defective memory of the action demanded. No. 10 confessed, "If I can't get the hands exactly where I want, I lose grasp, I get thinking"; and No. 8 said, "I can't make out the difference between *past* and *to* six; I don't know from which side to approach it."

Inability to recognise significance or to appreciate intention is at the root of these semantic disorders. It is not surprising, therefore, that the hand, eye and ear tests were badly executed, necessitating as they do accurate choice between three pairs of possible actions. When the patient imitated movements made by me sitting face to face, or carried out those represented on a picture held in his hand, the errors were gross. Oral and printed commands were badly executed and he usually had difficulty in recording in writing an action carried out by me. Eye and ear might be confused; he not infrequently failed to recognise that the movement was crossed and he was liable to give up the attempt before completing his task. No. 10 said, "My initial difficulty seems to be right and left; it confused me; I forget the rest of what I've got to do."

In all normal persons, and with other disorders of symbolic formulation and expression, movements reflected in a mirror can be imitated with much greater ease and certainty than when patient and observer sit opposite to one another. This also applies to the same actions, when given in the form of a pictorial command. The patient finds the task an easy one "because I have only to imitate you or the picture." But in the semantic group, though the number of errors may be less when the movement is reflected, there is not that conviction that the action is extremely easy. No. 8 explained a bad record as follows: "Somehow or another I didn't seem to be able to get the right part of the picture; sometimes I seem to look at one, sometimes at the other. I have to reason out the meaning of the whole picture." Dr P. (No. 24) was confused instead of helped by reflection in the mirror; he had an idea that he must make a movement opposed to that which seemed the natural one and complained, "It's more puzzling in the mirror; I see it's a left hand mirror; I don't think there is anything abnormal about that; I have to remember that it's the opposite to what I see in the glass." Seeing one of the picture cards on the table he said, "I see that's the right (correct), but it would be left in the mirror." This is a good example of the way in which these patients become confused over the general principles underlying some act or idea.

The act of counting was easy and the numbers were perfectly pronounced; but simple arithmetical operations were a trouble to all of them. They were subject to curious lapses such as $6 + 8 = 10$ in a simple addition sum, otherwise solved correctly; sometimes an integer was carried over, sometimes it was forgotten. No. 10, who had been an accountant, could neither add nor subtract; he said, "I seem to get tangled up in the process." No. 18 started all addition and subtraction from the left-hand side working to the right; he discovered that he was wrong, but could not make the necessary correction. Later, however, in the course of the same sitting, he suddenly exclaimed, "I've discovered where I went wrong in the sums. I started from the wrong end. I've been wondering what I had to do with the figures at the end, with the figures I had over and didn't know what to do with. I wondered and it suddenly struck me that I hadn't started right." He added, "I think I could get them right this time; I was always good at arithmetic before I was wounded." I therefore laid the same problems before him again and he solved them all correctly. Here it was not the detailed significance of numbers that was at fault, but rather the general conception of the acts of addition and subtraction. Once this had been corrected in his mind the problems were solved easily.

In every case coins were named correctly, but there was profound difficulty in formulating their relative value as a direct statement, although the final answer arrived at by a form of calculation might be accurate. Thus, when a sixpence and a two-shilling piece were placed on the table before him, Dr P. said, "One in two...two shillings...one in four," and with a sixpence and a shilling, "One in twelve...one in two." No. 10, puzzled by the juxtaposition of a sixpence and a half-crown, replied, "Let me see...twenty-two...I thought it was twenty-four, but it's not."

It is scarcely necessary to add that all these patients found difficulty in calculating the change they should receive after making a purchase and most of them adopted elaborate measures to circumvent this inconvenience. When No. 10's tobacco cost him a shilling an ounce, he would ask for two ounces, placing a two-shilling piece on the counter. If he wanted a box of matches in addition, he waited until the first transaction was over and then took a penny from his pocket, so as to avoid the difficulties of change. Should he happen to have nothing less than a ten-shilling note, he would ask the tobacconist to give him florins only; these he counted and knew that four was the right number. But, if he was given change in shillings, he was lost, and he much disliked half-crowns[1].

This want of ability to relate things to one another came out when testing memory for the position of objects in the room or on the table. In familiar surroundings, with his eyes closed, the patient had no difficulty in pointing to the window, fireplace, door, chest of drawers and other pieces of furniture. But, asked to say how the wash-hand stand stood in relation to the fireplace or the latter to the door, he failed entirely although, when allowed to say "The fire is there and the door there," he pointed with complete accuracy. He knows where they are; he is certain he can "see them in his mind," but he cannot express their relative position.

Told to draw a ground-plan these patients usually fail completely; the various objects are marked down in false relation to one another and in impossible positions. They may attempt to reproduce the shape of each individual piece of furniture and yet fireplace or windows are omitted and the diagram has no outlines. The general conception is faulty, although details may be remembered.

As a rule orientation is more or less gravely affected. No. 10 was completely unable to find his way alone. He never took his bearings

[1] See also Vol. II, p. 169 for his difficulties with change when the tobacco cost less than a shilling an ounce.

and, if he was going to a place for a second time, did not recognise land-marks or appreciate that he was passing over the same ground again. He did not know which way to turn and, if he took the opposite side of the road, became confused and was ignorant in which direction to walk. Given the number of a turning to the right or left he could never find it correctly; but told to take "the next on this side" he was able to do so. Left and right puzzled him greatly; he tried to work them out on each occasion and frequently arrived at a wrong conclusion.

So long as No. 25 could pass automatically from place to place she could reach her destination; but, as soon as she was compelled to think, she became confused. Thus she had firmly associated the Marble Arch with Montagu Square and this again with my house. But one day she alighted in error at the previous station on the Underground Railway and not seeing the Marble Arch was completely lost. The number on an omnibus conveyed to her nothing of its destination; but "when I see one with 'Barking' on it, I see Barking Park and then I know that's where I want to go."[1] Dr P. (No. 24), after many visits to me, made his daughter ring the bell at 4 Montagu *Street*; misled by the sight of the number "4" and the word "Montagu," he failed to notice the absence of my brass plate on the door or to appreciate that the appearance and surroundings were fundamentally different from those of my house. His local associations and memory were insufficient to correct an erroneous act based on incomplete verbal observation.

This tendency to confusion comes out perpetually in the operations of daily life. Thus No. 8 complained, "When I'm going to shave, I can't collect my things; I have to look hard at them all and then I am sure to miss some of them"; and yet once started he could shave perfectly. In the same way he was slow at table in picking out the object he wanted; he could see all the things on the table but did not "spot" them. "When I want the salt or the pepper or a spoon, I suddenly tumble to its presence." After his belt had been cleaned the runners were displaced and "I could not for the life of me think how to bring them into place." This young officer was an ardent and expert fly-fisher. He demonstrated to me a series of fishing knots saying, "I've done them ever since I was a child." But he was not familiar with a reef-knot and after I had shown him how it was tied, he failed time after time to reproduce it. It was startling to notice the ease, rapidity and precision with which he tied the familiar fishing knots compared with the slowness in making one which he was not in the habit of using.

[1] Cf. also the journey to Sweden, Vol. II, p. 386.

Since his discharge from the army many attempts had been made without success to train No. 18 for some useful employment. He complained, however, "I have difficulty in following out whatever I am doing; it makes me very confused. They put me on a course of sign-writing. You've got to keep your eye on a certain spot whilst you are doing a letter. I used to put the brush perhaps between the lines where I should be working." He was put to cabinet-making and told to work from drawings, which he was unable to understand. "I could have made an article if they had given me one and said 'make one like that'; I could put together a chest of drawers from the bits, but I used to take a long time over it."[1] He added that a piece of furniture must be put together in a certain order, but "I used to go the wrong way about from the commencement; before now I've put the frame of the cupboard together and then had to take it all to pieces again to get in the panels. Several times I hinged a wardrobe door so that the hinges came on the wrong side."

I gave him all the necessary utensils and asked him to lay the table for breakfast. He set the saucer in front of him with the fork to the left, the knife to the right and the large spoon above; the tea-spoon was laid alongside the knife. Then he became confused and gave up further attempts leaving the cup, plate, salt-cellar and pepper-pot untouched.

No. 10 failed in exactly the same way to carry out this test; he placed the cup, saucer and plate correctly. He then became confused and explained his difficulty as follows: "There was something missing, something unusual. I got the knife and the fork, I couldn't find...let us say the bacon and eggs. Then the spoon puzzled me; I wasn't quite sure why it was there. If I was laying my own breakfast table I should know because I always take porridge. If I saw the spoon I should look for the bowl for the milk and so on; but there seemed nothing like that and so I thought the best way out of the difficulty was to place the spoon in a position in which it might be convenient for any purpose."

When Dr P. was given a pair of scissors in which the joint had been loosened he was able to cut with the right hand, but not when they were held in the left, as is the case with all normal persons. This test interested him greatly owing to his scientific training and he was anxious to discover on what this difference depended; but it was impossible to explain to him the effect produced by loosening the joint, even after repeated practical demonstration.

These patients cannot play games such as chess, draughts or cards.

[1] Cf. No. 10 and the bee frames and pieces of a hive (Vol. II, p. 170).

Nor can they put together "jigsaw" puzzles; No. 8 complained, "I can see the bits, but I cannot see any relation between the bits; I could not get the general idea." This was revealed by his attempts to play billiards. He could hit a second ball directly and could pocket it with ease; but if he attempted to put his ball into the pocket off another, he not infrequently struck it on the wrong side. For the same reason he was unable to make a simple cannon and was incapable of bringing off any stroke from the cushion. He said, "I have so much difficulty in thinking out the scheme of it."

With No. 10 I tried the following striking experiment. A basket was placed at the end of the room and he was able to throw balls of paper into it even more accurately than I could. But when I placed a screen in front of it without otherwise changing the conditions, his shots became extremely bad and he said, "When I could see the basket, I could follow the line of vision; when it was covered I didn't seem to feel so confident it was in the same place, I don't know why. I'd seen the basket before you put the screen there; I knew you hadn't changed the position, but in some odd way I didn't feel perfectly confident in my own mind that it was in that position."

Drawing, even from a model, shows this want of consecutive memory and intention. These patients do not, as a rule, block out the drawing, but tend to begin at some one point and follow round the outline of the object; this is also evident when they attempt to reproduce it from memory. Told to draw an elephant No. 10 and No. 5 could not form a coherent figure of any kind; No. 8 succeeded in producing a four-legged creature with no trunk and ears. He then said, "I'd like to draw a landscape; you wouldn't think it, I've got a reputation for painting." After making a few meaningless scrawls on the paper he explained his difficulty as follows: "I want the thing in front of me. I don't know how to build it up. I can see it in my mind but I can't put it down." .

This form of aphasia is characterised by want of recognition of the ultimate significance and intention of words and phrases apart from their direct meaning. But other functions suffer that have no immediate bearing on verbalisation; for there is loss of power to appreciate or to formulate the logical conclusion of a train of thought or action.

The patient has no difficulty in forming words and can repeat what is said to him. But in general conversation his sentences tend to tail away aimlessly, as if he had forgotten what he wanted to say. Reading presents no serious difficulty; but the full meaning is liable to be misunderstood. These patients can write, but the results tend to be inaccurate and confused; for semantic defects are more liable to disturb the connected sequence of what is written rather than its verbal form. They can count correctly, but have much difficulty with arithmetic and in recognising the relative value of money. Even drawing from a model shows considerable lack of constructive ability. They are completely unable to find their way alone; for they do not take their bearings and fail to recognise familiar landmarks.

Semantic disorders interfere seriously with the activities of daily life. The patient's defects make him useless for any but the simplest employment; yet his memory and intelligence may remain on a relatively high plane. He has, however, lost the power to coordinate details into a general formula for internal or external statement.

CHAPTER V

THE EFFECT PRODUCED BY THE DEGREE OF LOSS OF FUNCTION ON THE FORM ASSUMED BY AN APHASIA

OF the many aspects of behaviour, comprised under the term symbolic formulation and expression, some are affected in one case some in another, and the form assumed by the clinical manifestations depends primarily on these qualitative defects. But the characteristic changes also vary profoundly according to the amount to which any one group of functions is disturbed. At first the patient may be unable to speak, to read or to write; but with the lapse of time he may regain sufficient power to carry out all these actions, and yet the manner in which they are performed shows that he is still suffering from the same specific variety of aphasia.

This quantitative aspect of these disorders of speech, on which von Monakow has so repeatedly insisted, has been almost universally ignored. The question is asked, "Can the patient understand what is said to him, can he speak, read or write?" and he is placed in one or other group according to the answer. Each such categorical combination of signs and symptoms is then erected into a "morbid entity" or "syndrome," e.g. "alexia" or "agraphia," and attempts are made to associate it with some structural change in a particular part of the brain.

No attempt is made to obtain records of the depth of the specific affection by means of tests of the same order but of graduated difficulty. I have already given examples to show that a patient can exercise some particular aptitude in a simple form, but fails to be able to do so, if the task is rendered more complex. Thus it is useless to assert only that he could speak, read or write; we must enquire, with the help of graduated tests, how much power he has of performing these acts.

Moreover, it is a fundamental error to look upon the clinical manifestations at any one moment as if they were permanent and could be directly associated with demonstrable anatomical changes in a restricted area of the brain. The condition of the patient is not static; from the physiological point of view every case must be regarded as a disorder of function, which is in process of changing. It is either increasing or decreasing, and the extent and severity of the aphasia fluctuates from time to time.

Most patients who come to post-mortem examination are for this reason entirely unsuited for the purposes of anatomical localisation. They suffered from some progressive disease of the brain and the clinical signs were profoundly influenced by the wide-spread functional effects of diaschisis.

On the other hand, if the lesion remains completely stationary and mental and physical vitality are high, the power to use language returns to a remarkable degree. Quiescent anatomical changes are associated with a gradual restoration of function.

But anything which produces neural shock, such as an epileptiform attack, or even the lowered vitality consequent on fatigue or worry, may profoundly reduce the power to use words. This can pass away so rapidly that it cannot have been due to any increase in the gross structural changes.

In the present chapter I shall examine the records of graduated tests taken from patients at various stages of recovery to discover the effect produced on the clinical manifestations by changes in the severity of the disorder of function. The same principles, in a converse sense, are applicable when the disturbance is increasing; but here the general debility and progressive mental deterioration render detailed examination impossible or unsatisfactory.

The more nearly any symbolic action, used as a test in aphasia, approximates to a frank proposition, the greater difficulty does it present. Conversely the more closely it corresponds to direct matching the less likely is it to suffer.

A patient may be able to execute a printed command to hold up his hand, although he is unable to carry out an order to touch with it his eye or his ear. The addition of the second factor has rendered the task too difficult. The larger the number of possible alternatives presented by the order, the more certainly will the desired action be defective. It is possible in this way by suitable tests to grade the patient's disability. First, he is required to carry out a series of movements, such as "lift your hand," "shut your eyes," etc., which name one part of the body only. Then the right or left hand is specified, and the task is gradually increased in severity until finally it is brought up to the multiple alternatives of the full hand, eye and ear tests. Somewhere on this ascending scale of difficulty, most aphasics will break down.

By bearing these principles in mind we are able to compare the severity of the disturbance of function in any two patients belonging to the same class of aphasia and to determine the degree of recovery or deterioration in a single individual at different periods. Because a man, who was unable to read or write, regains his power to carry out these acts, there is no reason to suppose that the situation or extent of his cerebral lesion has changed materially. The clinical manifestations may have altered in character solely in consequence of the diminished degree to which some particular language function is affected.

§1. A CASE OF ACUTE VERBAL APHASIA FOLLOWED THROUGH VARIOUS STAGES OF RECOVERY

The following example illustrates the effect produced on the manifestations of verbal aphasia by the acuteness and severity of the disturbance. So little permanent injury was produced in this patient by an operation for the removal of an intracranial tumour that recovery of function was rapid and could be recorded by means of graduated tests[1].

The patient was a middle-aged woman who for six years had suffered at rare intervals from seizures beginning in the right hand; six of these were sufficiently severe to be accompanied by loss of consciousness. From time to time she had also had slighter attacks which began with a "numb feeling" in the right thumb followed by involuntary flexion of all the digits. On May 20th, 1922, she experienced these symptoms without loss of consciousness; but, after the seizure was over, she was alarmed to find that she could not speak for several hours.

Ten days later, when she first came under my observation, speech was perfect and I could find no abnormal physical signs of any kind, except loss of the reflexes over the right half of the abdominal wall.

At the operation, on June 20th, a smooth lobulated growth was exposed springing from the dura mater on the left side; this had severely indented the substance of the brain in the region where the inferior frontal meets the precentral fissure. It was so carefully extracted by Mr Wilfred Trotter that not the smallest fragment of cortical tissue adhered to the tumour after removal.

This operation was followed by complete verbal aphasia and flaccid right hemiplegia accompanied by the usual changes in the reflexes on the affected half of the body. At no time was sensation in any way disturbed.

She improved rapidly day by day both physically and in her powers of speech. Her general condition was so unusually good that I was able to follow her recovery by means of serial tests, which yielded invaluable records illustrating the relation to one another of the various forms of verbal formulation and expression and of the order in which they were restored.

[1] No. 20, fully reported in Vol. II, pp. 295 to 319.

At first she was speechless except for "yes" and "no" and even "no" was at times wrongly employed. She seemed to understand simple orders, but frequently failed to comprehend the full significance of questions and was profoundly puzzled by her inability to express her wants. Told to touch her nose or give her hand she could do so, but became confused if I specified the right or the left.

When tested on the seventh day with a set of familiar objects in the usual way, she could point with ease to the one on the table, corresponding to that which she had seen or held in her hand out of sight; the act of matching was evidently performed with ease. She also chose correctly, though more slowly, to oral commands and made two mistakes only, when the order was given in the form of a printed word. She named these objects in ten out of eighteen attempts and most of her failures were due to defective word-formation; for the sounds she uttered bore an evident relation to the names she was seeking. When she attempted to write them down without saying them aloud, writing and spelling were defective; and this was the case even if she copied the words from print. But she was able to repeat them after me although her articulation was imperfect. Three weeks later all these tests could be carried out, but she still had difficulty in writing down the names of objects shown to her; each word corresponded to the usual nomenclature, but the spelling was poor and the letters were badly formed. Four months after the operation she could write the names perfectly and this test was the last of the group to show complete recovery.

The alphabet formed a most instructive guide to the order in which her powers of verbal formulation and expression were restored. On the seventh day after the operation she could not say the letters in proper sequence, but repeated them after me and read them aloud correctly. If she attempted to write them down without saying them aloud, many were badly formed and the order was imperfect. Even when the letters of the alphabet were displayed before her, she tended to copy them in capitals and could not translate them into cursive script.

Ten days later she said the alphabet without a mistake. But, when I gave her the twenty-six block letters and asked her to arrange them in order, she was unable to do so; and yet she could read them perfectly aloud. She transcribed printed capitals into cursive handwriting very imperfectly and wrote the alphabet badly even to dictation.

Improvement steadily continued and four months after the operation she could execute all these tests, although, when she wrote spontaneously or copied the letters they still showed slight defects of form.

The hand, eye and ear tests not only gave an insight into the nature of her defect but admirably illustrated the mode of her recovery. At first, although she obviously understood simple statements, she was liable to become confused if the words implied an order. She could touch her nose with her right or left hand; but, when asked to bring one or other hand into contact with either the eye or the nose, she frequently failed to do so.

On the tenth day after the operation I was able to carry out a more complete series of tests on these lines. There was no question that she now understood in general what she was asked to do; but a series of oral commands to touch one or other eye or ear with the right or left hand were imperfectly executed. To orders given in print she failed to exactly the same extent.

She had not the slightest difficulty in imitating these movements made by me, when they were reflected in a mirror; this is an act of almost pure imitation as far as this form of aphasia is concerned. Sitting face to face she failed in eight out of sixteen attempts. Asked to describe my movements in writing, she was unable to do so; she put down right or left to correspond to the hand I had used, omitting any indication of which eye or ear I had touched. Moreover, the words were badly formed and, towards the end of this series, her writing became illegible.

The first of these tests to show recovery was her response to oral commands, which were correctly carried out twenty-six days after the operation. At this time printed orders were imperfectly executed. A week later the only forms of this test in which she failed were imitation of my movements sitting face to face and writing them down on paper. Four months after the operation the latter task was the only one that was not performed correctly.

I have selected these three groups of tests for comment because the records were characteristic of the mode of recovery; all the other serial methods yielded similar results. Each task suffered according to the degree of verbal formulation and expression required for its accurate performance. Simple matching was carried out perfectly throughout; she chose with ease the object corresponding to one she had seen or held in her hand and set one clock in accurate imitation of another. Oral commands were executed slowly; she chose familiar objects correctly, but made many mistakes with the more complex hand, eye and ear tests. The power of doing what she was told was the first to recover, because orders given by word of mouth demand little spontaneous verbalisation; the words are pronounced by the observer and the patient has simply to remember them long enough to execute the movements required. Next in order of difficulty and therefore of recovery came translation of printed commands into action; for here the words must first be deciphered before they can form an effective order. Imitation of movements, when observer and patient sit face to face, demands a considerable degree of accurate verbal formulation, even though no word is spoken; this test was therefore severely affected and was not correctly carried out until a late stage in recovery. To write down such movements implies a still greater power of symbolic expression and was imperfectly executed even four months after the operation. In fact writing showed the most persistent defects, apart from those of enunciation.

In spite of rapid and profound recovery of articulated speech these abnormalities in verbalisation were still obvious to the end. She talked easily, her pronunciation was greatly improved and the pauses occurred at longer intervals; yet, in principle, the defects were of the same kind as before and she was conscious that her speech was still lacking in freedom.

In this severe example of verbal aphasia the acts of speaking, reading and writing were all affected at first; even the power of understanding what was said to her was somewhat disturbed. As she regained her capacity to use language those aptitudes returned first, which were least dependent on accurate word-formation. To the last, however, although she recovered her power to speak, to read, and to write, she was still a characteristic instance of verbal aphasia. For it is evident that the slight difficulties in articulation and in writing which remained resulted from a want of facility in verbal formulation and expression. Clinically she had been transformed from a severe example of this disorder into one so slight that it might have been mistaken on less complete examination for an articulatory disturbance only.

The course assumed by the recovery of function in this case is a striking confirmation of von Monakow's[1] description of the order in which the symptoms pass away in what he calls "motor" aphasia. First, internal speech becomes freer and the comprehension of spoken or written words may return completely. Then the loss of power to evoke words ("dumbness") yields gradually; the patient learns to utter those in common use and can repeat them to order. But speech is uncertain, the voice monotonous, intonation defective, syllables are slurred and there is a tendency to perseveration. Emotional expressions are uttered with greater ease and certainty. Then follows a period in which short sentences evoked spontaneously and words in common use can be said without

1 [107], p. 591.

difficulty; at this stage the patient may remain for many weeks or months.

It is interesting to notice that the physical signs followed the same rules of recovery as the aphasia. Those functions which stood least in direct relation with the injured parts of the brain were the first to recover; thus, power returned to the lower extremity within four days whilst the movements of the right angle of the mouth were not restored until a fortnight had elapsed. The last to become normal was the reflex from the lower half of the abdomen on the right side, the only sign that was defective before the operation. On the other hand it is an important fact that sensation was never affected even at the height of the hemi-plegia; for no sensory functions stand in direct or indirect relation with parts so far forward in the brain as the site of the primary lesion.

§ 2. OTHER EXAMPLES OF THE CLINICAL FORMS ASSUMED DURING RECOVERY

It is seldom that opportunity occurs to watch recovery step by step from so acute and severe a form of aphasia. But several of my patients with gun-shot wounds of the head showed profound improvement in their capacity to perform the various tests during the period they were under observation. Each different disorder of language led to some distinct and characteristic form of abnormal behaviour; but the clinical manifestations varied greatly, in cases belonging to the same specific group, according to the amount of the disturbance of function.

Shortly after the injury the patient may be grossly aphasic and unable to execute the serial tests without mistakes. With return of power, the records steadily improve and finally recovery can take place to such an extent that he is able to speak, to read and to write. But, in spite of this profound restoration of function, defects which betray the original aphasia are still evident; the patient is conscious that he cannot perform all acts of language with normal ease, and at the same time the observer notices a definite lack of freedom in some aspect of symbolic expression. The characteristic disorder is still present to a minor degree.

Each specific form of aphasia depends on a predominant disturbance of certain aspects of symbolic formulation and expression. As recovery occurs those functions are first restored which have suffered least, and in this way it is possible to obtain a further conception of the essential nature of each variety of disorder of speech. Moreover, it is only by watching the various stages of recovery that we are enabled to understand those "partial" cases where the defects in the use of language were slight from the beginning. I shall therefore select one or more examples from each group to illustrate the changes in the clinical picture produced by recovery or by diminution in the severity of the affection.

(a) *Verbal Aphasia.*

No. 6[1] was at first speechless and silent; he could not even utter "yes" and "no." But his power of finding words rapidly improved and, in less than a month after he was wounded, he could say the alphabet and the days of the week, although both letters and words were extremely badly pronounced. An attempt to give the words in order led to a string of incomprehensible sounds.

He understood what was said to him and commands requiring a single choice were carried out accurately; thus, he had no difficulty in putting out his tongue, shutting his eyes or giving his hand, when asked to do so. But, as soon as two of these orders were combined, his response became hesitating and he was liable to fall into error.

Given a newspaper his comprehension of the printed phrases was obviously defective; he could, however, reproduce accurately the simple words of the man, cat and dog tests.

He wrote his name and address, but, when asked to direct a letter to his mother, with whom he lived, failed completely. Writing was grossly affected and, although he showed considerable power of putting down on paper what he had seen, in the form of single words, he was unable to write consecutively. Simple phrases were badly written to dictation, but he could copy them from print in cursive handwriting.

This severe degree of aphasia rapidly passed away and seven months after the injury he had already recovered considerable powers of speech. Verbal formation, still obviously defective, was betrayed by faulty enunciation and spelling. When he attempted to say the alphabet spontaneously, many of the letters were mispronounced and the order in which he gave them was incorrect; similar faults appeared in writing and he could not even construct a complete alphabet out of the twenty-six block letters.

It is not surprising that writing in general was gravely affected; the form of the words was faulty and his errors in spelling followed the same lines as his defective utterance. In fact, spoken words and written speech showed the same kind of faults.

Throughout all the tests, simple or complex, he was able to carry out

---

[1] Vol. II, p. 76.

oral commands; for, during this method of evoking a choice, the word is presented ready formed by the examiner. No verbal formulation is necessary on the part of the patient; he has but to understand and to act accordingly. With printed commands the task is not so simple; he is compelled to read the words before he can convert them into an effective order. Thus, although he chose common objects or colours and set the clock correctly, he failed with the more complex choice of hand, eye and ear.

Seven years later he had regained his power of carrying out all the serial tests perfectly, except that his spelling was faulty; but he still remained a typical example of verbal aphasia. He hesitated in finding words to express his thoughts, the pauses were unduly frequent and prolonged, and enunciation was defective. He could read aloud intelligibly, but stumbled over the longer words and complained that, when reading to himself he was obliged to go over the same passage twice before he could grasp its meaning. For, as he said the words to himself silently, he was liable to mispronounce them and this confused him and destroyed his fluency. In the same way, although he could write an excellent letter unaided, he was slow and required "plenty of time." Asked to read a short paragraph and to put down on paper what he had gathered from it, he produced a coherent though somewhat shortened account; he was able, however, to say definitely what he had omitted. The sequence of ideas and grammatical structure were good; but he wrote slowly and with obvious effort.

The only tests which still gave a definitely abnormal result were those with the alphabet. Asked to say the letters in order, the sequence was defective, he wrote them imperfectly and even hesitated in putting together the twenty-six block letters. But he could read them aloud, repeat them after me and write them to dictation.

This patient was a characteristic example of want of capacity readily to formulate or express thought in words. Articulated speech and particularly writing suffered severely, because they demand accurate verbalisation; they were the last acts to recover and were still defective seven years after the injury. In the earlier stages repetition was affected, because of the difficulty in remembering the form of words. On the other hand, oral commands could be carried out from the first; for in all such tests the words were presented to the patient ready formed by the examiner and could be understood without difficulty. Simple printed orders were well executed, but not the complex choice of hand, eye and ear; for this demands accurate reproduction of the printed symbols in verbal form.

With No. 17[1] recovery took place along the same lines and, within five years from the date of his wound, he was able to carry out all the serial tests correctly. He could express what he wanted to say, read aloud or to himself with comparative ease, and write coherently. None the less he still showed evidence of considerable verbal aphasia. He talked slowly, with frequent pauses occupied by meaningless sounds. He knew exactly what he wanted to say, but had great difficulty in finding means to express himself. Articulation was faulty and some of the words were shortened or slurred, although each one corresponded in meaning and nominal significance to what he wanted to say. He understood perfectly all that was said to him, could read to himself and carried out oral and printed commands. Writing showed the same defects as articulated speech; thus, the written account of a short story he had read was full of corrections and verbal inaccuracies.

All the patients I have described so far suffered at first from a severe degree of verbal aphasia; as this gradually diminished the power of executing certain tasks returned, whilst others still revealed more or less gross abnormalities. Yet in spite of wide-spread restoration of function, the essential nature of the manifestations remained unaltered; the use of language was still defective in the same way, but to a less degree.

Sometimes injury or disease, even at the height of their influence, cause a comparatively slight disorder of language. The nature of these "partial" aphasias can only be discovered by studying the phenomena of recovery in the more severe varieties; for somewhere on the upward grade a combination of signs and symptoms will be found, which corresponds to the form we are desirous of placing into its proper category. It is not the gravity of the affection, but its specific qualities, that determine the group to which an aphasia belongs.

Thus, from the first, speech was comparatively little affected in No. 4[2]. To all who examined him superficially with the usual clinical tests, or listened to his conversation and watched his general behaviour, he seemed to be suffering from a slight "anarthria." But more extensive observations showed that his defects of speech were not purely articulatory, even in the highest sense of the term; they depended on faulty verbalisation both external and internal. He talked fluently, but was liable to slur the longer words. He complained that his vocabulary was limited and that he did not possess sufficient words to express his thoughts. On superficial examination he seemed to understand everything said to him and was able to carry out complex oral commands. But he confessed

[1] Vol. II, p. 257.   [2] Vol. II, p. 55.

that he could not gather the meaning of all the words spoken in the course of conversation, especially if they were said quickly.

He carried out printed commands without fail and understood a test paragraph he had read to himself; yet he complained that he had difficulty in remembering exactly the contents of a chapter in a book. This was due to the tendency, obvious when he read aloud, to miss some of the words; such want of verbal exactitude was liable to lead to confusion. He wrote well, except that his spelling was faulty, and he tended to omit a word here and there, exactly as when speaking or reading aloud. He carried out simple arithmetical exercises correctly, but found he had lost the power of adding up columns of figures in his head.

All the serial tests were executed correctly, except the choice of hand, eye or ear. When we sat face to face, or he held the picture in his hand, many of the movements he made in imitation were erroneous; for in both instances it was necessary to express, through some formula of internal speech, the nature of the act to be imitated. On the other hand, the same movements were executed perfectly to oral or printed commands, because the verbal form was then presented to him ready made.

From the first this young officer was in that condition of "partial" aphasia, reached after years of recovery by patients who were more severely affected. He could speak, read and write and yet his defects in the use of language pointed to a specific loss of capacity to form words for internal or external use, the distinctive characteristic of what I have called verbal aphasia. The use of words as names, once they had been evoked, was unaffected. He understood and remembered what he had heard or read to himself, provided he was not confused by the omission or defective internal reproduction of some significant word. Moreover, he wrote with comparative ease, although his spelling gave evidence of defective internal verbalisation.

(b) *Syntactical Aphasia.*

Rhythm, verbal balance and grammatical structure are mainly affected in this form of aphasia and, when I first saw No. 13[1], his speech was jargon. He talked rapidly, but slurred the words and tended to omit articles, conjunctions and prepositions. His pronunciation frequently resembled that of a child who, though fluent, has not learnt to form its phrases. These defects of enunciation and syntax frequently became so gross that it was impossible to understand what he said. If, however, he was made to talk slowly and to break up his answers into short

[1] Vol. II, p. 199.

phrases, words emerged used correctly and with a definite meaning; and yet, on a first hearing, he seemed to be talking incomprehensible nonsense.

The rhythmic beat of his phrases and of polysyllabic words was faulty; he could not "touch off" the sounds correctly so as to produce a coherent sequence of properly articulated words or syllables. Simple words and phrases, such as those of the man, cat and dog tests, were repeated after me better than he could say them spontaneously in response to pictures. But, with longer and more complex sentences, he tended to become confused and to lapse into jargon, even during the act of repetition.

He was perfectly familiar with the names of common objects and had no difficulty in evoking isolated words; but his mispronunciation of the less usual ones, especially if they formed part of a phrase, rendered them unintelligible without a knowledge of the context. Thus, the names he gave to a set of geometrical figures corresponded to their shape, though all but the simplest words were badly pronounced.

He understood what was said to him and chose familiar objects or colours correctly, when asked to do so. He even set the clock and carried out the hand, eye and ear tests without fail to oral commands.

He could undoubtedly comprehend the meaning of what he read to himself and executed printed commands perfectly. But it is impossible to reproduce exactly the sounds he emitted when he attempted to read aloud. Each sentence was said "in one break"; then after a momentary stoppage he dashed off again. With the original before me, I could recognise the words he was saying; but many of them approached so closely to jargon that I should have been unable to do so without this key.

He wrote his name and address correctly and composed a well written letter to his mother. Moreover, he put down on paper accurately the names of common objects or colours and the time shown on a clock, omitting the word "minutes." In the same way, when writing from pictures, he left out the conjunctions and the articles and reversed the order, reading from right to left instead of in the normal direction. To dictation he wrote extremely badly, reproducing the same kind of errors that were so evident in speaking. But he copied even long phrases and paragraphs perfectly.

When he said or wrote the alphabet, the order of the letters was defective; but he could read them aloud fairly and copied them perfectly in cursive handwriting. Obviously it was rhythm rather than form that was most severely affected.

Five years after he was wounded he had recovered sufficiently to return to his work at an Insurance Office. He was supposed to be normal; but the defects in his use of language, though less severe, were identical in character with those discovered on my first examination. He talked rapidly; single words were well pronounced as a rule, but he tended to shorten those of more than one syllable. Speech was jerky because he frequently omitted connecting words. Some phrases were run off glibly; others were shortened so as to be said in one breath. When a word was mis-pronounced, he did not go back like a verbal or nominal aphasic, but dashed on in the hope that he would be understood. If checked and asked to repeat what he said, he usually became confused and, the more he was pinned down to making his meaning clear, the worse became his speech. Moreover, his memory for the form of a sentence was defective; if he did not say it at once he forgot the words of the phrase. He complained "I say it to myself and it's gone again; don't hold it long enough."

He never used words of wrong significance and the names he gave to familiar objects and to colours were accurate; but those of more than one syllable, such as orange and violet, were badly pronounced.

He understood what was said to him and carried out oral commands perfectly, provided they did not demand the power of recalling some phrase of considerable length. When sent with a message from one department of the office to another, he could perform his task with ease, if he did not think about it; but if, as he went along, he said the message over to himself silently, he could not deliver it clearly and his speech became confused. Owing to the insecurity in phrasal formulation and expression it was difficult for him to go back over the ground freely at will, either aloud or in silent thought, and he avoided every occasion that compelled him to do so.

He carried out all forms of printed command accurately provided the text remained before him for reference. But, when translating pictures into words, as during the man, cat and dog tests, he still tended to read them from right to left instead of in the normal direction.

He wrote with great rapidity and apparent ease; single words were usually written correctly, but he tended to shorten the phrases and complained, "When find it difficult to pronounce a word, it much harder to write." Writing to dictation was still troublesome to him, although he copied perfectly.

In spite of the comparative ease with which he could now speak, read and write, he still failed to carry out some of the simple tests with the alphabet. He had recovered his power of saying or reading the letters aloud and was able to copy them accurately; but he could not write them down in order to arrange the block-letters in sequence. He still made mistakes in imitating movements made by me when we sat face to face, or in carrying them out in response to a picture held in his hand. He complained, "Your sitting opposite to me, that helps make the thing a bit mystery. Say to myself, then it's gone again; I lost it, don't hold it long enough." But he found no difficulty in imitating either my actions or those represented pictorially provided they were reflected in a mirror. Asked whether, under such conditions, he said them to himself, he replied, "No, simply come automatically; quite simple."

For ordinary purposes this patient was a normal man and had recovered to a great extent his powers of speaking, reading and writing. Yet he still showed a profound disturbance of rhythm and syntax. His capacity to form correct and well balanced phrases was diminished and even single words of more than one syllable were wrongly stressed or shortened. The qualitative aspect of his affection of speech was unchanged, and in spite of the amount to which he had recovered, he still remained a characteristic example of syntactical aphasia.

(c) *Nominal Aphasia.*

No. 7[1] was wounded on the 15th of October 1917 and, when he came under my care nearly six weeks later, was so grossly aphasic, that it was impossible to obtain from him any coherent information. The few words he uttered were, however, comprehensible and, if he succeeded in producing a short phrase, the syntax was perfect and the syllables were touched off correctly. But he could not express himself either in speech or in writing, and had obvious difficulty in discovering a method of formulating his meaning. Throughout, the character of his disabilities remained the same, although he rapidly regained sufficient facility to allow of more extensive observations.

He failed to say his name and address or the days of the week and the months correctly. He could not name familiar objects and colours and was unable to tell the time shown on the face of a clock. His power of repetition was gravely affected, though the sounds he uttered usually bore some remote resemblance to the words said by me.

He showed obvious defects in comprehending the significance of spoken words and phrases. Oral commands were badly executed; he chose common objects or colours after great hesitation and he frequently gave up the attempt altogether. He failed to set the hands of a clock, carried out the coin-bowl tests badly, and made many mistakes in the

---

[1] Vol. II, p. 89.

more complex choice between hand, eye and ear. Simpler commands of the same kind were performed with one exception correctly, showing that he still retained some power of appreciating verbal significance.

He had considerable difficulty in understanding the meaning of single words put before him in print and selected familiar objects and colours slowly with obvious effort. He set the clock badly to printed commands, confusing "past" and "to" the hour. In the same way he failed to place the proper coin into the right bowl and made many mistakes with the more complex, hand, eye and ear tests. Even simple orders, such as "shut your eyes," "put out your tongue" were misunderstood, when given in print.

Shown any two pictures of the man, cat and dog, he found difficulty in evoking the names correctly. If he attempted to read these mono-syllabic phrases from print, the results were even worse and he struggled ineffectually to find the correct expressions. Asked to read aloud the orders of the coin-bowl tests, he converted them all into numbers and "the second into the third" became "two into three"; but even this simplification did not materially improve his answers.

With great effort he succeeded in writing his name imperfectly, but he could not add his address and failed entirely to compose a letter. He was unable to write down the name of any of the colours shown to him and transcribed the time badly, although he employed numbers only. Writing to dictation was almost impossible; but he was able to copy correctly, using cursive script, interrupted occasionally by irrelevant capitals.

These defects came out clearly when he was tested with the alphabet. Asked to say the letters in order he was unable to go beyond H; he repeated them after me slowly with obvious effort, but read them aloud almost correctly. He was unable to write them spontaneously, had great difficulty when they were dictated, but could copy them in capitals.

He found it almost impossible to state the relative value of any two coins placed before him. Yet in spite of his confused replies, he un-doubtedly recognised their monetary value, provided he was not com-pelled to express the relation of the one to the other in words; for he was able to put together the equivalent of any one of them from amongst a heap of money on the table.

Drawing to order was grossly affected; he drew an elephant without trunk, tusks, eye or ear and was unable to produce a ground-plan of the ward in which he lay; and yet he could indicate one by one the position of the various objects visible from his bed.

Nearly five years after he was wounded I again had the opportunity of making a further complete series of observations and was able to estimate the extent to which he had recovered. His power to use all forms of language had improved profoundly; but, although he could speak, read and write, he remained as definite an example of nominal aphasia as before.

He managed to execute correctly all the serial tasks in which he had failed so lamentably during the six months following his injury. He could name common objects and colours, tell the time precisely and carry out oral and printed commands. But closer examination showed that any test, which demanded prompt nominal formulation or recognition of differences in meaning between two or more words and phrases, was performed slowly and with some difficulty. An oral or printed order. given in a single word was executed quickly; but he hesitated and was much less certain in his response if it necessitated accurate appreciation of the complex phrases of the hand, eye and ear tests. Above all, however, he found trouble in writing. He could write his name and address and compose a short letter with some effort and expenditure of time. But, when he wrote the names of common objects, the words might be badly spelt and in his letter to me capitals were interspersed amongst the cursive handwriting in an arbitrary manner. He said, "Well the... writing or spelling is the worst for me...any long words I can't say."

These faults were obvious when he was tested with the alphabet. Although he was a good scholar before he was wounded, he was still unable to say the letters spontaneously in order and made similar errors in writing them down on paper. He could write them to dictation and copy them from print; but in both cases he tended to lapse from cursive script into capitals. He even found difficulty in putting together the twenty-six block letters. But he could read and repeat the alphabet perfectly.

His powers of speech were obviously defective to the ear of an observer and he himself complained that he had difficulty in finding names and that this confused him. He said, "I can say the names...unless they might be...er...big words...big names...or I can say them all if I have a good look at them...read them over...have a good look at them and say them over." He did not make repeated attempts to find the right sound of some word he had articulated badly, but paused as if he had been unable to express his meaning. Syntax and grammatical construction were not otherwise affected. These difficulties were equally evident, when he attempted to formulate to himself the significance of what he had heard or read.

He had recovered his power to draw an elephant to command, but was still unable to construct a ground-plan of the room in which we worked. If, however, I drew a quadrilateral on paper and asked him to indicate the position of each object in turn, he did so accurately. He knew where they were, but could not relate them to one another.

He was able to state the relative value of two coins correctly, but added, "It used to be awful...I couldn't count the change...not correctly... it is much better...now and again I make mistakes...if I try to do it quick, I make mistakes."

This man had recovered to a considerable degree his power of using language and could speak, read and write sufficiently to carry out all the serial tests. But in spite of this profound restoration of function he still remained a characteristic example of nominal aphasia.

In the case of No. 2[1], who had received a much more severe injury, recovery followed exactly the same lines. In the course of three years he gradually regained the power of carrying out all the tests with common objects and colours. But he still found difficulty in telling the time, in writing it down and in setting the clock to oral or printed commands. At this period all forms of the hand, eye and ear tests were severely affected, except when reflected in the mirror.

Two years and a half later he was able to execute all the serial tests without mistakes, although he still hesitated over those forms of examination, in which he had previously failed. Thus he named colours slowly and wrote down the time and the names of common objects laboriously and with faults in spelling. During the hand, eye and ear tests he imitated my movements, or those shown on a picture, with some difficulty and made his choice slowly to oral and printed commands. When the task was rendered still more severe by asking him to transfer to paper my actions as we sat face to face, he failed in three out of sixteen attempts, the only actual errors he committed in the whole of these serial observations.

Here again the patient recovered his power of speaking, reading and writing; but he still betrayed the nature of his aphasia by the slowness with which he found appropriate names, the defects of writing and spelling, and the want of ease in making a choice to the more severe forms of oral or printed command.

[1] Vol. II, p. 14.

(d) *Semantic Aphasia.*

No. 8[1] was wounded on June 4th, 1916, and came under my care a month later. At that time he was intelligent, but his memory was extremely poor and he easily became fatigued by any mental effort. He could talk and write, although he complained that he was not able to "reason things out" or keep his mind on what he thought or read.

It was not until seventeen weeks after his injury that I was able to carry out a complete series of tests. Articulated speech was unaffected; the words were well formed and the grammatical structure of the sentences was perfect. He could count and say the alphabet, the days of the week and the months in due order. He repeated them after me exactly without a mistake. Nothing abnormal could be noticed in ordinary conversation beyond a tendency to become confused and to forget what he wanted to say. He had no difficulty in comprehending the meaning of single words or even of short phrases, choosing common objects and executing the hand, eye and ear tests correctly to oral commands.

In the same way he understood and carried out a printed order given as a single word or even in a sentence of some complexity. But, when asked to reproduce the contents of a paragraph selected from a book or newspaper, he shortened it down, saying, "I find difficulty in grasping the general idea of the thing; in reading the newspaper I have to letter out each thing and it does not convey so much to me as it should."

He wrote his name, address and the letters of the alphabet spontaneously and put together a short account of the events of his last Medical Board, which was coherent and contained no verbal errors. If, however, he attempted to reproduce in writing some passage he had read silently, he eliminated many of the details, complaining that he failed to obtain the "general idea." He wrote easily to dictation, but said, "I can't be sure if I've written it rightly or not."

Thus the crude acts of speaking, reading and writing were not materially affected; he could understand what was said to him and carry out most oral or printed commands. But he was liable to fail in any task which demanded for its performance precise formulation or expression in words or action of a general aim and intention. Thus he had difficulty in reproducing in speech or writing the full significance of a passage he had read to himself; he could remember isolated details, but could not arrange them in order so as to convey their general meaning.

[1] Vol. II, p. 108.

Like all aphasics of this class, the clock tests gave him relatively the greatest trouble; for, although he could tell the time and express it in writing, he was unable to set the hands correctly to oral or printed commands. Moreover, he hesitated and was uncertain, even when setting a clock in direct imitation of one placed before him; he would move one or other hand all round the face to reach a position, which might have been attained by a single backward displacement. Although in the end his response might be correct, he did not foresee and adopt the easiest method of reaching the goal.

For similar reasons, during the hand, eye and ear tests, he failed even to imitate my reflected movements. Usually this is extremely easy, because the action to be performed by the patient corresponds exactly to that of the observer as seen in the mirror. But, like most semantics, No. 8 tried to reason out what he was required to do and repeatedly came to a false conclusion. He grew confused and sometimes imitated me directly, whilst at others he reversed his movements, as if we had been sitting face to face. Precisely the same mistakes occurred when he attempted to carry out these acts from pictures reflected in the glass.

Arithmetic gave him considerable trouble and, in spite of his education, he made several mistakes in the simplest addition and subtraction sums.

He had no difficulty in naming any coin shown to him; but, when any two were placed before him, he could not express their relative value with certainty. This led to much confusion in the monetary transactions of daily life.

A simple, straightforward picture was appreciated readily; but, as soon as it conveyed a command, he failed to recognise its full significance. So long as the point of a joke was comprised within the limits of a picture, he could understand it; if, however, for its complete comprehension, he was compelled to combine it with a printed legend, he failed to recognise its full meaning.

He had always been extremely fond of drawing and possessed a considerable reputation in his family for his sketches; but since he was wounded this faculty had deserted him. Asked to draw an elephant he moved his pencil about aimlessly, saying, "I can't get the idea." Ultimately he succeeded in drawing a figure with an eye, tusks and four legs, but he omitted the trunk.

All sense of direction was lost and, although he could find his way about the house, he complained, "I haven't a clear idea of the whole house, how one room opens into another and that sort of thing."

When at table he found difficulty in picking out the object he required, such as the milk jug. In the same way, during his preparations for shaving, he could not collect the things he required and, when the slides on his belt were displaced, was unable to think how to restore them to their right position.

As might have been expected, all games were impossible and he failed to put together the portions of a puzzle. "I could see the bits," he said, "but I could not see any relation between them; I could not get the general idea."

This patient improved profoundly and, six years after the first examination, could carry out all the serial tests without a mistake. But he still showed in a minor degree all those disabilities, which had made him so characteristic an example of semantic aphasia; for, although his replies were correct, those actions in which he had failed during the earlier stages were still performed slowly and with hesitation. Thus he could tell the time quickly and write it down with comparative ease, but was less certain, when setting the clock to oral or printed commands; it was this group of tests that had given him trouble at first. On the contrary, during the choice of hand, eye and ear, he had no difficulty with orders given by word of mouth or in print, but was slow in imitating movements made by me sitting face to face or shown on a picture held in his hand. For it was in these tests more particularly that he failed during the first five years.

He still showed extraordinary want of power to coordinate detail in thought and action; this easily led to confusion and made him appear stupid, in spite of his general intelligence and education. Thus, he wrote down beforehand a series of questions with regard to his future plans, but could not correlate my reply to each one in turn with that to the subsequent question on his list. I was forced to let him ask all his questions seriatim and then to answer the whole of them in a single statement, which he wrote down to dictation. He had regained his power of carrying out simple arithmetical exercises and, on his journey to the East, managed his pocket money and kept accounts of his personal expenditure. But he could not estimate the amount of money required for an expedition and was unable to decide on routes or look up the trains; these he was forced to leave to his companion.

Here again the patient recovered his power of speaking, reading, writing and carrying out all the serial tests; and yet he still found difficulty in comprehending and retaining the general intention of a task set him, or of formulating to himself the goal of some action he was about to perform.

§ 3. THE RELATIVE ORDER IN WHICH THE VARIOUS ACTS OF
LANGUAGE RECOVER IN DIFFERENT FORMS OF APHASIA

Every case of aphasia is the response of an individual to some want of
power to employ language and represents a personal reaction to mechanical
difficulties in speech. No two patients exhibit the same signs and
symptoms; still less do the phenomena of recovery follow exactly the
same course. But by comparing on broad lines the manner in which
function is restored in cases of each particular variety of aphasia, it is
obvious that some acts of speech are recovered sooner than others, and
we thereby obtain an insight into the essential nature of the clinical
phenomena. Moreover, comparison of the sequence of recovery in
various groups of disordered speech throws light on the differences
between them; for certain aspects of behaviour are not only more severely
disturbed, but remain affected over a longer period than others.

Thus, for instance, as a severe and acute *verbal aphasia* gradually
passes away, power to execute oral commands and comprehension of
spoken words are first of all restored. But, although the patient can choose
familiar objects correctly in response to an order given by word of mouth,
he may be unable to set the hands of a clock or carry out the hand, eye
and ear tests; these frequently yield defective records, even when he
seems to understand everything said to him in general conversation.
Thus, capacity to perform any of these tasks to oral commands is
restored in the order to their normal difficulty.

At about the same period the patient becomes able to comprehend
printed matter and can carry out a command read silently. But here
again the easier tasks can be executed long before it is possible to perform
those of greater complexity. He can choose a common object at a time
when he is unable to set the clock to printed commands, and the last
tests to become normal are those of hand, eye and ear.

To name an object or colour in spoken words is at first impossible on
account of the extreme verbal defects and not because the patient is
unable to recognise its usual designation; for he can make a correct
choice in response to either oral or printed commands. Moreover, he
can frequently carry out a still harder task and select without fail a
printed card bearing the name of an object or pictorial combination
shown to him. Even at a time when he can scarcely say a word, the
sounds he utters in his attempts to name an object, frequently bear some
obvious resemblance to its usual designation.

Articulated speech is severely affected in verbal aphasia and the acts of repetition and reading aloud suffer in proportion to the amount and nature of the articulatory loss. Both are restored with the capacity to form words for external speech; but the power of repetition and reading aloud, judged by the character of the performance and the severity of the task, is always in advance of spontaneous speech. For, when he repeats or reads them aloud, the words are presented to him ready made; he is not compelled to formulate them unaided, but has simply to express them in comprehensible articulate sounds.

The characteristic features of this variety of aphasia depend on defective verbal formation, not only for external, but also for internal speech. Spontaneous writing is therefore severely affected and recovers slowly step by step with the power of correct enunciation. Even when the patient appears on superficial examination to have recovered completely, slight defects in word-formation are evident as he talks, and errors of a similar kind appear in writing and spelling.

When asked to write to dictation or to copy print in cursive handwriting, most persons, especially of the uneducated class, say the words to themselves silently; sometimes the lips can be seen to move and perhaps a whisper is audible, but usually no sound is uttered. It is not surprising, therefore, to find that both these acts are somewhat disturbed in verbal aphasia; the letters are poorly formed, words are mis-spelt and occasionally omitted. Provided the patient is highly educated, the power of copying and writing to dictation recovers somewhat more quickly than that of spontaneous writing; but in persons who have attended an elementary school only, all forms of writing may remain equally defective, although external speech has recovered sufficiently for daily use.

Counting and the power to employ numbers suffer severely and these patients are frequently compelled to express themselves in a sequence of single numerals; thus 110 becomes "one, one, oh." But the meaning of numbers, presented orally or in print, is not disturbed; even if the patient says the wrong one, he acts as if he had said it correctly. Thus it is not surprising that counting and the use of numerals are recovered pari passu with the power of verbal formation, both in articulatory speech and writing.

In verbal aphasia articulatory speech and the power of writing correctly continue to be more or less defective long after other aspects of symbolic formulation and expression are normal. Comprehension of oral and printed commands is the first to recover and ability to name an object, apart from the difficulty in verbal formation, is disturbed in the severest stages only, if at all.

Syntactical aphasia consists essentially of defects in grammatical structure and rhythm. Any act which requires orderly balance and verbal coordination, either in external or internal speech, is liable to suffer, not only more severely, but for a longer period. Even after the patient has regained power to execute all the ordinary tests, his articulation still betrays evidence of these faults.

Repetition and reading aloud show the same defects to a less degree and consequently, in the course of recovery, are always somewhat ahead of voluntary speech.

The power of naming is little if at all affected, except in as far as the words are badly enunciated. Even if the sounds uttered are entirely incomprehensible, the patient may be able to designate familiar objects correctly in writing.

From the first he usually comprehends single words and can choose some familiar object to commands given orally or in print. But, if he attempts to carry out an order couched in a short sentence or combination of words, he is liable to become confused, because he has difficulty in formulating it to himself with accuracy. He fails to remember the exact order of the words and is troubled by internal jargon; moreover, with the man, cat and dog tests, he tends to reverse the order of the two pictures shown to him and reads indifferently from right to left and left to right. These defects may become manifest in general conversation and the patient fails at times to understand exactly what is said to him, although it may have a direct bearing on some subject started by himself. So long as the talk consists of short phrases or questions, they are usually understood correctly; but, as soon as they are sufficiently extended to require verbal registration on the part of the hearer, they are liable to be misunderstood. Internal speech fails from lack of orderly coordination.

The power of writing exceeds that of articulated speech throughout, and the patient may be unable to read aloud what he has written spontaneously. He can usually write down the names of objects, even though the words he utters are incomprehensible. But, when he is asked to convey in writing the meaning of what he has read or heard, he is liable to be betrayed into jargon; the words are badly spelt and the phrases imperfect. This may be the case, even when the sentences are dictated; but, from the first, these patients can copy from print, although they are unable to read correctly what they have written.

These difficulties persist and, so long as articulatory speech shows any evidence of syntactical defects, the patient does not regain his power to reproduce to order, with freedom and correctness, what he has heard or read; and yet he can write the names of objects and may even be able to compose a short letter spontaneously.

Such patients can count freely; the numerical order is accurate and the name given to each numeral, however badly pronounced, corresponds recognisably to its proper designation. It is not the meaning of numbers, but the enunciation of the words which is defective, and this is recovered simultaneously with the use of articulated speech.

With *nominal aphasia* the patient can neither find names nor understand the meaning of nominal expressions presented to him either orally or in print. Articulatory speech is at first severely affected, but recovers rapidly and the patient gives long and elaborate accounts of why he cannot express himself or understand what he hears or reads. It is not words which he lacks, but distinctive designations for what he wants to say or think.

Repetition and reading aloud, though at first severely affected, are quickly restored and to repeat or read an order aloud is a material aid to its execution.

Writing suffers severely throughout; for, as the patient has grave difficulty in finding the nominal expression he requires, this is greatly increased, when he is compelled to transform it into written symbols. Even after articulatory speech has recovered, so that the defects are scarcely noticeable, spelling tends to remain astonishingly bad.

Writing to dictation and copying print in cursive script are affected in the earlier stages of nominal aphasia, because of the difficulty in finding the correct letters required to form the words demanded by the task. But both of these acts are easier than spontaneous writing and consequently recover earlier and more completely.

Throughout all forms of writing these patients not only select wrong words and correct themselves with difficulty, but show a tendency to interject irrelevant capitals; these appear even in the middle of words, mingled with the small cursive letters.

The power to carry out oral and printed commands, together with that of naming objects and telling the time, may all be ultimately restored. But, even in such circumstances, spontaneous writing remains imperfect; spelling is poor and the patient complains that he cannot write with ease and certainty. The double operation of finding a symbol for a symbol is a harder task than simple naming, and the act of writing suffers accordingly.

Semantic defects in the use of language consist in want of power to comprehend the general meaning of detail, or the aim and intention of an act carried out spontaneously or to order.

Articulatory speech is not materially affected; the patient can find words to express his thoughts, but his talk tends to die away aimlessly without arriving at its natural conclusion. He has no difficulty in naming common objects, or choosing them correctly to oral and printed commands.

He can usually tell the time and may be able to write it down correctly from the beginning. Should either of these tests yield at first defective results, the power to execute them is rapidly restored.

But any attempt to set the hands of a clock in response to oral or printed commands is liable to lead to intense confusion; the long and short hands are wrongly employed, "past" and "to" the hour are mistaken, and the records exhibit every possible error. It is not the isolated words of the order that are misunderstood, but they do not convey the precise intention of the act to be performed.

In most cases of aphasia the simple act of setting the hands of one clock in conformity with those of another is performed with ease. The semantic patient, however, carries it out clumsily; he reaches the goal by a roundabout way instead of by the shortest and most direct method. Thus, in order to shift the long hand from 50 minutes to 45 minutes, he may move it all round the clock unable to appreciate that he could have arrived at the same result by shifting it backwards five minutes.

It is interesting to find that in this form of aphasia it is easier to perform the hand, eye and ear movements to oral and printed commands than to set the hands of a clock. From the first the patient may be able to carry out the former test; even if it is defective in the severer stages, the records obtained to orders given by word of mouth or in print become normal long before the clock can be set correctly.

But the hand, eye and ear tests reveal another significant peculiarity. To copy movements made by the observer, or their pictorial representation, when reflected in a mirror, is for most persons a simple act of matching. The patient does not think whether he must use his right or his left hand to touch one or other eye or ear; he simply imitates what he sees in the glass. But, with semantic defects, he fails to recognise that the act he is asked to perform requires no reasoning. He attempts to argue the matter out just as if he were sitting face to face and consequently arrives at wrong conclusions. Even these are inconstant, for at one moment he reverses the movement, at another carries it out correctly and even mistakes eye for ear or vice versa. This form of error may appear in all very severe forms of aphasia; but in the semantic variety it tends to persist, until the whole set of hand, eye and ear tests can be executed without mistakes. For the patient does not appreciate that there is a fundamental difference in principle between the request to imitate my movements sitting face to face and the reproduction of those he sees in the mirror. It is his general conception that is at fault.

The power of writing spontaneously is restored early in the course of the case; but the patient writes with great rapidity as if afraid of forgetting what he wants to say. The letters are often badly formed and spelling may be defective in the severer stages; these faults disappear rapidly as he improves.

Orientation and the power of recognising the relation of external objects to one another are always gravely affected; they are recovered late, if at all. In the same way drawing to order, at first almost impossible, remains affected in most cases so long as any signs of this disorder persist.

The patient can count and recognise numbers with ease. But he has profound difficulty with all forms of calculation. Simple arithmetic may be impossible and he is unable to reckon how much change he should receive, except in the simplest terms. These disabilities remain and form a fundamental manifestation of this variety of aphasia.

Any form of behaviour which requires recognition of general significance or intention tends to suffer, and such defects persist more or less to the end. I have seen no case in which they disappeared entirely.

§4. REGRESSION

So far I have considered solely the phenomena associated with recovery of speech; but those which accompany its progressive degradation are equally instructive, especially if they are temporary. Everyone who has examined patients with aphasia systematically, must have been struck by the way in which they vary from time to time even during a single sitting. This is particularly true of those elderly individuals, who form the material for the study of this subject in civilian practice; in them fatigue or loss of temper may obliterate all power of responding to an otherwise easy test.

For instance, No. 19, an example of severe verbal aphasia, usually had no difficulty in carrying out oral commands. Whenever he left the hospital to visit my house, it was the custom of his wife to meet him in order that they might spend some time together. One day she wrote him a note, which he found on arrival, excusing herself on the ground of a business engagement. This disturbed him greatly, for he had recently been growing jealous and anxious about her conduct. The records I then obtained to oral commands were marred by several unusual errors. Asked what troubled him, he burst into tears and confided his suspicions to me. These I was able to allay and the sitting was suspended until the afternoon, when I obtained another series of records to the same tests, which were entirely free from errors of any kind.

Sometimes, in consequence of fatigue, all capacity to carry out some particular task dies away in the course of a set of observations. Mrs B. (No. 20) had regained her power of writing to a considerable degree. But, during a series of attempts to record exactly the movements made by me in the hand, eye and ear tests, she broke down at the twelfth observation and her writing was reduced to an illegible scrawl. An identical failure occurred with the same test, when she was examined during the period of her relapse.

Any increase in the organic destruction of tissue, especially if it occurs acutely, produces a profound degradation of function, which radiates into parts at a distance from the diseased focus. This is the "diaschisis" of von Monakow and, whatever theoretical conception we may form of its nature, it is an undoubted clinical fact. But in this section, under the term "regression," I wish to lay stress on those temporary variations in function, which occur in consequence of other than increased structural changes.

Such phenomena occur frequently in the daily life of normal persons. When we are tired or worried, we are liable to forget words and names, to make unaccustomed mistakes in spelling, to interject some absurd jargon word into our conversation, or to forget the point of a story in the telling. If this can happen with an intact brain, these defects of function are more easily produced and assume an infinitely more severe form, when there is an organic lesion.

But it must not be forgotten that with brain injuries such temporary loss of power is not confined to speech; it occurs in every part where the functions are in any way diminished. Thus, fatigue not only makes it more difficult to find words, but may at the same time evoke abnormal sensations in the face and hand. Regression may appear in the activities of any mechanical system from the high-grade aptitudes of speech down to the condition of the superficial reflexes. There is no hard and fast line between psychical and somatic reactions; both kinds of response tend to suffer if the capacity of the central nervous system is lowered, and all forms of regression may occur simultaneously.

Nothing is a more potent cause for regression than an epileptiform attack. Thus, a verbal aphasic (No. 17) complained that, for a considerable period following a Jacksonian convulsion, he had increased difficulty in finding words in which to express his thoughts; at the same time power was perceptibly diminished in his right arm and leg. Even when the attacks were reduced to a feeling of "dizziness," accompanied by no loss of consciousness or convulsive movement, he said, "I can read through the dizzy attack, but I can't speak so well for about ten minutes afterwards; I can speak, but not so well; I can understand what I read, but it is an effort." During an attack of this kind his right hand seemed to disappear and he was no longer conscious of its existence. Under ordinary conditions, in consequence of the loss of sensibility produced by the cerebral lesion, it seemed a numb, dead object attached to his upper extremity. Here we find speech, sensation and motor power all affected together in consequence of a minor epileptiform seizure.

No. 14, a case of syntactical aphasia, was watched throughout an attack from start to finish. He was answering questions in his usual manner, partly in speech and partly in writing, when the pencil dropped from his hand, which fell powerless on to the bed. He ceased to talk for nearly three minutes, but did not seem to be completely unconscious, nor was he convulsed. Later he explained that a "tingling feeling" passed down his right side and he lost power in the arm and leg. At the same time he could not speak and was powerless to think. For a considerable period after this attack the characteristic aphasic manifestations were distinctly increased.

Should epileptiform attacks recur and become a feature of the clinical manifestations, recovery of power may be arrested and the condition of the patient slowly deteriorates. Thus, No. 15, a case of syntactical aphasia due to gun-shot injury of the temporal lobe, showed every sign of improvement until he developed characteristic seizures. He had long suffered from recurrent hallucinations, which he described as "Nasty smell in mouth make you sick like"; but it was not until six years after he was wounded that they were followed by loss of consciousness and convulsions. His speech, at first typical jargon, somewhat improved; but, with the advent of these attacks, he fell back to the condition found eighteen weeks after the injury. He had less power of repeating to himself or aloud exactly what he was told to do and frequently failed to understand and execute with certainty a command given in the course of conversation; he could, however, still make a correct choice to an order in the form of a single word. But his power of carrying out the more complex hand, eye and ear tests to pictorial commands was distinctly diminished and he imitated my movements more slowly than before. Throughout, his responses had become less prompt and he was more liable to be confused by his own jargon.

Mrs B. (No. 20), from whom we removed an extra-cerebral tumour, furnished the most astonishing example of regression, mainly due to worry and fatigue. The operation was followed by gross verbal aphasia and flaccid hemiplegia; but, at the expiration of four months, the paralysis had passed away and she had regained to a great extent her powers of speech. She could carry out oral and printed commands and was even able to write down the movements made by me in the hand, eye and ear tests, making three slight mistakes only in sixteen observations. In fact, except for her defective articulation and difficulty in forming words whether for speech or writing, little remained of her previous aphasia.

Then followed a period of much domestic and business worry. Her sleep was disturbed; she began to feel exhausted and her powers of speech deteriorated. Suddenly one evening she experienced an abnormal "feeling" in the right hand and the same side of the mouth, which momentarily affected the right leg. This lasted for a few minutes only and was not accompanied by loss of consciousness or any form of convulsion; but she was terrified and "next day I hardly knew what I was speaking about."

When I saw her three days later and put her through a complete examination, I found that she had regressed to a condition equivalent to the state discovered four weeks after the operation. During spontaneous speech her phrases were shortened, the pauses were longer and occurred more frequently and she had greater difficulty in evoking the words she required to express her thoughts. She was slower in comprehending exactly the action she was asked to perform, although she still chose common objects and colours correctly to oral commands. Her writing had greatly deteriorated and, towards the end of a series of hand, eye and ear tests, she gave up all attempts to write down the movements made by me. Even imitation of my actions, when we sat face to face, was so defective that she made eight mistakes in a series of sixteen observations, although previously all these tests had been carried out correctly. She failed to place the block letters in alphabetical order and was unable to solve three out of the six arithmetical problems.

In consequence of my representations the most severe causes of her anxiety were removed and, when she again visited London five months later, she had almost completely recovered. She was gay, cheerful and had regained her power of speech to a remarkable degree. She still had obvious difficulty in finding words with which to express her thoughts and articulation was somewhat imperfect. But she was fluent and the pauses were shorter and less frequent. Her writing had enormously improved; she even wrote down my movements in the hand, eye and ear tests without a mistake of any kind. She chose common objects and colours to any form of command and wrote their names correctly. The man, cat and dog and all the clock tests were executed perfectly and she failed once only to imitate my hand, eye and ear movements when we sat face to face.

In this case a woman, who had almost recovered from a traumatic aphasia, was thrown back demonstrably in her capacity to execute a series of graded speech tests. She began to have abnormal "feelings" in the right half of her face and body, reminiscent of the aura of the fits which preceded the removal of the tumour, a condition that had not occurred otherwise since the operation. Psychical readjustment caused all these symptoms to pass away and she was restored to a condition more nearly normal than any she had so far attained.

The behaviour of No. 10, a profound case of semantic aphasia, illustrates the evil effect on the functions of the nervous system produced by mental confusion. So long as he remained in the Empire Hospital, where he occupied a room to himself, he progressed favourably. The wound in the left parietal region was healed, he had suffered at no time from fits or other attacks and, beyond his affection of speech, I could find no abnormal signs of any kind.

Four months after he was wounded he was moved to our Convalescent Hospital in the neighbourhood of Richmond Park, where there was a large training camp. Bands played, men marched in and out and the sound of explosions from the bombing school was distinctly audible. He wandered about unhappily and complained that there was "too much going on, it puzzles me. They are always going by with a band and I want to think what they are. It bothers me." He suffered from headache unaccompanied by nausea or vomiting. The discs were normal and there were no fresh physical signs; but, after he had been there a month, he developed a definite epileptic convulsion. He was moved back to the Empire Hospital and his condition steadily improved. A trivial operation was performed on the scar and a minute fragment of bone removed; but this can have had little or no effect on his subsequent progress. All headache disappeared, he had no further attacks and his powers of speech increased greatly.

Finally, some six years after the injury, he took a cottage in the West of England in order to carry out his business of bee-keeping. At first all went well and he was happy; but gradually the strain and worry of the hard work began to tell upon him. The little house was badly constructed and the winter storms beat upon the galvanised iron roof like hail, preventing him from obtaining a sufficient amount of sleep. The new hives, ordered from the makers to an exact measure, deviated from scale and could not be readjusted; this troubled him greatly. Finally the bees turned out to be infected with disease; they had to be destroyed, and all the capital and labour expended were lost. Throughout this year he steadily degenerated and, six years after his first seizure, he had a second epileptiform attack in bed. This was followed by greatly increased "nervousness" and tendency to confusion. He became so much less able to carry out his daily work, that he gave up all attempts at bee-keeping and retired to live with relatives. I did not see him until six months after the attack, when he had again recovered somewhat; but at that time the serial tests gave almost exactly the same results as on the previous occasion. There was none of the recovery of power that might have been expected had he not passed through a period of serious regression.

Whenever the powers of speech gradually deteriorate, those tests suffer first which were originally affected most severely. Regression retraces the lines along which recovery has advanced. But any violent or explosive change, such as an epileptiform seizure, is liable to produce simultaneous loss of function at different physiological levels. Thus, in No. 17, a Jacksonian attack was not only associated with increased difficulty in speech, but at the same time he lost all sense of the existence of his affected hand. Dr Saloz[1] noticed repeatedly how his powers of speech and the condition of sensibility in the affected limbs came and went together.

These phenomena of regression are of fundamental importance and have been too little studied by physicians. This is especially the case with such high-grade functions as speech and sensation. For a loss of power is not necessarily a sign of advance in organic destruction; it may be due to a general diminution of neural capacity in those parts which were subjected to injury. No study of aphasia can make any pretension to completeness that does not include the phenomena both of recovery and of regression.

[1] [111].

CHAPTER VI

THE EFFECT PRODUCED BY DISORDERS OF SYMBOLIC FORMULATION AND EXPRESSION ON VARIOUS FORMS OF BEHAVIOUR SUCH AS SPEAKING, READING, WRITING AND THE USE OF NUMBERS

IN the past it has been the custom to distinguish one form of aphasia or amnesia from another by the patient's ability to speak, to read, or to write. Disputes raged round such questions as whether "motor" aphasia was of necessity associated with "agraphia" and the categorical value of "alexia." But in the light of the facts detailed in Chapters IV and V, all such conceptions are absurd. Speaking, reading and writing may be affected more or less with any form of disordered use of language, and the extent to which they suffer depends not only on the nature, but even more on the severity of the disturbance.

Speaking, reading and writing are purely descriptive terms applied to certain modes of behaviour, each of which may include acts that differ intrinsically in nature and origin. Thus, a patient may be unable to designate a familiar object because he cannot form the necessary word, or because he fails to discover its appropriate nominal equivalent. In both instances he suffers from a disorder of speech, a true aphasia; and yet the two morbid conditions are fundamentally different. To read aloud and to read silently are both included under the term "reading" and inability to carry out either of these acts is called "alexia," although the two procedures may suffer independently. For to carry out a printed command silently requires complete comprehension of verbal significance, whilst to read it aloud demands the correct translation of written symbols into sound apart from their meaning. Not infrequently a man, who cannot execute an order read silently, can do so if he is permitted to say the words aloud; for he thereby gives himself an oral command.

Like "walking" and "running" and a host of similar expressions, such terms as "speaking," "reading" and "writing" designate certain forms of behaviour as they appear to the observer. They are purely descriptive and do not correspond to any distinct functional categories, mental or physical.

This applies equally to the words "aphasia," "amnesia," "alexia," "agraphia," "agnosia," "apraxia," and other terms of a like nature.

They are convenient shorthand descriptions for varieties of abnormal behaviour, each of which may comprise morbid phenomena of a totally different nature and origin.

A man who has hurt his foot may be unable at first to stand, to walk, still less to run. As the effects of the injury pass away, he recovers his power of standing and can perhaps walk in some characteristically abnormal fashion, although he cannot run. But we gain nothing by stating that the patient has recovered from his "astasia" and still suffers from some "abasia" and total "adromia."

The use of language is acquired during the life of each human being and consists of a vast number of ways in which the individual meets his imperious desire for expression. He develops diverse facilities, conscious and automatic, all directed to enable him to face a certain situation by the assumption of a distinct attitude. The orator confronts his audience, not only with words, but also with appropriate gestures. So the words I write are the active expression of my attitude of mind towards the subject under discussion.

The various disorders of speech produced by injuries of the brain manifest the ways in which the organism masters a situation, demanding the use of language, with a defective mechanism. A certain form of behaviour becomes necessary as a sequel to certain external or internal events; some normal facility is disturbed by the presence of the lesion and the orderly exercise of a series of functions suffers in consequence. A new attitude must be assumed; for the patient has to face a familiar situation with an imperfect apparatus. It is as if he were compelled to play lawn-tennis with a broken racquet; many of his favourite strokes will become impossible and he will have to vary his conduct in accordance with the defective instrument in his hand.

The movements he adopts in consequence of these unusual conditions do not form integral parts of his normal method of playing the game. A man who has a pain in his toe walks differently from one whose heel is affected. But neither gait reveals the elements out of which normal walking is composed. Both are due to the assumption by the individual of a new functional attitude in face of abnormal conditions.

All aptitudes, comprised under the term symbolic formulation and expression are acquired, some earlier some later, during the life-time of the individual. First of all comes articulatory speech and the power of comprehending what is said by others. From this moment the power to manipulate symbols of all kinds with ease and freedom steadily increases and in truly educated persons is terminated only with death or disease.

The earlier a faculty is acquired the more strictly does it become organised; it tends to depend more and more on automatic processes, which require a decreasing amount of voluntary effort to set them into action. Any disturbance of function, if sufficiently grave, will tend to affect such modes of behaviour in a more or less specific manner; recent acquirements, on the other hand, are more likely to be disturbed as a whole. Thus, although the mother tongue suffers from some characteristic form of aphasia, power to employ some familiar foreign language may be abolished completely.

In this chapter I shall contrast the results produced by disorders of symbolic formulation and expression on certain forms of behaviour such as speaking, reading, writing and the use of numbers, in the hope of establishing a hierarchy of these manifestations of mental activity.

§ 1. ARTICULATED SPEECH

Before a man can express his thoughts in articulated sounds he must be able to call up the appropriate words and enunciate them perfectly. They must be strung together grammatically into groups to form phrases and sentences, which are comprehensible to an auditor; this demands accurate rhythmic adjustments and the proper use of pauses. Finally the speaker must hold firmly in his mind the aim and intention of what he wants to say so that the form and content of its various parts are directed towards the expression of his general meaning.

All disorders of symbolic formulation and expression tend in some way or another to affect articulated speech. But the most profound loss, amounting almost to dumbness, may be produced by those *verbal defects* which deprive the patient of all power to use words other than "yes" and "no" or a few emotional ejaculations. Even those words which can be employed voluntarily cannot usually be repeated to order.

As the capacity to speak returns, the true nature of this disorder is apparent. Words are badly pronounced, although their nominal value is appreciated; for on attempting to designate some familiar object or colour the sounds emitted usually correspond more or less closely to the correct name, although enunciation may be so faulty that the word is scarcely recognisable. Verbal formulation and expression are defective and not the power of employing words as appropriate symbols; there is no tendency to substitute expressions with a different meaning.

Such patients talk slowly with frequent pauses, which interrupt the flow of the sentence and may divide it into a string of widely disconnected sounds; polysyllabic words are split up, shortened or slurred. The patient gropes for suitable expressions, repeating "er...er..." like an un-practised public speaker. But the grammatical form of the phrases is maintained, except in so far as he is compelled by want of words to change the construction with which he started the sentence. He knows perfectly what he wants to say and struggles to express it.

Finally, as recovery advances, he may be able to talk fluently, although he is liable to slur or mis-pronounce the longer words. But closer in-vestigation shows that these difficulties are not purely articulatory; for he complains that his vocabulary is limited and that he does not possess sufficient words to express his thoughts. To the last, speech retains traces of that verbal hesitation and syncopated rhythm so characteristic of this form of aphasia.

Syntactical defects produce an entirely different disorder of articulated speech easily distinguished because the patient tends to talk jargon. The verbal aphasic speaks slowly and with difficulty; each word is produced with an effort. But, when the disorder of language is purely syntactical, speech is usually voluble and words are emitted with great rapidity; sometimes each one is comprehensible, however difficult it may be to gather the full meaning of the phrase, whilst in other cases the sounds uttered are apparently without significance. The words tend to be strung together with omission or slurring of articles, conjunctions, and other structural components of a perfect sentence. The most characteristic feature of this form of disordered speech is its want of grammatical coherence; each phrase is made up of a stream of more or less discon-nected verbal sounds, many of which may be unrecognisable.

In extremely severe examples the patient is unable to name common objects and colours in intelligible terms. But this is not a true nominal defect, for he can write the name correctly, if it is not too complicated, and choose with ease a printed card which bears the word he is seeking.

The same set of defects in enunciation and formation of the phrases appear, though to a less degree, when he is asked to repeat what is said to him; the words are emitted rapidly, the rhythm of the longer ones may be slurred and the grammatical structure of the sentence be im-perfect. Given three definite statements he can repeat each one ac-curately, although he is unable to reproduce all three in sequence.

At first articulated speech may be completely incomprehensible; but as recovery takes place it becomes easy to understand what the patient intends to convey, although the structure of the phrase still shows dis-orders of rhythm and syntax. Capacity to form well-balanced sentences is diminished and even single words of more than one syllable may be wrongly stressed. There is no tendency to use names of wrong significance and familiar objects and colours are designated correctly, although such words as orange and violet may be badly pronounced.

Nominal defects are associated with a fundamentally different disturbance of articulated speech. We are no longer dealing with a difficulty in reproducing words and phrases for external or internal speech, but with an inability to discover verbal symbols of appropriate significance. During the first few weeks the patient may be almost dumb, with little or no power of spontaneous speech, and it may be impossible to obtain from him any coherent information. But the few words he utters are comprehensible and, if he succeeds in producing a short phrase, the syntax is not materially affected and the syllables may be touched off correctly.

As speech improves it becomes obvious that this form of aphasia depends essentially on want of power to use names correctly and to select words of appropriate meaning. Not only does the patient fail to name objects placed before him, but he has difficulty in employing with ease and certainty any part of speech which acts as a distinctive nominal indicator. Such words as "high" and "low," "up" and "down," "right" and "left," "to" and "past" the hour, tend to be wrongly applied and misapprehended, thus causing confusion in an otherwise correctly constructed phrase.

Asked to name an object placed before him, the patient gropes for a suitable expression. Sometimes he selects a word of similar sound such as "pencil" for "penny"; at others he answers with a more or less descriptive phrase or movement. Thus "orange" may be "something that has a bit of red in it," or a key is "what you use to do this," making the motion as if to lock the door. Occasionally the reply may be frankly metaphorical, as for instance "what you do for the dead" in place of "black."

These patients frequently give long, slowly enunciated explanations of their difficulty in finding words with which to clothe their thoughts. They talk in broken phrases and frequently retrace their steps in the attempt to discover some better expression; when seeking a name, they try one word after another until they succeed in finding the right one, or give up the task in disgust. These defects break up the rhythm of the sentence and even single words may be deformed during efforts to capture the right designation.

Long after the patient can carry out all the ordinary tests, these faults are obvious to the ear of the observer and the patient complains that he still has difficulty in finding names. This is liable to confuse him, both when he talks voluntarily and if he attempts to formulate the significance of what he has heard or read.

All these defects of symbolic formulation and expression, verbal, syntactical or nominal, tend to make articulated speech more or less incomprehensible and, at one time or another, all these various disorders have been classed by different observers under the heading of "jargon." But I want to confine this term strictly to that form so characteristic of syntactical aphasia. For, if sufficiently severe, the patient's utterances are a flow of gibberish, truly unintelligible or meaningless talk, whilst the slighter forms reveal that this failure of speech is based on a disorder of rhythm and grammatical structure.

Sometimes the efforts at verbal expression of a patient with nominal aphasia have been classed as "jargon"; for, if he is of a lively temperament, he may emit a series of apparently inconsequent words or phrases in his attempt to express his meaning or to discover an appropriate name. A woman under my care, when asked her name, replied, "Yes, it's not Mount Everest, Mont Blanc, blancmange, almonds to put in water...you know, you be clever and tell me." On my supplying the word "Blanche," she said "Yes, Mont Blanc, yes blancmange, yes." This was not jargon in the strict sense of the word, but the attempt of a voluble person to find the correct designation; all the words she strung together had some distinct connection with the name she was seeking. In the same way she spoke of me as "Dr Hairpin" or "Topknot."

The slow, painful utterances of the verbal aphasic, though frequently unintelligible, cannot be classed as true jargon. They are badly articulated sounds, which result from ineffectual attempts on the part of the patient to form the words he requires to express his thoughts.

On the other hand, even in those who suffer from less severe degrees of syntactical aphasia, the form assumed by articulated speech can rightly be described as "jargon." For although the individual words may be comprehensible, they are strung together without those parts of speech necessary to transmit to an auditor the full meaning they are intended to convey. Anyone can think out logically, or state some proposition to himself in strings of unconnected words and images; but he cannot convey his full meaning to others unless his phrases are arranged in some grammatical form. Given a knowledge of the subject under discussion most of the statements of No. 15 could be understood. Thus, when he wanted to explain to me how he developed an inguinal hernia, he said, "I got that rupture, after left hospital, when dark, no lights;

when airships came over; couldn't see, smashed the wall, the house like, smashed into wall, couldn't see; had a pain, saw doctor, pushed it up," etc. Here all the words are perfect and convey the meaning desired; but they are strung together in such a way that if the subject of conversation had been less easy to understand, or the rhythm more gravely disturbed, they would become incomprehensible. Sometimes a patient who talks easily in this manner may, if pushed or flurried, lapse into complete gibberish[1].

Semantic defects produce little or no disorder in the mechanism of articulated speech. The patient has no difficulty in forming words or in finding appropriate names and he can repeat what is said to him correctly. But, when he attempts to narrate some more or less complex story, either spontaneously, or as a sequel to something he has heard or read, many of the essential elements are omitted. He cannot retain firmly in his mind that total conception necessary to impart the general idea underlying a series of episodic details.

These patients talk rapidly as if afraid of forgetting what they intended to say; at times this actually happens and the conversation tails away aimlessly and is brought to no definite conclusion. There is no difficulty in pronunciation and, although the sentences may be somewhat short and jerky, syntax and intonation remain undisturbed. Any defect in articulated speech that may occur is due to confused appreciation of the general significance of details and of the ideas necessary for the orderly use of language.

§2. COMPREHENSION OF SPOKEN LANGUAGE

In order to determine whether the patient understands what is said to him, he is usually asked to perform some simple action, such as to shut his eyes or to put out his tongue. Occasionally we are informed that, although he could carry out these orders, he did not comprehend the tenour of general conversation, or that he seemed to be more or less "word-deaf." But there is no aspect of these disorders of language in which it is more important to graduate the tests employed and it is useless to record simply that the patient could or could not understand spoken words. Thus, the oral commands I have habitually employed can be arranged in the following order of difficulty; choice of some familiar object, selection of a colour, setting the clock, and the hand, eye and ear tests. Even though the patient comes through the easier

---

[1] Cf. No. 13, Vol. II, p. 201 and p. 209.

forms of examination triumphantly, he not uncommonly responds slowly and with hesitation, or actually fails completely with a test of greater severity.

Moreover, in the course of recovery, the same patient may pass through various stages with regard to his capacity to execute oral commands. At first one or more of the simplest tasks may be performed accurately, although he fails grossly with those which are of higher propositional value. As power to use language returns, even those which present the greatest difficulty may be executed without mistakes; and yet, from the nature of the response to other methods of examination, it is obvious that the specific form of the aphasia has remained unchanged.

With extremely severe *verbal defects* of symbolic formulation and expression, as for instance in No. 1, even the simplest oral commands were badly executed; but recovery of power in this direction was so rapid that within five months there was not one of the tests that could not be carried out correctly to orders given by word of mouth. In the case of Mrs B. (No. 20), where the aphasia was due to acute operative injury, common objects were from the first chosen with ease to oral commands; but she set the clock badly and made many mistakes with the hand, eye and ear tests. Moreover, there was no doubt that she had occasional difficulty in understanding ordinary conversation, especially if it included a request to act in some particular manner. But, within three months of the operation, all these tests could be executed faultlessly; in fact the earliest and most profound signs of recovery were evident in her power of comprehending spoken words.

It is not surprising, therefore, that in three instances of verbal aphasia, where the patients came under my care some considerable time after they were wounded, orders given by word of mouth were promptly carried out, even at my first examination. But all these young men recognised that in the earlier stages the power to understand spoken words had been defective, and No. 4 complained of occasional failure to grasp the exact meaning of a conversation, especially if the phrases were uttered rapidly or the subject under discussion took an unexpected turn.

In No. 9 I was able to obtain a superb series of graduated responses, showing how capacity to execute oral commands depends on the nature of the task. This patient could carry out all the serial tests to orders given by word of mouth, except those with the hand, eye and ear. He had no difficulty in putting out his tongue, shutting his eyes or giving his hand on demand; but, when two of these orders were combined, as for example "Give me your hand and shut your eyes," his responses became uncertain. As soon as the difficulty was still further increased by giving him the more complex orders of the full hand, eye and ear tests, he made many mistakes. Had the examination been confined to the simpler actions, this patient would have been declared capable of understanding all that was said to him; and yet a more difficult test revealed gross failure in executing oral commands.

With verbal defects of symbolic formulation and expression the power to understand spoken words is habitually less affected and recovers more readily than any other aptitude concerned with the use of language. For patients of this class are unable to find the words they require for speech and, in all tests based on oral commands, these verbal symbols are presented to them ready made by the examiner. If the disease is not progressing, they can therefore understand the greater part of what is said to them; but we are not justified in asserting that in this form of aphasia capacity to appreciate the significance of oral speech remains unaffected.

With *syntactical defects* the want of understanding of spoken words is more subtle and less easy to determine precisely. The patient may be able to carry out all the serial tests to oral commands and yet show curious lapses of comprehension in the course of general conversation. The key to this puzzling condition is given by the behaviour of No. 13, especially at the last examination, when he was supposed to have recovered completely. He understood what was said to him and could carry out oral commands, provided they did not necessitate the recall of some phrase of considerable length. When sent on a message from one department of the office in which he worked to another, he could perform his task with ease, provided he did not think about it; but if, as he walked along, he said the message over to himself silently, he could not deliver it clearly and his speech became confused. In the same way, although he repeated one by one three short sentences said by me, he failed in his attempt to say them in consecutive combination. Owing to this insecurity of phrasal formation, his internal speech became untrustworthy and he could not recall exactly what he had been told. His memory for the form of a sentence was defective; he complained, "I say it to myself and it's gone again; don't hold it long enough."

At this period of recovery, his power of retaining what he heard was sufficiently good to enable him to perform even the hand, eye and ear tests to oral commands. But he was liable to fail in general conversation, because he could not elaborate the form of his phrases in silent speech sufficiently clearly for full logical comprehension. For, in order to understand exactly what is said in daily intercourse, we must not only comprehend the significance of each word and phrase, but be able to repeat the essential parts to ourselves silently at will. This is a familiar experience when asking the way; we are to "take the second to the left, keep straight on and then take the third to the right." This conveys nothing to most people until they have said to themselves internally, "second to left, straight on, third to right."

Should these defects in the use of silent speech be severe, as in No. 14, they may lead to grave difficulties in appreciating what is said. He could choose common objects correctly, when the order was given as a single word, although he was somewhat uncertain in his choice if they were replaced by simple geometrical shapes; moreover, the complex commands of the hand, eye and ear tests were imperfectly executed. But the most profound disability appeared in the course of general conversation; he could not follow up a remark made by me, although it proceeded directly out of some intelligent and apt statement he had formulated in his halting, agrammatical speech. Spontaneous thought was rapid and correct; but the power of exact recollection and internal recall of what he had heard, necessary for complete appreciation of spoken words, was obviously defective.

In this state patients with syntactical aphasia are unemployable; for, although they may be capable of carrying out simple direct commands, they cannot respond effectively to orders given in the form of a complete sentence or to suggestions made in the course of conversation.

The most profound inability to understand the significance of spoken words occurs with *nominal defects*; for it is the significance of the word which is affected and not, as in verbal aphasia, its structural formation. Choice of action in response to oral commands may be severely restricted and much confusion can arise in the selection of common objects and especially colours. Thus, although these patients are usually classed as "word-blind," one of their most obvious disabilities is want of verbal appreciation, especially for the purposes of action.

When an order is given in the form of a single word, the hand of the patient hovers in the air, whilst he ponders over the choice to be made in response to what he has heard. Captain C. (No. 2) explained that it took some time "to get his brain straight" before he could interpret my words into "pictures," his habitual expression for images. When I mentioned a name, he was obliged first of all to evoke the appropriate image and then to fit this to one of the objects or colours lying before him on the table. Suppose, however, that I said some word, which did not correspond to anything in sight, he had much greater difficulty in understanding to what I alluded. This loss of power to grasp the significance of spoken words depends essentially on inability to fit a verbal symbol presented orally to its appropriate object.

Even though single words may yield a sufficiently accurate meaning to lead to correct choice from amongst a limited number of objects, more complex commands are always badly executed. When attempting to place a certain coin into a definite bowl, the lips of the patient move silently; he is repeating the order to himself and yet, not knowing exactly what it means, he hesitates or comes to a false conclusion. No. 2 said, "If I do it myself I can do it as quickly as you like; but, if you tell me to do it, I have to think what it means, even if I say it to myself." When he attempted to formulate an order silently, he failed to appreciate the meaning of the words, though more nearly automatic responses, made "without thinking," were usually correct.

This failure of exact verbal appreciation is liable to lead to want of understanding in the course of ordinary conversation. Expressions, which bear an opposite meaning, such as "right" and "left," "to" and "past" the hour, etc., are misunderstood or confused, if presented in contrast to one another. Thus, when the patient is asked whether he wishes to go out or stop in, he may reply "either," to hide his want of comprehension; but, should each alternative be presented to him separately, he can express his unhesitating desire to go out. During a conversation on the contrast between the rule of the road in this country and that which obtains elsewhere, No. 2 became confused about right and left; yet, by tapping the edge of the pavement with his stick accompanied by appropriate gestures, he was able to demonstrate that in England vehicles keep to the left whilst elsewhere they travel to the right of the roadway.

As recovery proceeds, the power to execute oral commands and to understand general conversation increases step by step with other actions, which depend on exact appreciation of nominal significance, such as silent reading and the capacity to carry out orders given in print. But, throughout, defective recognition of verbal meaning forms an essential feature of nominal aphasia.

Semantic defects in the use of language consist essentially of a failure to combine a series of relevant details into a single coherent mental act. Power to form a general proposition is diminished from both the emissive and receptive aspects; the patient cannot formulate the aim or intention of what is in his mind, whether the thought has arisen spontaneously,

or is the direct consequence of something said to him. He can understand single words or phrases and usually selects with ease familiar
objects and colours to oral commands. His difficulty lies in comprehending the ultimate or general meaning of a series of words, phrases
or other symbols in contradistinction to their immediate significance.
He therefore fails grossly to set a clock to orders given by word of mouth,
confusing the hands, mistaking "to" and "past" the hour, unable to
understand or retain in his memory the ultimate aim of the act he is
asked to perform. The power of executing the hand, eye and ear tests
is usually less severely affected; for from the point of view of general,
as opposed to verbal meaning, it is simpler to distinguish between right
and left, eye and ear than to set the hands of a clock, each of which stands
in a different symbolic relation to the numbers and their position on the
face. It is not so much the individual words of the order which are
misunderstood; but doubt arises when formulating the full nature of
the act demanded.

It is scarcely necessary to add that defects of this class are most
apparent in general conversation. The patient talks fluently, words and
phrases are correctly understood and all seems to be proceeding normally,
when it becomes evident that he has missed the point. Not only has
he failed to appreciate something that has been said to him, but his own
ideas have become so confused that he draws some erroneous or absurd
conclusion. Sometimes he pauses and leaves a sentence unfinished,
having forgotten what he intended to say.

Thus any form of aphasia, if sufficiently severe, may lead to some want
of capacity to appreciate the full significance of spoken words; but each
variety affects the use of language differently and in its own particular
manner. Verbal defects must be very grave before they deprive the
patient of power to appreciate what is said to him or to carry out oral
commands. This is also true to a less degree of syntactical disorders,
which are peculiarly liable to interfere with comprehension of general
conversation. The most extensive affection is found with nominal
aphasia, where recognition of the significant value of words and other
symbols is mainly at fault. On the other hand, semantic defects interfere
with that logical conception of the aim and intention of some action
suggested by oral commands or necessitated by the statements of others.

§3. READING

When a patient chooses some familiar object, which corresponds to a word presented to him in print, the act is one of immediate recognition. But, as soon as he experiences the slightest difficulty, he sets about the task in two stages. He studies the symbols on the paper until he succeeds in deciphering the verbal pattern, not infrequently saying the word aloud or moving his lips silently. Then he looks at the objects on the table before him to discover which of them corresponds to the name on the printed card. Either one or both of these actions may be badly performed and the resulting mode of behaviour varies accordingly.

Again, most persons, when reading to themselves, skim over the words without becoming acutely aware of their actual structure and arrangement. But, should any difficulty arise, the doubtful word or phrase must be analysed and dissected into its constituent parts; although an educated man does not habitually "spell out" what he reads, he must always be able to do so, should the combination of symbols appear in any way unfamiliar or their meaning obscure. This demands capacity to perform two distinct actions. Words and the letters which compose them must be endowed with a significant form and sound values for external speech. On the other hand, the meaning of these verbal patterns must be duly appreciated before it is possible to obtain an idea of the contents of the printed page.

The act of reading is further complicated if the words are said aloud. Normally our attention runs far in advance of what we are saying; we appreciate the meaning before the sounds pass our lips and verbalisation is almost automatic. But, in the uneducated and those who suffer from some defective use of language, the words are deciphered and are translated into sound, or at any rate into movements of the lips, before their meaning is completely apprehended. Moreover, an aphasic may be unable to understand a printed order until he has uttered the words aloud or in a whisper and so reinforced what he has read by a self-given oral command.

But it must not be supposed that these various procedures, unlike as they are to one another, can be recognised as integral parts of any one defective act of reading. For the patient, faced with a difficulty, employs every available means of carrying out the task set him and may end in solving the problem by some method unusual in normal speech. If he cannot recognise at once the meaning of a word shown to him, however simple, he says it under his breath or aloud, looking backwards and forwards repeatedly from the paper to the object, to discover whether the sound he has uttered corresponds in significance to what he sees. Should the figure "5" convey nothing to him directly, he counts up to that number on his fingers. Handed a printed card with the order to place "the second penny into the third bowl," he succeeds in spite of his disability by saying to himself "second into third" or even "two into three."

Thus, analysis of the way in which an act of reading is performed under pathological conditions does not reveal the functional elements out of which it is normally composed. The value of such analysis lies in the light it throws on the varieties of aphasia and the means adopted by the individual to overcome his disability.

Most patients with *verbal aphasia* can make a simple choice to printed commands given in a single word, although the response may be slow and hesitating. No. 21, who was almost completely deprived of external speech, was said to be totally unable to read. Yet he not only chose colours with fair accuracy to printed commands, but, shown any one of them, selected the card bearing the appropriate name in nine out of sixteen attempts. Moreover, when he was given any two of the man, cat and dog pictures, he picked out the printed card, which exactly expressed the combination he had seen; he even paid attention to the order in which they stood, reading from left to right.

But as soon as the difficulty of the task is increased, the answers become slow, hesitating and are marred by gross errors. The hands of the clock are set badly, especially to orders given in railway time, and the records obtained with the hand, eye and ear tests to printed commands contain many mistakes. Evidently the patient is unable to formulate the words and retain them sufficiently correctly in his memory to lead to perfect responses.

Power to carry out even these complex tasks is, however, rapidly restored, though articulatory speech remains extremely defective. Thus No. 19, who could scarcely speak at all, learnt to perform all the movements of the hand, eye and ear tests to printed commands.

It is not surprising therefore that patients, in whom the verbal aphasia had assumed a less severe form, and those who had partly recovered before they came under my observation, could read to themselves and carry out all these tests from the beginning. Some of them could read a book with pleasure, although they confessed that they read slowly and had difficulty in gathering an exact knowledge of its contents. This was mainly due to a tendency to miss some of the words, if they read to themselves, exactly as when they read aloud. Such want of perfect internal verbalisation leads to confusion, when they attempt to recall the words they have read. No. 17 complained that he could not read a book silently with pleasure "because I'm bothered when I say the words to myself. I can get the meaning of a sentence, if it's an isolated sentence, but I can't get all the words. I can't get the middle of a paragraph; I had to go back and start from the preceding full stop again." But it is remarkable how correctly these patients may appreciate the meaning of what they read in spite of these verbal defects.

Since the main difficulty in such cases centres round correct verbal formation, reading aloud suffers profoundly. It is affected in the same way as spontaneous speech; words are deformed and separated by abnormal pauses, articulation is slow and hesitating and phrases are broken up into fragments of varying length, strung together by the proper grammatical links. Provided the patient can speak at all, he can read aloud comprehensibly; for the defective words bear a definite nominal relation to those he is striving to utter.

These difficulties are due to defective verbalisation, both for external and internal speech, and do not occur solely when printed symbols are translated into words. For, with the man, cat and dog tests, the results are equally bad, whether the patient reads the printed phrases or attempts to express in words a combination of any two pictures shown to him. Provided the verbal aphasia is sufficiently severe, the task is poorly performed in both cases.

Syntactical defects consist essentially of a disturbance in the rhythm and grammatical structure of syllables, words and phrases. This form of aphasia is not accompanied by any inherent loss of verbal meaning, particular or general, and printed orders given in a single word can always be executed correctly. In one only (No. 15) of my three cases was there any serious hesitation in carrying out even the complex hand, eye and ear tests.

But as soon as the patient attempts to read aloud, the words are deformed, particles are omitted and his utterance may be incomprehensible jargon. This tends to confuse him and hinders comprehension of what he has read. Should the sentence contain some simple command, the act required may be duly performed; but the patient is frequently puzzled by the abnormal sounds he utters and is liable to jump to some erroneous explanation of what he has read aloud.

This tendency to jargon also leads to confusion when the patient reads to himself, though to a much less degree. A highly educated man like Major X (No. 14) could not only follow all the events of the war from the newspaper, but was also able to read French to himself with understanding. Now and then, however, it was obvious that internal speech was not perfect and he was liable to fall into error, especially if he attempted to formulate silently what he had gathered from his reading. This was much more evident in the case of No. 15, who, though intelligent, was poorly educated; for he was unable to read a newspaper or a book with pleasure and failed to reproduce accurately what he had read to himself.

These syntactical defects of speech do not primarily affect comprehension of the meaning of what is read silently or aloud; but the patient may be misled by the abnormal form assumed by external and, to a less degree, by internal speech.

Inability to recognise the meaning of words is a characteristic feature of *nominal aphasia* and, in consequence, the power of executing printed commands suffers severely. Familiar objects and colours are badly chosen and none of the more difficult serial tests can be performed accurately. Numbers suffer less than words or short phrases and the patient can usually set the clock somewhat better to a printed order in railway time (e.g. "6.50"), than when it is given in the ordinary nomenclature (e.g. "10 minutes to 7").

No. 2, a most intelligent officer, explained his difficulty in making a correct choice in response to a printed word as follows: "When you give me KNIFE I can't see the picture in my brain. All these things (passing his hand over the objects on the table) have no names at all, until I read K N I F E and say 'knife' to myself; then I can say (indicate) what it is." In fact he was first obliged to read the word on the card and then to find the object on the table which fitted it. Should no corresponding object lie before him, recognition of the significance of the printed word was delayed or perhaps became impossible. Thus, I handed him two cards one bearing the word MATCHES the other WATCH; on the table lay a match-box, but no watch. He pointed to the former and holding up the other card said, "Nothing here." Asked what is the difference, he replied, "They are both written (printed); this one is here (pointing to the matches), the other there is nothing. I focus this one because it is here, I can't focus this (watch) because it is not so clear." But as soon as he caught sight of my consulting room clock, he recognised the meaning of the card he held in his hand. Evidently he was helped to understand the printed word by seeing the object to which it referred in front of him; to imagine it and give a meaning to the name on the card was a distinctly harder task.

It is not surprising that these patients have great difficulty in appreciating the significance of what they read to themselves; they cannot understand the newspaper and are scarcely able to decipher a letter. In the vain attempt to narrate the meaning of some paragraph read silently, they fall into the wildest errors and usually end in a complete state of confusion.

Single words are read aloud badly and any attempt to spell them out letter by letter usually adds to the difficulty and hinders recognition of their meaning. Even when the patient succeeds in spelling out correctly all the letters of some simple phrase, he may be unable to reproduce the words aloud. As recovery proceeds, he can, not uncommonly, read aloud a series of consecutive sentences; but, should he fail to evoke the exact verbal equivalent of the same printed word, it may spoil his comprehension of the whole sentence. Apart, however, from this cause of misunderstanding, he generally gives a very confused account of what he has read aloud.

But during simple choice of an object or colour in response to a single printed word, reading the order aloud was of distinct assistance. Thus, at a time when No. 2 was responding badly to printed commands read silently, he made a perfect series of answers to the colour tests on reading the names aloud. A similar result occurred even with the more complicated manoeuvres of hand, eye and ear.

It is interesting to find that the phrases of the man, cat and dog tests can be reproduced aloud from pictures, although the patient is unable to read them correctly from print. He does not lack the simple names required; but it is easier to evoke them from a pictorial representation of the objects, than from their printed symbols.

In *semantic aphasia* the difficulty lies in comprehending the general significance of some group of statements or complex order. The patient appears at first sight to understand everything and carries out the choice of common objects to printed commands correctly. But he is particularly liable to mistake colours, not in the gross manner already described with nominal aphasia, but more subtly; thus he confuses yellow and orange, violet and blue, which have some similarity to one another.

Given a printed command, it is not so much the actual words which puzzle him as the general intention or method of carrying out the act demanded. In the graver forms of this disorder he fails to set the clock and to carry out the hand, eye and ear tests. But as recovery progresses, and in the less severe cases, he may use the correct hand to touch eye or ear and yet be entirely unable to set the hands of a clock to printed commands. Here again, however, the response to orders in railway time is better than to those given in the usual nomenclature. For in the former case the number of the hour stands first and is followed by the figures representing the minutes, whilst in the ordinary nomenclature the minutes precede the hour and in between stand the confusing expressions "to" and "past"; it is easier to comprehend the meaning of " 5.40 " than of " 20 to 6."

These patients can read to themselves, but are particularly liable to be puzzled with regard to the general meaning of what they have read silently. Memory for details may be remarkable. If a number of facts connected with some event are arranged in sequence and presented in print, the patient may reproduce them all correctly, provided he is allowed to say them in any order he chooses; but, when they are combined with a coherent narrative, many may be omitted. Given a series of sentences which lead on by consecutive steps to a general conclusion, he frequently fails to appreciate what he has read. This makes it impossible, in the severer forms of this disorder, to read a book with pleasure.

The patient can read aloud rapidly and as a rule without serious mistakes. Single words or short phrases convey their full meaning; but in the course of a longer narration, sentences correctly pronounced seem to him questionable and he may fail to reproduce their meaning as a coherent statement. It is not words or their verbal significance that are lacking, but the power of welding them into a whole and deducing from them some general conclusion.

§4. WRITING

Writing is a delicate art, acquired at a period of life when the powers of speech are developed and any defect of symbolic formulation and expression, if sufficiently severe, can disturb this complicated act. The phrases may be incomplete, spelling bad beyond all normal limits and the shape of words and letters defective.

Since capacity to write is closely associated with the condition of internal speech, the nature of this disturbance in writing may vary in accordance with the other aphasic manifestations. Apart, however, from these more or less specific changes, the power of writing is liable to be diminished as a whole by any condition which interferes with the efficient use of language. If a task is too difficult, the patient gives up all attempt to execute it and appears to be unable to write; yet, if it is simplified, he can carry it out correctly. The "agraphia" is not absolute but relative. Even in those cases where writing was at first impossible, recovery of function is rapidly accompanied by capacity to perform one or more of the easier tasks. Then the records begin to show specific differences according to the essential nature of the various forms of aphasia.

Moreover, the degree to which the power of writing is lost depends greatly on the facility with which the patient was able to express himself in this medium and the urgency of his desire to do so. Everyone is anxious to talk, but there is not the same necessity for expression in writing. Here the previous state of education has a profound effect; however intelligent, the labourer and private soldier suffered more severely and in a less specific manner than men of the educated classes to whom writing was habitual.

Throughout my clinical observations writing was tested under three headings: the power to write spontaneously, to do so in response to dictation, and to copy print in cursive handwriting. But these three tasks differ widely in severity. To write spontaneously demands that the thoughts to be expressed must be clothed in perfect verbal forms, which in turn are translated into written symbols, and to write the name of an object indicated requires the discovery of its appropriate designation, before the word can be transferred to paper. Writing to dictation, on the other hand, is somewhat less difficult, because the words are presented ready made to the patient by the observer. Copying is still easier in most cases; for all that is required is the power to transform print into cursive script and to place the words on paper.

Any interference with the capacity to write tends to affect these three modes of behaviour according to the difficulty they present as psychical acts. In most forms of aphasia spontaneous expression of thought in writing suffers most severely; writing to dictation is somewhat easier, whilst copying is affected to a still less degree. During recovery power to carry out these three tests is restored in the converse order. First of all copying becomes easier and more accurate; then reproduction of the same passage to dictation improves, whilst spontaneous expression of thought in writing may continue to show characteristic defects to the end.

Verbal aphasia, if sufficiently severe, may destroy all power of writing. So grave a loss of function was rare amongst my traumatic cases, though common as the result of vascular lesions. Even No. 1, who was at first completely unable to write, rapidly recovered sufficient power to copy the simple words of the man, cat and dog tests, although he still had some difficulty in writing to dictation and even more when he wrote in response to pictures. The woman from whom we removed an extra-cerebral tumour (No. 20) could copy these monosyllabic words from print accurately sixteen days after the operation; but she reproduced them with difficulty to dictation and still worse, when she was shown two pictures in combination.

To write one's name is easier and more automatic than any other form of spontaneous writing[1]. It is consequently the last to disappear and the first to be restored during the progress of recovery, and in many severe examples of verbal aphasia it may be the only comprehensible written word.

To subscribe the address considerably increases the severity of the task and many patients who can write their names cannot add where they live. Sometimes a man can write his name and address correctly, but cannot give that of his mother with whom he lives; the unfamiliar beginning renders the act less automatic, heightens its propositional difficulty and it suffers accordingly. In the same way No. 19 could write his name and the place where he lived after his discharge as a wounded man from the army. At a later period, when he was again in hospital, he changed his home and, although he spent all his free time there, he was unable to write the new address. Whenever he wrote his name, he tended automatically to continue in the old habitual way. With severe syntactical aphasia, although the name is written correctly, the address may be given in a curious syncopated style closely resembling that of a telegram. Nominal defects, if sufficiently severe, destroy all power of writing the address, although the patient can produce a good signature followed, in the case of a regular officer, by his rank and regiment.

Any grave diminution in the capacity to write interferes with the power of composing a letter spontaneously. This is especially the case with verbal and nominal aphasia. Even syntactical defects, if sufficiently severe, may make it impossible to produce a letter, although single words or short verbal combinations can be written correctly. On the other hand, semantic disorders interfere more with the composition than with the form of words and phrases.

---

[1] But it must not be forgotten that to write the phrases of the man, cat and dog tests from pictures is one of the easiest tasks in spontaneous writing. It may happen, therefore, that a poorly educated patient finds it easier to evoke the names from pictures than from print; if so, he can also write them with less difficulty from pictures than when they are dictated to him (No. 22, Vol. II, p. 338).

Amongst the various forms of writing to order, which I have employed habitually as tests, one of the simplest is to write down the names of the man, cat or dog in response to pictures. For these three mono-syllables are extremely familiar, easily evoked and amongst the earliest words a child is taught to write. The full test consists in writing "The man and the cat," or some analogous combination, according to the pictures exhibited before him. Not uncommonly the patient simplifies his task by leaving out the particles, writing "man cat," although he well knows what he is expected to do. This is particularly liable to occur with verbal aphasia, when he has so much difficulty in evoking the form of the words that he adopts every possible device to render the task easier.

Syntactical defects, on the other hand, are associated with a tendency to write the words correctly, but in a reversed order; they are reproduced sometimes as they stand from right to left, at others from left to right. But this fault is not peculiar to writing; it runs all through these tests and is just as liable to appear when he reads aloud from pictures.

With severe nominal aphasia the patient frequently substitutes a com-bination of names which differs from the one exhibited; thus instead of "The man and the dog" he may write "The dog and the cat." At the same time there is a tendency, so common in children, to write "God" for "Dog"; and yet he reads what he has written as if it was spelt correctly.

Semantic aphasia, even in its most severe form, has no material effect on the capacity to write the phrases of the man, cat and dog tests in response to pictures. The actual writing may be unduly hurried and the letters carelessly formed, but each sentence corresponds to the combina-tion shown and is grammatically complete.

These specific changes become still more apparent if the patient is asked to write down the name of some object or colour shown to him, especially if this test is applied in the slighter cases of aphasia or during the progress of recovery. Characteristic differences appear in the way the patient overcomes his disabilities and the new attitude he assumes may reveal the nature of the disorder.

In verbal aphasia he cannot evoke the proper articulated word and consequently has still greater difficulty in translating it into correct written symbols. It is not naming that is at fault; for many of the scrawls he makes on the paper correspond sufficiently to the usual name of the object to be recognisable. But he writes laboriously; words may be incomplete or badly formed and spelling is grossly defective. This is particularly evident in the slighter cases, where the faults may be solely those of verbal formation and the meaning of the written words is obvious.

Syntactical defects must be very severe before they destroy the power of writing the name of an object indicated. In fact, the patient can usually write words he cannot evoke for external speech, and No. 14 used to carry about paper and a pencil to help him out of his conversational difficulties.

On the other hand, nominal aphasia is associated with profound inability to evoke the name of an object and still more to write it down. Even when considerable power of correct naming has been restored, writing remains defective, showing faults of the same kind though less gross than those observed in the earlier stages. For to find the appropriate nominal symbol is difficult, but to convert it into its written symbol is a still harder task.

The only abnormalities revealed by this test in cases of semantic aphasia arise from the rapidity with which the patient is compelled to write in order that he may not forget what he intends to put down on paper. Letters may be badly formed and spelling imperfect; but the actual significance and form of the words he writes are otherwise correct.

In order to observe these specific differences in a still more definite form, the test must be greatly increased in difficulty and applied in cases of comparatively slight loss of symbolic formulation and expression. For, if the task is too severe for the patient's powers, he is totally unable to execute it. But if the loss of function is less grave he attempts to solve the problem set him and the records he produces may then show characteristic differences according to the form of the aphasia.

A printed paragraph, containing if possible something of interest to the patient, is laid before him; he is asked to read it silently and to write down what he has gathered from it. Any form of aphasia is liable to lead to faults in spelling and to a degradation in the calligraphic aspects of writing; but apart from these general abnormalities the final result reveals certain more or less specific abnormalities.

Thus, in verbal aphasia the writing shows defects analogous to those of articulated speech, consisting mainly of faults in word-formation and spelling. The sentences are written slowly and with great effort, although they are on the whole grammatically correct and logically consecutive. No. 17, a highly educated officer, said in explanation, "I always have to spell out every word, even the little ones. I have to say 'of'; I know it is a preposition, but then I have to think is it 'to,' 'from' or 'of.' It's not the long words that stop me. When I am puzzled over a word like 'help,' I have difficulty in knowing whether the l or the p comes last. My spelling of Latin derivatives is better than that of other words. I can't spell; I think I can write if I have tried on the blotting paper. I have difficulty in writing the words, because I speak the thing out when I write it." But in spite of all these faults the contents of a paragraph of considerable length were reproduced with remarkable fidelity.

Syntactical defects greatly hamper the due performance of this test. The patient becomes confused by his internal jargon and is liable to give up in disgust all attempt to write down what he has read. If, however, the disturbance of function is less severe, his writing shows faults analogous to those of speech; the longer words are syncopated or slurred and particles are omitted. Even when No. 13 was supposed to have recovered completely, he failed to write down the contents of a printed paragraph read silently. To dictation his writing was better, but showed the same kind of faults; and yet he copied the whole without a mistake of any kind.

This test reveals the characteristic disabilities of nominal aphasia in a striking manner, provided the loss of function is not too severe. Words, badly chosen, are erased and the patient makes more or less successful attempts to write them correctly. Thus No. 2, a highly intelligent Staff Officer, after reading an account of the prize fight between Carpentier and Beckett, wrote as follows: "Carpanter the Hevey champion of [Phrance] France met Beckett the English Hevey waite at the Holborn [Sadeon] Stadion on Thursesday the 4th. Dec after 74 minutes fight [with] Carpomter [nockered] knocked out Beckett with a right hand nunch in the [gor] jaw."[1] (Carpentier the heavy-weight champion of France met Beckett the English heavy-weight at the Holborn Stadium on Thursday the 4th December. After 74 minutes' fight [an error for seconds] Carpentier knocked out Beckett with a right hand punch in the jaw.) The noticeable features of this account are the difficulty he found in writing the names, the extremely faulty spelling, the intrusion of irrelevant capitals and failure to mark the end of one sentence and beginning of the next.

Semantic defects are more liable to disturb the intellectual content and logical sequence of what is written than its verbal form. Thus Dr P. (No. 24) reduced a long paragraph about the planting of a garden in Italy to the following incoherent phrases: "I have Italy as my country

---

[1] The words in square brackets are those he wrote at first and then erased.

and mimosa, 4 bushes." Not infrequently the written account tails away inconsequently, exactly like the spoken narration on the same subject. But apart from these faults in sequence and intention, spelling may be grossly defective and the letters imperfectly formed. Thus No. 10 wrote carelessly with extreme rapidity and employed the same curious sign to represent several different letters. The character of the handwriting depends on the ease or difficulty of the task; thus, Miss S. (No. 25) copied the paragraph excellently, but any attempt to express her thoughts spontaneously led to profound deterioration in her handwriting. Her spelling suffered in the same way; the harder the task the worse it became until the faults reached a degree unknown in an educated person.

Thus, any want of capacity to use language with freedom and certainty may affect the power of writing as a mechanical act of verbal expression. It is rendered as a whole more difficult and less automatic. Words are written with undue effort, spelling is defective and the form of the letters may be faulty. The gravity of such abnormal changes varies profoundly according to the severity of the disorder, but they are not obviously characteristic in the different forms of aphasia.

On the other hand, when the written words are considered from the point of view of their aptness as expressions of thought, specific differences appear in accordance with the other morbid manifestations. Verbal aphasia disturbs the formative aspect of internal speech and makes it still more difficult to write the words required by spontaneous thought. Syntactical defects destroy the structure of the phrase and the rhythmic balance of the longer words; the patient tends to write the same kind of jargon that he talks. With nominal aphasia the principal fault lies in the choice of wrong words and inability to find those which express the exact meaning required. Substitution in thought of some word of wrong significance is liable to lead to further confusion and the patient may fail to write an accurate account of something he has read aloud correctly. Semantic disorders produce a greater effect on the way in which a series of details are communicated in writing than on actual verbal formulation; the structure of the words and the power of choosing those of the correct significance are little if at all affected. Thus the clock tests and the printed paragraph, which reveal the difficulties in articulated speech, also show in writing to an even greater degree the nature of this form of aphasia.

§5. THE ALPHABET

At first sight it might seem as if the various tests in which the alphabet was employed traversed much the same ground as that dealt with in previous sections of this chapter. For, when carried out systematically, the patient is asked to say the letters in order, to repeat them after me, to read them aloud, to write them spontaneously and to dictation, to copy them in cursive handwriting and finally to arrange the block letters in alphabetical order. But, long after he appears on superficial examination to have recovered his powers of speech, such tests may reveal grave incapacity to perform these apparently simple acts and they form a valuable method for recording not only the nature, but the extent of the defects in symbolic formulation and expression.

When a normal man is asked to say the alphabet aloud spontaneously, he begins with great rapidity and, after uttering a certain number of letters, pauses for a varying period. Then he starts the next series, which in turn is followed by a pause and so he continues, to end with a rapid run, consisting as a rule of the final three or four letters. These groups appear to be purely individual and in many instances seem to be due to causes operative at a time when the alphabet was acquired in childhood. Sometimes they are the relics of a primitive verse or sing-song measure; at others they depend on the way in which the letters were displayed on the page of the book or table from which the alphabet was learnt. But, whatever the grouping of the letters, they always tend to show a distinct rhythm.

Now it is remarkable that even highly educated persons depend on these habitual rhythms, when saying the alphabet aloud or to themselves. Moreover, the various groups differ greatly in the degree to which they are formulated automatically; this is particularly evident from the records obtained in all forms of aphasia. To say "A B C" requires scarcely more thought than an exclamation; but somewhere in the region of G H I J, more care must be expended, if the sequence is to be continued with normal rapidity and accuracy. N and M are liable to be transposed and Q forms a point of difficulty, because of the close resemblance of its sound to that of the letter U; it is not uncommon for the patient to jump from P to U and so on to the end of the alphabet. The final three letters, like the first, are again uttered almost automatically.

Any defect in articulatory speech, whatever its nature, can disturb the mechanical precision of these habitual acts; the patient hesitates, becomes confused and may fail to proceed beyond the first few letters. The most profound disorder is produced by verbal aphasia; for, if it is difficult to formulate and pronounce the individual letters, it is obvious that the power to say them in orderly sequence will be gravely diminished. Long after recovery of speech has so far advanced that each single letter can be articulated more or less correctly, the patient may be unable to say the alphabet without gross mistakes.

Syntactical defects also reduce the capacity to say the letters of the alphabet in their proper order. Not only are they badly pronounced, but the sequence is given incorrectly and some are omitted altogether. These faults may be still apparent in spite of profound recovery in speech.

Severe degrees of nominal aphasia also tend to disturb the power of saying the alphabet spontaneously. The patient may begin rapidly but, becoming confused, either ceases altogether or jumps to the final letters, which he says correctly. On the other hand, with a less severe disorder of speech, and if he belongs to the highly educated classes, he may carry out this task to the end with perhaps some hesitation, but no actual errors.

When the aphasia assumes a semantic form, the patient rattles off the alphabet with unusual rapidity, as if afraid of forgetting what he wanted to say. Pronunciation of the individual letters is not affected, except in so far as they are unduly hurried and semantic disorders of speech are not as a rule accompanied by any constant disturbance of this test.

But these defects are not evident only when the alphabet is said aloud; for if the twenty-six block letters are laid before the patient and he is asked to place them in order silently, he frequently finds extreme difficulty in arranging them in due sequence. Indeed, with verbal, nominal and syntactical aphasia the records obtained with this apparently simple test are usually worse than those when the letters are said aloud; the fact that the patient has to pause to select each one from the heap on the table, seems to hamper internal verbalisation and so to diminish the normal facility of choice. Semantic defects alone produce no material disturbance in this form of the test.

Thus, inability to say the alphabet aloud or to arrange the letters in sequence may be a consequence of most forms of aphasia, if sufficiently severe, and is not a distinctive feature of any one variety. Any defect of speech, which diminishes the ease and fluency of verbal formulation, tends to hinder the perfect performance of these acts and we cannot determine the specific nature of the disorder without taking into consideration other abnormal forms of behaviour.

There is, for instance, one essential difference between nominal and verbal aphasia. In the former condition the patient can repeat each individual letter more or less correctly as it is said by the observer, because the symbol he is seeking is presented to him ready made. On the other hand the verbal aphasic cannot repeat the letters with ease on account of the difficulty he finds in pronouncing them correctly. The same difference is apparent when the alphabet is read aloud. But provided the disturbance is not excessively severe, the power of repetition and of reading aloud is always in excess of spontaneous verbalisation and both these acts are restored at an earlier stage of recovery.

Any want of facility in reproducing the alphabet aloud becomes still more evident when the letters are written spontaneously in silence. For, as we write them in sequence, we say them to ourselves before transforming them into their written equivalents. If it is difficult for any reason to find the correct verbal symbol, it is a still harder task to translate it into writing.

Thus all four groups of aphasia are associated with difficulty in writing the alphabet, although for different causes. With verbal defects, want of facility in finding the correct articulatory form of the letters disturbs the free flow of internal speech necessary for proper reproduction of the alphabet in writing. Similarly the tendency of syntactical aphasia to destroy rhythm and order may cause gross imperfections in the written alphabet. If nominal aphasia is sufficiently severe to diminish the power of saying the alphabet aloud, the patient may be unable to produce a complete written sequence of letters. Even though semantic disorders do not materially reduce the power of saying the alphabet aloud, writing usually suffers gravely; the shape of the letters is frequently defective and the patient hesitates over the order in which they should follow one another.

It is always somewhat easier to write the alphabet to dictation, because the order in which the letters should follow one another is formulated by the observer. In many instances, where the alphabet could not be written spontaneously, it was reproduced fairly correctly to dictation and power to perform this task is regained earlier than that of writing without such guidance.

Any patient who can write at all can copy the letters in printed characters; this is a simple act of imitative drawing. But translation of print into cursive script requires a certain capacity for symbolic formulation, although it is usually easier than writing to dictation. Verbal defects disturb this test more gravely than any other form of aphasia and if the loss of function is severe may destroy all power of translating printed capitals into normal handwriting. Nominal aphasia is frequently associated with a tendency to employ cursive script intermixed with capitals indiscriminately. Syntactical and semantic disorders produce a less severe disturbance and the only abnormality may consist of a certain hesitation and want of ease in copying some of the letters.

But it must not be forgotten that the extent of the patient's education has a profound effect on the results of all these alphabetical tests which necessitate writing. It is always easier to say the letters aloud in proper order than to write them down silently; but the relative loss of power to perform these two acts varies with the normal ease of expression in writing.

These tests with the alphabet exemplify in a striking manner the principles which emerge from the study of aphasia. Any condition which diminishes the ease of verbal formulation and expression tends to destroy the power of forming a complete alphabet in words, with the block letters, or in writing.

These three tasks are usually affected to a different degree and in the reverse order to that in which they have just been enumerated. Thus, the alphabet when written is more imperfect than that said aloud spontaneously; somewhere between them lies the power of putting together the block letters in due order.

So long as the disturbance is severe it is impossible to discover from the defective records of these three tests any distinctive difference between the various forms of aphasia. We can only say that the patient was unable to perform the task set him; but as soon as we examine the form assumed by the responses in slighter cases it becomes evident that the failure may be due to several different causes. Verbal aphasia is shown by hesitation and want of ease in articulation, together with a perceptible increase in the number of intervening pauses. Syntactical disorders are associated with slurring and indistinctness of utterance, with somewhat jerky enunciation. The nominal aphasic becomes confused and makes many attempts to discover the correct sequence; he is particularly liable to omit whole groups of letters. Semantic disorders as a rule simply quicken the rate at which the letters follow one another, but does not disturb their order or prevent the patient from completing the alphabet.

But, when we examine the written results of this test, no such distinctive differences can be discovered. Articulated speech as the oldest and most primitive acquirement shows specific changes, whilst the less highly organised powers of writing tend to be disturbed as a whole.

Throughout these observations with the alphabet it is evident that the harder the task from a psychical point of view the more gravely will it be affected. But any one individual test does not present a problem of equal difficulty in all forms of disordered speech; repetition and reading aloud, for example, suffer severely with verbal aphasia, but are not materially influenced by nominal defects. This is another instance of the law that each test is affected in accordance with the severity of the intellectual task it presents under certain definite conditions.

§6. NUMBERS AND ARITHMETIC

To count up, at any rate as far as ten, is one of man's earliest achievements, upon which he depends perpetually in daily life. At the same time he learns not only to utter the numerals in serial order, but to understand the significance of any one of them presented to him singly.

The apprehension and formulation of the relations of numbers is an intellectual act of a higher grade acquired later than their employment as names or the comprehension of their numerical significance. A child can count his toy soldiers and divide them to command into definite groups, long before he can solve the simplest problem in formal arithmetic or state the relative value of two coins. Similarly, when adding together two low numbers, it is easier to reach the answer by counting than by means of a direct proposition; many aphasic patients can add 6 and 3 by saying to themselves, "Six, seven, eight, nine," although they are unable to formulate $6 + 3 = 9$.

The various methods of employing numbers are so diversely affected by these disorders of speech that I shall consider the subject matter of this section under four headings; counting and the nominal use of numerals, comprehension of their direct significance as symbols, simple arithmetic and lastly the power of stating the relative value of two coins to one another together with the use of money in daily life.

(a) *Counting and the nominal use of numerals*

The disorder of speech must be very severe before it destroys the power to count up to ten; but with verbal aphasia it may be impossible to formulate the words necessary even for so simple an act. For instance No. 21, when asked to count, said, "One, two, three, four, fifth, sixth, seventh, eighth, ninth, tenth, elevenpence"; after several attempts, he reached "thirteenth, fourteenth, fifteenth, sixteenth, seventeenth, ninth," and then ceased all further efforts to say the numerals in order. He was unable to repeat after me any of them beyond ten, showing how greatly his difficulty in counting was due to defective word-formation.

When I suggested to No. 1, who was an extremely severe example of traumatic aphasia, that he should count, he struggled vainly to do so, but emitted no sound. He still made no response, when I said, "One, two, three," and asked him to repeat the words after me. But ten minutes later, whilst I was preparing a completely different form of test, he suddenly burst out, "One, two, three, four, five, six." Then he went back to the beginning again, counted correctly up to thirteen, added "twenty-one, twenty-two," and ceased from all further attempts.

No. 9 counted correctly up to ten and the words were fairly well pronounced. He continued "eleven, twenty" and then ceased. After a pause he began again "eleven, twelve, ten, twelve...no, sir"; and yet he used the figures 20, 30 and 40 correctly in writing to express the number of minutes shown on the clock face.

No. 19 overcame his difficulties in verbal formation by changing the nomenclature. Except that he could not say seven, he counted correctly up to ten; from this point he continued "one one," "one two," etc., up to "two and oh" (20). By this means he was able to reach "six and nine" (69) successfully; then he exclaimed, "Oh! you've got me." I suggested the word "seven"; he replied, "I know, that's what I want...sed" and continued "sed-one, sed-two," etc., but broke down at seventy-seven before he reached the close of the decade. The double occurrence of the difficult word "seven" prevented all further progress; but, when started again with "eight," he continued successfully up to "nine, nine" (99) and "one, no, no" (100). This demonstrates how greatly these disorders depend on defective verbalisation rather than on the fundamental conception of number.

Mrs B. (No. 20), whose verbal aphasia resulted from the removal of an extra-cerebral tumour, could count up to a hundred as soon as she recovered even a moderate power of forming words; but from fifty onwards she became progressively slower and her enunciation was slurred. This was particularly evident when she regressed again some nine months after the operation in consequence of domestic worry.

This want of ease and a tendency to slur the high numbers remain amongst the last signs of verbal aphasia; they are present even in patients who have otherwise recovered the power of counting with correctness and certainty.

A patient suffering from syntactical defects of speech may be able to count correctly, but his utterance is rapid, the words are slurred and the rhythm defective. Thus No. 13 counted freely up to a hundred and showed none of that hesitation in finding the correct word, present in some other forms of aphasia. The numerical order was accurate and the name given to each numeral corresponded recognisably to its proper designation, although many were badly pronounced. Three became "free," but otherwise his articulation was fairly correct up to fourteen; then he continued "hif-teen, sick-teen, seven-teen, eight-teen, ni-teen, twenty." From twenty onwards he said "henty-one, henty-two, henty-free, tenty-four, penty-fi, twenty-six, twenty-seven, twenty-eight, penty-nine." Thirty was sometimes pronounced correctly, at other times it became "sirty"; in the same way fifty was "pissy," "pifty" or "pisby." The remaining decades were "sickty," "sempy," "eighty," "ninety," "hundred." Throughout, there was that want of consistency in the use of denominative terms, so common a manifestation of syntactical aphasia.

Should these defects become severe, as in the later stages of No. 15, the patient may cease to be able to count above seventy. At first his utterance was rapid and a little slurred; but, when he regressed after developing epileptiform seizures, he counted correctly, though slowly and deliberately, up to thirty-nine. Then, instead of saying "forty," he began again at the thirties reaching "forty-four" without a mistake. From this point he became uncertain, saying, for instance, "sixty-two, sixty-four, sixty-six, fifty-seven, fifty-eight, fifty-nine, sixty." He was perpetually thrown out of his stride and tempted thereby into some false sequence. At seventy he broke down altogether, saying, "No, I can't think more."

In severe examples of nominal aphasia the patient starts quickly, but rapidly slows down and ends in confusion. For instance No. 7 counted as follows, "1 2 3 4 5 6 7 9 7 8 9 9 10 10 12 14." He began again, "1 2 3 4 4 5 6 7 9 10 11 10 12 4 4 12 14 7 7 17." Starting from thirty he said, "thirty, twenty-one, thirty, thirty-two, twenty-two, twenty-thirty, twenty, no, thirty-two, twenty-three, thirty-four, twenty-six, twenty-five, twenty-seven, thirty, thirty, thirty-eight, thirty-seven, thirty-six, no, thirty-nine." On the whole the words were not ill-pronounced, but throughout there was that tendency to confusion and inability to discover the correct term, so characteristic of this variety of aphasia.

In slighter examples of this disorder of speech counting is not materially affected and it is noticeable that the numerals are not badly articulated.

Semantic defects alone produce no noticeable disturbance in counting or in the pronunciation of the various units of a numerical series.

(b) *Numerical significance*

Four coins are laid on the table in front of four bowls and the patient is told to number them consecutively from left to right. He is then asked, either orally or in print, to place a certain coin into a definite bowl and the command is graduated in difficulty from the complete phrase, such as "The first penny into the third bowl," down to "first into third." Moreover, if the order is given in print it may be written out fully in words or presented to the patient in a simplified numerical form, e.g., "1st into 3rd."

This is the only direct means I have employed for testing comprehension of numerical significance; but much additional information has been gained from the use of the clock tests, especially when the order is expressed in figures or so-called "railway time."

Verbal aphasia, unless it is extremely severe, produces no disturbance in the extremely simple coin-bowl tests, which demand appreciation for purposes of action of the first four numerals only. Moreover, since the defects lie more in verbal formulation than in meaning, presentation of the order in printed words, rather than in figures, does not materially add to the difficulty.

Such patients are capable of using for the purposes of thought numbers which they cannot express. Thus No. 21, who could not utter or repeat after me any numeral beyond at most seventeen, was able to set the hands of a clock correctly, when the figures 1.55, 3.40 and 11.20 were shown to him in print.

The power of understanding and acting correctly in response to numbers which have been wrongly uttered is a characteristic feature of slighter cases of verbal aphasia. Thus No. 17 explained, "When I am scoring in a game, I say twenty-eight, when I mean forty-one. But this makes no difference to my score; I count forty-one though I say twenty-eight. I do the sum right, but get the figures wrong." He added, "When I first began to look at reference books, like the Army List, I couldn't say it was 982, when I looked the page up; but if I didn't try to say it, I could look up the page without difficulty. Silent thought was easy but vocal thought was muddling."

Verbal defects, if sufficiently severe, are associated with inability to evoke numerical symbols for use in external and internal speech, whilst appreciation of their significance is little if at all affected; nominal aphasia produces an almost exactly opposite condition. Asked to place one of four coins into some particular bowl the patient becomes confused and fails to execute this supremely simple task, because he is evidently puzzled as to the meaning of the words in which the command is couched.

If an order is given in print, the rapidity and accuracy of the response depends on the manner in which it is presented. The patient chooses less quickly and is more likely to fall into error, if it is set out in full, e.g., "First penny into third bowl," than with the shortened form, "First into third." For, puzzling over the meaning of the words "penny" and "bowl," he becomes less certain of the numerical significance of "first" and "third." When however the command is still further simplified to figures, as for example "1st into 3rd," his choice may be rapid and accurate. In the same way, with the clock tests, the response may be better to orders expressed in railway time than to those given in the ordinary nomenclature; figures convey their meaning more easily than words.

Told to pick out five objects, the nominal aphasic carries out the operation in the usual way by counting. But numbers may have little or no significance unless they are reached by serial enumeration. Thus, when No. 2 was asked to add five to any written number, he wrote 5 and then made five dots on the paper which he counted; this he did with all numbers up to ten. Above this no number had any meaning for him unless he had arrived at it by counting. Like a child he tended to count on his fingers, or by means of dots on the paper, instead of using figures as direct numerical symbols.

Neither syntactical nor semantic defects interfere with the direct appreciation of numbers, or so simple a numerical task as the coin-bowl tests. The profound difficulties, which occur with the latter form of aphasia, when the patient attempts to set the hands of the clock to oral or printed commands, arise from other causes than want of direct appreciation of the meaning of numbers.

(c) *Arithmetic*

Throughout these tests for counting and direct comprehension of numbers, the nature of the defects differed according to the character of the loss of speech. Each variety of aphasia was associated with some distinctive form of disorder. But, when, as with arithmetic, the tasks set demand the exercise of higher propositional powers, this is no longer the case. Any severe degree of aphasia may disturb the solution of simple problems in addition or subtraction; and yet it is impossible, by examining the crude records of these tests alone, without further observations on the patient's behaviour, to determine the specific form of the disorder of speech.

My arithmetical tests were carried out systematically in the following manner. The patient was asked to add together two numbers each of which consisted of three figures. In the first example the sum of no single pair of them exceeded ten and it was not necessary to carry over from one column to another. The second problem set to the patient demanded one such operation, whilst the third required that it should be performed twice. This was followed by three exercises in subtraction graduated on exactly the same principle; in each series the third was the most difficult and the second was harder to solve than the first.

Whatever the form assumed by an aphasia these tests are affected in the order of their severity as propositional acts. Except in the gravest cases, the first addition could usually be solved correctly; with each subsequent task the patient responded more slowly and less accurately, until perhaps he would give up all attempts to solve the problem. Whether or no he could execute some operation in simple arithmetic depended on the intellectual difficulty it presented; an aphasic, who at first sight appeared to be completely unable to manipulate numbers, might be able to add or subtract, if the task was sufficiently simplified.

Power to perform these simple exercises is restored according to the relative ease of the problem they present. Thus a patient, who was at first unable to solve the third addition and the second and third subtraction, failed seven years later with the last one only. Captain C. (No. 2) was also puzzled by the third, fifth and sixth of these tests; but he steadily improved and five years after the injury had acquired the power of answering them all correctly, although he still hesitated over the last subtraction, which required the greatest intellectual effort.

After adding together two figures, which amount to more than ten, it is a common fault with all forms of disordered speech to write down the total sum instead of carrying over one to the next column. A patient suffering from severe verbal aphasia (No. 19) added two numbers thus: $\frac{864}{256}$; another with syntactical defects (No. 15) gave the following answer: $\frac{3\ 8\ 5}{6\ 3\ 8}$, whilst a third, whose difficulties were nominal (No. 7)
$\frac{9\ 11\ 13}$

wrote $\frac{345}{868}$.
$\overline{11\ 10\ 12}$

The same want of certainty in carrying over is experienced to an even greater degree during the act of subtraction; the third problem of the series, which demands that this operation shall be twice performed, offers peculiar difficulties and it is here that the patient most often shows evidence of his defective powers. He frequently fails to bring out any answer to this problem, although he solves all the others correctly. Even when recovery has so far advanced that all these tests in simple arithmetic are performed correctly, there may be evident want of ease in carrying over from one column to another during both addition and subtraction. No. 4, who had been a bank-clerk, complained, "I can't carry over; I was in a bank and used to do figures in my head; I know about it, it's not difficult, only the carrying over from one column to the top of the next column."

Although the patient is aware of the processes involved in addition and subtraction, his method of carrying them out may be abnormal. Thus when Captain C. (No. 2) was about to add 8 and 6 he did not take these numbers as entities, but counted up to eight and then on for another six, saying finally "fourteen." This was a difficult task and required several attempts before he reached the answer; with 3 and 6 on the other hand he simply counted up to nine. By this cumbrous method he frequently forgot to carry over from the previous addition; if the answer was given correctly, as for example $7 + 5 + 1$ carried over, he called the 7 "eight," counted eight and then on for five more to "thirteen." But, when he came to add $8 + 2 + 1$ carried over, he counted eight and then two, thus bringing out the answer wrongly as "ten."

Occasionally the patient is puzzled with regard to the nature of the intellectual task he is required to perform. Thus, although No. 10 had been an accountant, he was unable to carry out the simplest arithmetical operation; he complained that he seemed "to get tangled up in the process." At a later stage, when he completed all but the last of the six tests correctly, he added, "I found difficulty in them all. I found the subtraction more difficult than the addition. When there was a carry, it seemed to be more difficult. What I feel about it is...if I were to begin my education, like a boy at school, I shouldn't know where to begin. In these sums you gave me I did the addition almost involuntarily, I think the result of former practice. The subtraction...the simplest one, I did in a more or less involuntary way...but with the more difficult I had to think what subtraction really meant."

Sometimes the patient adds the figures from left to right instead of in the ordinary manner, or subtracts the lower number of any column from the higher, irrespective of whether it is situated above or below.

All such instances of defective comprehension of the nature of arithmetical operations are more liable to occur, when the defects of symbolic formulation and expression assume a semantic form; but they are in no way specific or confined to any one variety of aphasia. The patient, who suffers from want of appreciation of the particular or general meaning of numerical symbols, is more likely to be puzzled as to the nature of the acts he is required to perform. On the other hand, want of power to formulate or express numbers with accuracy and ease adds greatly to the difficulty of manipulating them freely and the patient may fail to produce a correct answer, because he cannot carry out an operation the essential nature of which he comprehends.

Counting and appreciation of the significance of single numerals revealed specific defects, which varied with the form assumed by the aphasia. But, from the study of the actual records of the arithmetical tests, it is impossible to discover any such fundamental differences unless we take into account what the patient tells us and the manner in which he behaves during his attempts to solve the problems placed before him. Even then, more depends on the severity of the disturbance of speech than on its nature. These high-grade aptitudes tend to be affected as a whole rather than in some specific and peculiar manner.

(d) *Relative value of coins and the use of money*

To name the various coins as they are exhibited one by one and choose them correctly to oral or printed commands differs little from similar tests carried out with familiar objects of common use.

But to express the relative value of any two pieces of money to one another is an intellectual task of a fundamentally different order. After the patient has given a name to each single coin or bank-note, two of them are laid before him and he is asked, "How many of this go into that?" or "How many of this would you have to give me for that?" the observer pointing first to the one of lower value and then to the other.

This is essentially a problem in formulating meaning, rather than one of expression, and it is more particularly in cases of nominal and semantic aphasia that the patient fails to solve it accurately. On the other hand, with verbal defects he can frequently give a correct reply, although he is compelled by his speechless condition to express himself on his fingers. Thus, No. 21, who could not utter the name of a single coin, gave the relative value of a penny and a shilling by holding up five fingers; he then said "nover" (another) and finally indicated two more, making twelve in all. By the same means he was able to express the number of pennies that went into a two-shilling piece (24) and even into half-a-crown (30). It was evident that although he could not pronounce the names of the coins, he formulated to himself with accuracy their numerical relation. No. 19, who was almost wordless, answered correctly all such tests as to the relative value of sixpence and two shillings (4), sixpence and half-a-crown (5) and even a penny and a shilling (12); in the last instance he replied "one two," his habitual method of counting twelve.

If the disorder of speech assumes a syntactical form, the simpler relative values can be expressed correctly; but the patient may be puzzled when compelled to employ the higher numbers. For instance, No. 13 stated the relation of a penny to a shilling correctly as "twelve"; but, when the former coin was replaced by a half-penny, he shook his head and gave no answer. Twenty-four was too high a number to be evoked with certainty.

With nominal aphasia this test is profoundly affected. Even if the answer is given correctly, the patient hesitates, whispers under his breath, or calculates on his fingers. Yet he undoubtedly recognises the value of a coin laid before him; for he can build up its exact equivalent from a heap of money lying on the table. Although he is unable to express the relation of two coins in correct terms, he can construct a pile corresponding in value to that of the higher one.

Moreover, one of the commonest faults is to state the number of pieces, which must be added to the coin of lower value in order that it may equal the other, instead of expressing their relation as a multiple. Thus, if the patient is asked, with the coins before him, how many pennies make a shilling, he not uncommonly answers "eleven," evidently counting up from the lower to the higher. In fact, wherever possible he counts instead of multiplying or subtracting, using his fingers in the operation like a child.

This test usually produces intense confusion in a patient with semantic aphasia. Every coin is named with perfect ease; but, as soon as any two of them are presented to him and he is asked to express their relative value, he is puzzled and gives absurdly inaccurate replies. No. 10, who had been an accountant, stated that twelve pennies went into a sixpence and shown the latter coin and a shilling, said, "Twelve... yes, twelve, sixpence." Dr P.'s (No. 24) replies, even if correct, tended to assume a curious form; shown a sixpence and a two-shilling piece, he said, "one in two...two shillings...one in four." Miss S. (No. 25) went through elaborate calculations, which might lead to a correct answer or leave her completely puzzled. Thus, with a penny and a half-crown (two shillings and sixpence), she replied, "It's quite a bother to add 24 and 6 together; that is what I am trying to do; I try to do it by remembering that five sixes is thirty"; finally she gave up in complete confusion. Even in an advanced stage of recovery from semantic defects of speech, this test is still executed slowly and the replies vary greatly in ease and accuracy.

To determine, on making a purchase, what coins must be given or received in change is one of the most frequent exercises in mental arithmetic. Verbal and syntactical aphasia do not materially diminish this capacity to handle money in daily life. So long as the defects of speech are concerned mainly with verbal expression or appropriate formation of a phrase, the patient experiences little difficulty in making these calculations and can shop with ease; for, even if the answer is given wrongly, he acts as if the amount had been stated correctly.

But nominal and especially semantic disorders of speech are accompanied by profound difficulty in manipulating change. Thus No. 10 had extreme difficulty in calculating the change he should receive after making a purchase. I gave him a ten-shilling note and asked him to pile up its equivalent from amongst the coins on the table; this he carried out with some effort correctly. I then handed him the same note and, telling him I had bought something for "two-and-six," asked for change. This puzzled him greatly; for although he said "seven and six," he had great difficulty in collecting the coins to make up this hypothetical sum. I gave him the same note once more and said I had purchased something for "three-and-three"; this he was entirely unable to work out. He complained, "It is parts of a shilling that bother me and a halfpenny makes it worse; I get confused and lose the significance of the figures."

When his tobacco cost him a shilling an ounce, he would ask for two ounces, placing a two-shilling piece on the counter; if he wanted a box of matches in addition, he waited until the first transaction was over and then took a penny from his pocket, so as to avoid the difficulties of change. Should he happen to have nothing less than a ten-shilling note, he asked the tobacconist to give him two-shilling pieces only; these he counted "one, two, three, four" and knew that four was the right number. But, if he was given change in shillings, he was completely puzzled. Throughout, he had no difficulty in naming the coins, although he was unable to grasp the full significance of monetary operations he was asked to perform.

Nominal aphasia, if sufficiently severe, is also associated with want of capacity to calculate the correct change; but this arises from a somewhat different cause. The patient has difficulty in evoking the names of coins and in formulating their relative value. This greatly hampers all exercises in mental arithmetic. But even after Captain C. (No. 2) had regained the power of naming coins and expressing the relative value of any two of them correctly, he still experienced difficulty in the more complicated act of calculating change. This he explained as follows: "If I buy something at say one and nine...I give the man a two-shilling piece...at the same time I say that I can't be worried if it's two pennies or three pennies or four pennies...I look it up afterwards to see if he is an honest man." From frequent experience he had learnt that the railway journey from his home to my house cost "five shillings less twopence halfpenny" (i.e. four shillings and ninepence halfpenny); "that's what I expect to get...to see...I figure it up beforehand."

§7. GENERAL CONCLUSIONS

The capacity to speak and to comprehend spoken words is acquired by each individual in childhood and the vast majority of human beings do not progress to more complicated methods of symbolic formulation and expression. But, with the invention of reading and writing, man advanced to a higher stage and gave permanence to his verbal activities by means of symbols in which he could record his thoughts. Written or printed matter forms a further representation in visual terms of the symbols of articulatory speech; in order that it may be understood certain conventional signs must be correctly apprehended and translated silently or aloud into verbal forms.

With an increasing desire for expression and for means to register the complexities of thought, the functions of speech became wider and demanded the exercise of many aptitudes not originally connected with articulation and comprehension of the meaning of sounds. Perceptions and visual images came to be profoundly involved in disorders of speech, as soon as words were transformed into written, printed or any kind of ideographic symbols. Elaborate mathematical calculations were developed out of the simple acts of enumeration and comprehension of numbers. The clock, with all its complexities of meaning, was invented to indicate the time. Coins were endowed with an arbitrary significance and a comparative value. Drawing grew from simple imitative representation to a means of recording relations of objects to one another in space diagrammatically.

But, although these diverse forms of behaviour are closely associated with acts of speech and suffer in aphasia, they remain intact for other purposes of thought. A man, who has obvious difficulty in recalling visual images to command, may be able otherwise to use them freely. He complains that he cannot "see" an object indicated orally or in print, and yet he has no difficulty in doing so, when it is placed in his hand out of sight. He cannot draw an elephant to command, but spontaneously in the course of conversation, produces a spirited representation of a camel. In spite of profound difficulty in naming the hour and in setting the clock to oral or printed commands, the patient may recognise the passage of time and associate it correctly with certain events. Numerals, which are wrongly expressed, convey their right meaning. A number of coins can be gathered into a heap to correspond in value to a certain piece of money, although the relation between any two of them cannot be stated correctly. The patient may be unable to construct a ground-plan of a familiar room with its salient objects; and yet he can indicate with his eyes closed the exact position of each one of them in relation to the place where he is sitting.

Articulated speech and the comprehension of spoken words are the most primitive and mechanically the lowest of all acts of symbolic formulation and expression. Any such form of behaviour, which is acquired early and remains in habitual employment, tends to become increasingly automatic; it is highly organised, the response is stereotyped and the morbid manifestations are liable therefore to assume various distinctive forms. Should the normal perfection of a process of this kind be disturbed, the defects can be readily described in terms of articulated speech or verbal meaning and it is for this reason that I have classified the different forms of aphasia as verbal, syntactical, nominal and semantic.

But, as soon as these articulatory symbols are translated into printed words, they are raised in difficulty for propositional acts; more voluntary effort is required to employ them with freedom and accuracy. Written words are symbols of symbols and the act of writing is interposed between verbal formulation and expression. Again, although a child learns at an early age to count and to understand the meaning of numbers, an exercise in arithmetic demands not only that they shall be at his immediate beck and call, but that he can employ them in high-grade logical acts.

When such recent acquirements, demanding a high degree of propositional aptitude, are rendered difficult, the records do not exhibit so readily those specific differences, evident with more habitual and primitive modes of behaviour. The patient fails in a more general manner to execute the task set before him.

Passing in review the answers given by each particular patient, we find that some tests are not affected in any form of aphasia, unless it is extremely grave and is associated with definite mental enfeeblement. These are all acts of direct imitation, such as choice of an object or colour corresponding to that exhibited by the observer, which requires no symbolic formulation. Another task of the same order consists in selecting an object identical with one placed in the hand out of sight. Such simple exercises in matching do not suffer in uncomplicated cases of aphasia.

But every test which is definitely affected in these disorders of speech differs in severity according to the degree of propositional ability required for its perfect performance. It is obviously harder to execute an order demanding a triple choice than one which offers but a single possibility of error; power to execute the more difficult task is therefore affected more easily and returns later in the course of the disorder, whatever the form of the command.

Apart, however, from its absolute or inherent difficulty, each test may vary relatively according to the form assumed by the disorder of speech. It is, for instance, an easy matter for most verbal aphasics to select an object or colour to oral commands; but this form of choice is profoundly confusing to the patient with nominal defects. In the same way, with verbal aphasia, the clock can be set more easily to a printed order in the form "20 minutes to 6," than when it is given as "5.40." The exact opposite is true of the semantic patient, who finds more difficulty with the ordinary nomenclature than if the command is presented in railway time.

Whenever an otherwise simple task is rendered difficult by some disorder of speech, the patient is liable to adopt a more primitive method of solving it. If, on attempting to select an object or colour to printed commands, he does not at once associate the verbal pattern on the card with something before him on the table, he laboriously spells it out letter by letter, combines them into a word, which he says aloud or under his breath, and then proceeds to make his choice. When in doubt as to the meaning of words or phrases he is reading to himself, his lips move although he may not utter a sound. He adds or subtracts by counting on his fingers, as is the custom with poorly educated persons even in adult life. Given two coins and asked to express their relation, he counts from the less to the greater instead of stating how many times the one goes into the other; thus, given a penny and a shilling, he answers "eleven" instead of saying "twelve pennies in a shilling." All these methods of solving a problem represent a regression to a more childish method of thought.

Let us consider in this light the effect produced by a disturbance of symbolic formulation and expression on the various forms of behaviour discussed in this chapter. Articulated speech is profoundly affected in verbal aphasia, which may reduce the patient almost to dumbness. With syntactical aphasia words remain to him, but they are strung together as jargon and in severe cases his speech may be entirely incomprehensible. Nominal aphasia makes it difficult or impossible to find the correct name or appropriate words. Semantic aphasia does not materially diminish the power of verbalisation, but tends to destroy the capacity to express the general intention and logical conclusion of a train of thought arising spontaneously or induced from without.

When we turn to the comprehension of spoken words, the changes are equally distinctive, but the severity of the affection in the various forms of aphasia is almost exactly reversed. Verbal defects must be very grave before they produce any material want of capacity to execute oral commands. In the syntactical group single words can be understood, but the patient tends to miss the import of phrases or orders given in the course of general conversation; when he attempts to repeat to himself silently what he has been told, he becomes confused by internal jargon and fails to comprehend its significance. Nominal aphasia is associated with a profound loss of power to comprehend the meaning of words and figures in whatever form they are presented. Semantic defects, on the other hand, prevent complete appreciation of the general or ultimate significance of a series of detailed statements.

So far the clinical manifestations are distinctive and easily comprehensible. Should the disturbance of function be extremely severe, the patient fails to make any response; but, if he can reply to the test presented to him, his answers tend to assume different forms according to the nature of the disorder of speech.

To read a printed command aloud or to act upon it silently often requires translation of the symbols on paper into their verbal equivalents. It is true that the normal man, when shown a single word, such as Knife or Blue, does not of necessity spell it out and say it over to himself; he makes his choice immediately. Not so the aphasic; for, if he has the slightest difficulty in recognising the printed words, he says them over to himself aloud or under his breath, trying to find the verbal form which corresponds to the signs on the paper. Even a highly educated man, accustomed to snatch the meaning from a printed page without exactly appreciating the form of the words, if he encounters a difficulty, tends to fall back on to the childish method of "spelling them out," before he can appreciate their significance.

Under these abnormal conditions reading tends to become a double process, whether the words are said aloud or not. If the patient does not immediately apprehend their significance, he verbalises them silently, whispers them under his breath, or reproduces them in some articulated form and so gives himself what is equivalent to an oral command. In most cases this makes the task easier and approximates the results of the reading tests to those obtained, when the order is given by word of mouth. Occasionally, it is true, printed commands are executed somewhat better than those presented orally. With syntactical aphasia this is due to the fact that internal speech is less disturbed by jargon than articulation. Moreover, an order given in spoken words is transient and, if the patient fails to comprehend it at once, it cannot be recalled; whereas he can look back time after time to the printed card he holds in his hand.

Apart, however, from the increased difficulty caused by translation of the printed symbols into words, the records obtained with the reading tests tend to coincide with those yielded by any other task, which demands the comprehension of the meaning of words. In verbal aphasia the patient can execute printed commands correctly, unless the disturbance of function is extremely severe. He chooses common objects or colours without fail and can not only select pictures of the man, cat and dog from their printed names, but picks out correctly the card corresponding to the particular combination of pictures he has just seen. He may be almost dumb and incapable of reading aloud; and yet he appreciates the meaning of the words on the paper sufficiently for accurate choice.

Syntactical aphasia does not materially diminish the powers of reading to oneself or carrying out printed commands, provided the words are not articulated. But, when he attempts to repeat to himself silently the sense of what he has read, the patient is liable to be confused by internal jargon; provided, however, he does not try to do so, he can usually execute even complex printed orders correctly. As soon as he reads aloud his utterance is marred by more or less gross jargon. This spoils his comprehension of the meaning of the words and leads to greater mental confusion than if he had read them silently. This is the converse of the condition in most other forms of aphasia, where understanding of print is aided by saying the words aloud.

Nominal aphasia leads to profound difficulty in comprehending print, whether for purposes of thought or action. Presented with a card bearing the name of some familiar implement or colour, the patient hesitates, unable to associate the verbal pattern with an appropriate object lying before him on the table. He then tries to spell out the word, like a child with its first reading book; if he succeeds in evoking the name correctly, he looks up and down the row of objects until he finds the one, which seems to him to match the word he has deciphered. Should no corresponding object lie before him, recognition of the significance of the printed word is delayed or perhaps becomes impossible. Even if he remains silent throughout the process, his lips tend to move and, when he is allowed to say the word aloud, his choice is often considerably facilitated. He reinforces the words he has read by a self-given oral command.

The patient with semantic aphasia appears at first sight to understand everything he reads. Not only can he occupy himself with the daily paper or a book, but he chooses an object or colour correctly to printed commands. Yet as soon as he attempts to narrate what he has read, it is obvious that he has missed the point, although he may have appreciated most of the details. Moreover, he fails with the complex tests, especially when asked to set the clock to printed commands, because he becomes confused, mistaking one hand for the other and unable to differentiate "to" and "past" the hour. These patients can read aloud without serious mistakes; but they are liable to doubt whether they are doing so correctly and to puzzle over the meaning of sentences, which are perfectly enunciated. Not infrequently they enquire, "Is that sense? It doesn't seem so to me."

Thus, any test which depends on accuracy in reading, silently or aloud, suffers in a characteristic manner according to the form assumed by the aphasia. The more it disturbs the capacity to appreciate verbal significance, the greater will be the loss of power to grasp the meaning of printed matter, especially as the vehicle of a command. Nominal aphasia is therefore associated with profound defects in silent reading, whilst verbal aphasia produces little or no loss of aptitude unless it is unusually acute or severe. On the other hand, reading aloud, which demands perfect ability to evoke and articulate the exact word required, suffers gravely with any disorder of verbal formulation. But I was able to demonstrate that a patient with extremely severe verbal aphasia, unable to read a single word aloud, could appreciate simple phrases for the purposes of accurate choice. Silent comprehension of printed symbols was less affected than their translation into articulate words.

When the patient is asked to write words and phrases, which are the spontaneous expression of his thoughts, or the reproduction of something he has heard or read, these defects are less obviously distinctive in the various forms of aphasia. The power of writing easily and with accuracy can be disturbed by any disorder of symbolic formulation and expression, if sufficiently severe. Spelling suffers badly, the letters are incorrectly formed or are written with difficulty, capitals are interjected without reason amongst cursive script and the stops are wrongly placed. These defects are not distinctive; the calligraphic aspect of writing may be affected more or less indifferently with any form of aphasia.

If, however, the written matter is considered as a mode of expressing thought, specific differences become evident. Thus, with verbal aphasia, the patient knows what he wants to write and struggles against mechanical difficulties to find the words, in which to clothe his ideas or the names of the objects presented to him. He can ultimately produce a long coherent account of something he has read silently, although the spelling is incredibly bad; he is in doubt how to write even the simplest words; and yet he recognises his mistakes and can often correct them.

The syntactical aphasic writes the jargon he speaks. It is true that his capacity to put on paper single words, the names of objects and short phrases is usually in excess of his power of saying them aloud; this is due to the comparatively slight affection of internal speech. But, when he attempts to retail some longer narrative that he has heard or read, the sentences show the same sort of faults as his articulated speech. They reproduce in fact his internal jargon.

A patient with nominal aphasia has difficulty in evoking the correct words and names in which to express his thoughts. It is the meaning of the verbal forms that puzzles him, rather than their structure; he is also doubtful of the significance and proper use of the individual letters of which they are composed. His script not only shows the mechanical faults common to all varieties of disordered speech, but he tends more particularly to employ wrongly nouns, prepositions and words of opposed meaning, such as right and left, to and past the hour.

Semantic defects interfere with consecutive writing, because the patient loses the thread of what he wishes to communicate, or writes unduly rapidly for fear that he should forget. Not only is the writing careless and the sentences incomplete, but they are frequently inconsequent. The natural order of the statements may be changed and there is often a characteristic want of logical sequence.

Thus, the results of a written test of this kind can be looked at from two points of view. Mechanically, the act of writing as a whole may be disturbed and, from a calligraphic aspect, the records do not reveal truly distinctive differences according to the form assumed by the aphasia. On the other hand, when the written matter is considered as an expression of something to be communicated in writing, it shows defects, which vary characteristically in harmony with the disturbance of external or internal verbalisation and the comprehension of spoken words.

The alphabet stands in a peculiar position compared with the other tests I have used in aphasia. A child learns, as one of his earliest acquirements, to say the letters in order; but in later life this act is rarely performed, except when we wish to look up a name in a list or to consult a dictionary. We read by recognising the verbal pattern on the page and we write without thinking of the shape of the letters. Thus, although we early learn to say them in their proper sequence, we seldom do so at a time when our powers of symbolic formulation are most highly developed. This accounts for the otherwise astonishing fact that many aphasics, who can speak, read and write with comparative ease, are unable to carry out the tests with the alphabet.

To say the alphabet aloud, or to arrange the block letters in due sequence, requires the perfect exercise of an habitual rhythm; this can be disturbed by anything which diminishes the ease of verbal formulation and expression. The records obtained, when the patient says the alphabet spontaneously or arranges the block letters in proper order, show no characteristic differences in accordance with the various forms of disordered speech. Verbal aphasia produces the most profound incapacity to carry out these tests; in nominal aphasia the loss is less severe; syntactical aphasia, even after considerable recovery has occurred, is associated with grave defects; semantic aphasia alone produces no material alteration, beyond a tendency to say the alphabet with unusual rapidity.

Yet all four varieties of speech defect diminish the power of writing the alphabet spontaneously in silence. For, as we write the letters one after the other, we say them over to ourselves and, if for any reason it becomes difficult to evoke the verbal symbols, it is a still harder task to translate them into writing.

So far the records of these written alphabetical tests do not show obvious differences with the various forms of disordered speech. But some indications of such specific changes appear, when we set the patient a still easier task and ask him to copy printed capitals in cursive script.

Verbal aphasia may destroy all power of carrying out this test; the patient laboriously imitates letter by letter, but cannot transform them into their cursive equivalents. Nominal aphasia is accompanied by a tendency when copying to employ capitals and the smaller script indiscriminately. On the other hand, with syntactical and semantic aphasia the only abnormality may consist in a certain hesitation and want of ease in writing.

In the same way, when the patient is asked to repeat the letters one by one as they are said by the observer, specific differences appear in accordance with the various forms of disordered speech. This is an extremely easy task; for each word is presented ready formed to the patient and all difficulties with rhythm are avoided, since he is no longer compelled to determine the order in which the letters follow one another. Thus, with nominal or with semantic aphasia, there is no difficulty in executing this test, whilst any considerable degree of defective verbalisation may make repetition impossible.

With the exception of these comparatively slight differences, the various forms of aphasia are not associated with characteristic disorders of the alphabetical tests in any way comparable to those specific changes, so evident if the task set before the patient depends directly on articulated speech or the comprehension of spoken words.

Counting, being closely dependent on the power of internal and external verbalisation, suffers in a distinctive manner with the various forms of disordered speech. It is grossly defective in verbal aphasia and the patient may be compelled to overcome his difficulties of expression by using his fingers to indicate the number, or by changing the nomenclature; instead of saying "a hundred," which is impossible, he speaks of "one oh oh," as is customary when using the telephone. The meaning of numbers is retained; for even if they are said wrongly the patient acts as if he had uttered them correctly and he can employ conceptions of high numbers that he is unable to put into articulate words.

A syntactical aphasic may be able to count correctly, but the words are slurred and the rhythm defective. This leads to great variability in pronunciation and consequent confusion at the decades; he is perpetually thrown out of his stride and misled into some false sequence. But the significance of numbers is retained, except in as far as the patient is puzzled by his own defective utterances.

Nominal aphasia, if sufficiently severe, leads to profound confusion in numerical sequence and comprehension of the meaning of numbers. The patient not only counts badly, but has difficulty in recognising immediately the significance of any number presented to him.

Semantic defects produce no noticeable disturbance in counting, in pronunciation of the numerals, or direct appreciation of their meaning.

Thus, these numerical tests form a useful method of distinguishing the form assumed by any particular example of disordered speech. But the records of exercises in arithmetic do not exhibit these specific differences; it would be impossible by examining the answers to simple problems in addition or subtraction to determine the variety of aphasia to which the patient belonged. The harder the intellectual task the more likely is he to fail in solving it correctly; but there are not those profound differences according to the form assumed by the defects of speech, which are apparent in the acts of counting or recognition of numerical meaning.

Similarly, the manner in which coins are named varies profoundly in accordance with the different forms of disordered speech. On the other hand, when the patient is asked to express the relative value of any two of them, the erroneous answers are not obviously distinctive. In verbal and syntactical aphasia it is mainly words and suitable phrases that are lacking; the fundamental idea is intact. Consequently as the fault is mainly one of expression, the disturbance must be extremely grave and acute before the power to manipulate money or calculate change is affected. Conversely, the defective answers, which accompany nominal and semantic aphasia, are due to want of appreciation of the significant factors in the relation and the difficulties with money are frequently very severe; either of these disorders of speech is liable to disturb capacity to formulate the value of one coin as a multiple of another.

When we sum up the results of these tests based upon speaking, verbal comprehension, reading, writing and the use of numbers, we find that in no single case was there an isolated disturbance of any one of these forms of behaviour. In every instance certain modes of action were affected, which could not be classified under such terms.

Sometimes the morbid manifestations varied from case to case in a manner so distinctive that it was possible to separate these disorders of speech into various classes. Other tests were affected in a more general and less specific manner; they revealed a disturbance of symbolic formulation and expression, but justified no further conclusion.

The more definitely a task set before the patient approximates to an act of verbalisation, internal or external, and comprehension of verbal meaning, the greater the probability that it will be affected in a specific manner in accordance with other morbid manifestations. On the other hand, any form of behaviour, which demands a greater voluntary effort and higher propositional ability, suffers in a more general degree.

Thus, the more recently acquired and high-grade aptitudes, such as the act of writing, exercises in arithmetic, or the use of money tend to be disturbed as a whole. Provided they are affected, they reveal simply a lack of symbolic formulation and expression. But tests based on articulated speech, reading, writing in so far as it is the direct expression of thought, counting and the meaning of coins, suffer in different ways according to the nature of the case and it is by such means that the varieties of aphasia can be distinguished the one from the other.

CHAPTER VII

PICTURES, DRAWING, VISUAL IMAGERY AND MUSIC

IN the present chapter I shall describe in closer detail the response of my patients to pictures, their capacity to execute various drawing tests, the behaviour of visual images and finally the power to sing and to perform on a musical instrument.

Now it is evident that all these actions postulate crude appreciation of the significance of sights and sounds. If, when shown an object such as a knife, the patient can neither match it nor indicate its use, although he can do so when it is placed in his hand out of sight, he is evidently suffering from what Jackson called "imperception." This falls naturally into three forms, visual, auditory and tactile agnosia, according to the particular functions which are affected. Of these the two first are familiar under the terms "mind-blindness" (Seelenblindheit) and "mind-deafness" (Seelentaubheit).

A person suffering from visual imperception can see an object shown to him and yet fails to appreciate its character and meaning. Not only is he unable to name it, but he cannot show how to use it and does not remember that he has ever seen it before. In the same way a patient with auditory imperception, or "mind-deafness," cannot recognise the significance of sounds, although there is distinct evidence that he hears them.

But the actual clinical records of cases of imperception do not follow strictly these diagrammatically simple lines. Although there were obvious perceptual defects, the morbid manifestations were either too extensive, or fell considerably short of those which should theoretically have accompanied "mind-blindness" or "mind-deafness." Moreover, the lesion was frequently bilateral and always extensive, whilst the symptoms varied from time to time.

It is obvious that any want of visual perception must disturb the power to read and to appreciate pictorial symbols, whilst auditory imperception will be accompanied by inability to understand spoken words. These symptoms have been classed under the terms "word-blindness" and "word-deafness." But they have nothing in common with aphasia, amnesia, or similar high-grade disorders in the use of language. Any affection of speech that may be present is due to a deeper and cruder loss of function; as Jackson pointed out, defects of speech may exist with or without imperception. It is of fundamental importance clearly to understand the confusion that has arisen from erroneous application of these various terms and I have therefore dealt with the matter historically in Part I, pages 103 to 116.

None of my patients suffering from the wounds of war showed any form of imperception in the strict meaning of the word. This was probably due to the comparatively small extent of the cerebral lesions and to the fact that they were unilateral. This is in accord with all recent experimental evidence.

§ 1. APPRECIATION OF PICTURES

The capacity to recognise the meaning of pictures, possessed by patients with aphasia and kindred disorders of speech, is worthy of special and systematic investigation. To this I make no pretence; the exigences of clinical observation compelled me to treat the question in a somewhat cursory manner, but I have amassed sufficient material to draw certain tentative conclusions.

When we are shown a picture and are asked to make up our minds what it means, the task may comprise acts of the most diverse nature and difficulty. Sometimes it necessitates little more than crude recognition of similarity and difference; shown the picture of a dog, we know that it resembles in its general characters other representations or our preconceived ideas of this animal, and that it differs fundamentally from those of a cat. Such simple acts of discrimination were not disturbed in any of my cases, although they may apparently suffer in gross examples of visual imperception.

The meaning we gather from a picture depends on the details it contains; but we do not normally add one item to another to arrive at a conclusion by summation. We receive a general impression of the meaning as a whole and reinforce or correct it by closer attention to its integral features. When in doubt, we must be able, not only to recognise these details with accuracy, but to combine them into a coherent and reasonable whole. Not uncommonly a picture bears some secondary meaning beyond that indicated by its parts taken one by one; it may tell a story or illustrate some humorous situation. Sometimes its full significance cannot be recognised until the pictorial representation has been elucidated by combination with certain printed words.

So far we have considered the picture, with or without its illustrative legend, as a means of conveying an impression which can be employed as part of the general activities of the mind. Another aspect of pictorial appreciation is discovered by the man, cat and dog tests, in which a picture must be translated into its verbal equivalent and either articulated aloud or written down on paper. Here we are not testing the power of recognising the meaning of a picture, but the capacity to formulate it in words.

Finally, a picture may imply a command to act in some particular manner. If I show a patient the diagrammatic representation of a man touching an eye or ear with one or other hand and ask him to do the same, he is compelled, not only to recognise the details of the picture, but to discriminate them as the formulated elements of a command. He must distinguish without fail right from left and eye from ear.

These various modes of interpreting the significance of a picture present the most diverse problems in symbolic formulation and expression; in any one instance, they are affected independently and each form of aphasia tends to disturb them in a different manner.

(a) *Comprehension of the meaning of a picture with or without a descriptive legend*

In most instances of disordered speech the patient has no difficulty in appreciating the various constituent parts of a picture, or in recognising its meaning as a whole. But should the defects assume a semantic form, he may arrive at an inadequate or erroneous conclusion, because he has failed to perceive some significant detail or was unable to grasp the total import of the picture. For instance, No. 10 was given a coloured picture of a motor car standing before a large country house with a driver talking to two girls one of whom held a greyhound by the collar. Asked the meaning of this picture, he went over it in detail from left to right without the least evidence of constructive appreciation. Every detail was named correctly; but he did not weld them into a coherent whole and express the meaning of the picture in a set of general propositions. On another occasion he was handed a picture of a jetty with a small lighthouse projecting into the sea; moored close to the shore was a fishing boat occupying at least one third of the picture. He described what he saw to the smallest details, pointing to them one by one, but omitted the fishing boat. After the picture was removed from sight, he again enumerated the various objects even more minutely without mentioning this salient feature. The picture was then replaced in his hands and he suddenly exclaimed, "Oh! I left out the very large boat, fishing boat, sailing boat. I think I missed it from the beginning."

In addition to its primary or immediate significance a picture can bear a secondary meaning; it may tell a story or convey some humorous implication. Here again the semantic patient is liable to be at fault, because he fails to grasp the situation as a whole. In several instances of this defect in speech, I showed a series of sketches representing a spectator who, arriving late at the play, strips off inadvertently both his coats and is taking his seat in his shirt sleeves to the horrified amusement of the audience. When a young officer (No. 10) was asked what he saw in these pictures, he entirely missed the point. "There's an audience, possibly a concert audience. The audience is seated, waiting and...a man comes along wearing his coat. He has some difficulty in taking it off, whether real or assumed. The audience seems greatly interested. I'm not sure about it...I was trying to think it might have been part of the performance...or he might have got there and seem to be rather prominent. It often happens at a theatre that somebody comes late."

I showed Dr P. (No. 24) a ludicrous picture of a man drinking with gusto the sulphur waters of Harrogate to the astonishment of the rest of his fellow patients in the Pump Room. He failed entirely to see the point, even when allowed to read the legend, "The man who liked it." He said, "No, I don't see it. The man who liked it. The Pump Room. He's been to the beer house because he liked it." I asked, "Is it a beer house?" and he replied, "He's a man who goes into the public bars and drinks the pump...like Bath and these places." I said, "Suppose it was Harrogate?" He answered, "He's been drinking the Pump Room waters; they're mostly sulphur. I suppose the other man is laughing because he likes it. There, you see what difficulty I have."

Many pictures bear a legend or description in words, which is more or less necessary for their complete comprehension. Should the patient suffer from semantic defects of speech, this may form an additional complication rather than an assistance. For instance, I showed Lieut. M. (No. 10) a photographic representation of the tower with the leaning Virgin at Albert; at the top of the picture was printed, "When the end of the war will be; a prophecy." After examining it with care and reading the superscription, he said that it reminded him of something he had seen before. "In the other picture I saw there was a piece of statuary. I don't know if that is a confusion in my mind or not. It was a piece of old building tumbling down; like the leaning tower of Pisa. That building has fallen over much more than this; the local French people believe that the statue of the Virgin Mary...they believe that the statue has fallen and that then the war will end...just in that place the war will end." During the narration he looked away from the picture, evidently recalling some previous memory, and I therefore said: "What bearing has this picture on the story you have just told me?" He then looked at the picture again, passing his finger over the various details as he mentioned them. "This is simply a building, that has been bombarded, in ruins; one tower, as often happens, seems standing unmolested. I can now see the statue quite plainly; I can see the arms quite plainly. I think I might have been confused about the statue if I hadn't known the story." It was not until after he had recounted to me the familiar legend and recalled previous illustrations he had seen of the church at Albert, that he suddenly noticed the most salient feature in the picture before him.

Sometimes the legend not only fails to elucidate the meaning of a picture, but actually leads to further misunderstanding. No. 5 selected from a newspaper the picture of a man riding on a cow, headed by the words "Mayor's Curious Steed." After looking at it for some time he said, "That's a man riding on a colt...no, it isn't, sir, it looks more like a cow...or a young cow...no it isn't...heifer sir." After he had read the legend, I asked, "Who is the man?" and he replied, "A farmer, sir. No, Major...no, the Mayor curse sted...the Mayor curious stid. It's something you don't see every day...that stid...something very uncommon that animal. It's in a horse's place instead of where it is. I should think myself they are going to show that animal; it's uncommon, that stid, more so to see a man riding on it...you don't often see a man riding on a stid." When I asked, "What is a stid?" he replied, "It's something the same family as a cow." In this instance he appreciated that the picture represented a man riding a cow but, misled by the word "Steed," invented a fantastic explanation.

Should a picture simply illustrate a text without which it would be incomprehensible, the possibilities of misunderstanding are greatly increased. For example I showed Miss S. (No. 25) a picture from *Punch*, in which a tramp is being taken to task by a patriotic country gentleman who says, "It's about time you chaps started to do something; hard work never killed anybody." The mendicant replies, "You are mistaken, Sir, I lost three wives through it."

She said, "There's no joke in it; he lost three wives through the War. I suppose he lost three wives, but I don't know what by." About ten minutes later she exclaimed, "Oh! now I see it. It was the wives who were killed by work." She laughed heartily and added, "That's very characteristic; when once I've seen it, I wonder how I have been so silly not to have seen it at once."

At our next meeting she handed me the following luminous explanation in writing[1]. "It was not so much that I did not see the joke but that I did not see anything. This is most characteristic; I make my remarks upon it before I have read all the words, before I have really looked at the picture. The one word 'kill' calls up war associations. I jump to the conclusion that it is a war joke. As I do not see where the joke is I think it is a bad one and put the thing down. When Dr Head jogs my attention to it again, *then* I see I have missed something; *then* I see what the picture stands for. Then I put it altogether and see the joke. But the interesting part in this test is that Dr Head's jogging of the attention was equivalent to *interest* in subject matter when alone. Just as the one word 'kill' in this case turned me off the whole thing, so one word or sentence bearing upon something of interest will jog my attention in the same way and cause me to read a passage over and over again until I get its full meaning. But this *has* to be done; and if the interest is not there to 'jog,' the effort is not made because one is unconscious that an effort is needed."

All these forms of misunderstanding occur with semantic defects, because the patient fails to grasp the full meaning of a situation. No other disorder of symbolic formulation and expression disturbs direct appreciation of either the details or totality of a picture; but any want of perfect internal speech is liable to diminish accurate comprehension of the legend or description which accompanies it. Not infrequently this verbal inaccuracy is actually corrected by the salient feature of the picture, but occasionally it may give rise to some confusion or uncertainty. For instance, No. 15, a case of syntactical aphasia, concluded as the result of reading the legend to himself that the flowers contributed by passengers on the railway for the wounded soldiers in the infirmary were "for sale." When, therefore, he was asked to point out the various features in the picture, he indicated the station master, saying, "He's selling 'em." Such purely verbal misunderstandings are liable to occur whenever internal verbalisation is defective; but they are trivial and never pervert or confuse the total significance of a picture, except in semantic aphasia.

[1] Vide Vol. II, p. 386. The mistakes in verbal formation and spelling have been corrected in this version.

(b) *Translation of a simple picture into spoken or written words*

When a picture is placed before a patient and he is asked what it conveys to him, he may find extreme difficulty in rendering his impressions either in speech or writing. This can arise from two different causes. On the one hand perhaps he appreciates its meaning perfectly, but is unable to find words in which to express his ideas, either aloud or to himself; or his failure to describe what he has seen, even though he can talk and write with ease, springs from want of complete understanding of its significance.

To describe a complicated picture either in spoken or written words is a difficult task and I have therefore reduced this act to the simplest possible terms in the man, cat and dog tests. Two out of the three pictures are shown to the patient in various combinations and in different positions from left to right. He is asked to say what he sees in the form of a series of simple phrases, e.g., "The man and the cat," or "The dog and the man." He is told to write down silently each combination as it is shown to him in order. The value of this test lies in its extreme simplicity; all the words are monosyllables and the names of the objects represented are amongst the earliest acquired by a child. No normal person could fail to carry out this task with ease; yet in the various forms of aphasia it is capable of revealing the most instructive defects.

Should the main defect be verbal and speech be reduced to a few emotional expressions only, the patient may fail to execute this test because he cannot articulate even these elementary monosyllabic words. In such circumstances, he is usually unable to write them down silently in response to pictures. External and internal speech suffer together[1]. Moreover as recovery takes place power to perform these two apparently dissimilar acts is restored simultaneously (No. 20, Vol. II, p. 304).

But, although the patient can neither say nor write the names of the figures shown him, he may recognise them accurately in print. When No. 21 was shown two pictures of the man, cat and dog series, he could point out the corresponding printed card; he even paid particular attention to the order in which the words stood from left to right. This is more nearly an act of matching and requires less power of symbolic formulation and expression than saying the names aloud or writing them down in cursive script.

Syntactical aphasia appears to induce remarkable carelessness with regard to the order in which the words are arranged. Sometimes the

---

[1] The only exception was No. 19, Vol. II, p. 288.

names of the figures are said aloud or written as they stand from left to right, at others they are reversed. Both No. 13 and No. 15 tended to lapse into this peculiar error of sequence, whatever the method of expression. This is in accord with the view that syntactical aphasia is in the main due to defects in the rhythm of language.

Nominal aphasia is liable to affect the power of translating pictures into spoken or written words, because the patient cannot retain in his mind exactly which pair of figures have been exposed to his view. Shown the man and the cat, he may say he has seen the dog and the cat and occasionally he omits one of the pair altogether. If this is the case, the written is always worse than the spoken record; for the difficulty of finding and retaining the appropriate names for the pictures is heightened by the necessity for translating them into written symbols. If by chance, as in No. 22, a patient with nominal defects can reproduce the whole series of pictorial combinations in words, he is also able to write them down correctly.

Semantic aphasia, accompanied by inability to grasp the total meaning rather than the details of a situation, produces no disturbance of this simple test. The patient can not only express in words each combination of figures he has seen, but is able to write them down with ease.

From the point of view of pictorial significance this test is childishly easy and is not affected by semantic defects. But on the other hand it is imperfectly executed in any condition which interferes with perfect formal and detailed expression of simple visual impressions.

(c) *Pictorial commands*

So far I have been able to show that most of the disorders of speech, with the exception of the semantic form, do not interfere with appreciation of the details or the total significance of a picture, however greatly the power of expressing it in words may be diminished. But as soon as a picture is charged with a meaning that must be translated into action, this is not the case.

The test I have habitually employed assumes two forms, one of which can be executed with ease by all normal individuals, whilst the other may present difficulty and lead to mistaken responses even in persons of high intelligence and education.

The patient is handed a simplified picture of a man touching his eye or ear with the right or left hand. A line is drawn down the centre to mark the halves of the body and on each diagram the limb to be moved is alone represented. Hence it is obvious that, if the right hand touches the left eye, it must transgress this line, whilst if it is to be brought into contact with eye or ear of the same side no crossing occurs. Now, if a picture of this kind is placed before the patient, the right hand of the figure lies to his left and there is a natural tendency even in normal persons to reverse the action, when executing the movement required. Such "reversal" is a common fault in cases of aphasia and is reckoned a less serious mistake than other forms of error, such as failing to recognise that the hand must cross the middle line to execute the command conveyed by the picture. In order to obviate this misunderstanding careful instructions are given to the patient before beginning a series of observations; he is asked to lift one or other hand in response to that shown on a diagram and is corrected if he holds up that of the wrong side. In this way we can be certain that, at any rate at first, he has understood the nature of the action demanded, however grossly he may fail in carrying out the subsequent tests. Such commands are always difficult to execute; for even the normal man must formulate to himself that the movement he is required to perform is apparently the opposite to that he sees in the picture.

But as soon as the diagram is reflected in a mirror, this difficulty is removed. To execute the order correctly the patient has only to copy exactly what he sees; the hand of the reflected figure is now on the same side as his own and little symbolic formulation is necessary. In normal persons this is a purely imitative act and can be executed with ease and certainty.

So long as the disorder of speech consists mainly of defective word-formation and syntactical errors, these reflected pictorial commands can be performed correctly. On the other hand, the semantic patient frequently finds considerable difficulty in carrying out this test. For, in spite of preliminary explanations, he is liable to argue with himself as to the meaning of the task he is asked to perform; he cannot resign himself to direct unformulated imitation. Thus Dr P. (No. 24) complained, "It's more puzzling in the mirror; I see it's a left hand mirror; I don't think there is anything abnormal about that; I've got to remember that it's the opposite to what I see in the glass." Such confused reasoning led to gross errors in execution, even with this simple test.

Nominal aphasia consists mainly in want of exact comprehension of detailed meaning and, should this disorder of speech be extremely severe, it is liable to disturb the accurate execution of pictorial commands reflected in a mirror. The number of errors is considerably less than when the diagram is laid on the table face to face with the patient. But as soon as he begins to think whether it is the right or left hand, the eye or the ear, he lapses into error. So long as he simply obeys what he sees in the mirror without formulation, he can execute the tests correctly. This want of accuracy rapidly passes away with the recovery of power and in nominal aphasia is a manifestation of severe loss of function only.

Thus so long as the disorder is mainly concerned with accurate verbal or phrasal formation for the purposes of external or internal speech, pictorial commands reflected in a mirror can be carried out with ease and certainty. When, however, the aphasia affects mainly the appreciation of meaning or intention, even this test may be badly executed; but obviously this is more likely to occur with the semantic than with the nominal form, which must reach a severe degree before it can disturb so simple a task.

When the picture is laid on the table in front of the patient so that he is face to face with the figure delineated on the card, his responses tend to be faulty whatever the form assumed by the aphasia, provided it reaches a sufficient degree of severity. With this method of setting the test some translation is inevitable, even in normal persons. We say to ourselves "my right is his left," "everything is reversed," or adopt some general conception indicating the crossed nature of the movement demanded. Between the pictorial command and its execution stands some formula however abbreviated.

In every example of verbal aphasia this form of the hand, eye and ear tests was more or less affected. Capt. W. (No. 17), a case of comparatively slight defects of word-formation, carried out a series of sixteen pictorial commands with one mistake and two corrections only. Several patients[1], who at first gave faulty answers, recovered sufficiently to perform these tests correctly, showing that the previous gross errors were not due to normal incapacity. Evidently want of mastery over word-formation hindered that freedom of internal verbalisation necessary for the perfect execution of this somewhat severe intellectual exercise.

Syntactical aphasia also tends to interfere with the execution of pictorial commands and this forms another instance of the manner in which defects of internal speech hamper the actions of this class of patient.

As might have been anticipated, nominal aphasia profoundly disturbs the execution of pictorial commands. The patient confuses right and left, eye and ear; he fails to recognise that the hand of one side touching the opposite eye or ear has crossed the middle line of the body. Defective

[1] No. 19, No. 6.

power of formulating and designating in appropriate terms the act to be performed leads to the appearance of every possible error.

The patient with semantic defects of symbolic formulation and expression fails to carry out pictorial commands, presented to him face to face, for the same reasons that produced the mistakes, when the diagram was reflected in a mirror. He cannot obtain a clear general conception of the aim or intention of the order. He is unable to discover the meaning of the total situation presented to him by the picture, just as he was puzzled when it was reflected in a mirror.

Although I have indicated the different causes which underlie failure to execute this test in the different varieties of aphasia, it must not be supposed that the erroneous answers, as they appear on the records, are in any way specific. Whatever the nature of the disorder of speech, the mistakes which occur tend to assume the same forms; right and left are confused, eye and ear are mutually mistaken and the movement performed is frequently the exact opposite to that demanded by the picture.

There is a remarkable resemblance between these results and the records obtained when the patient imitates hand, eye and ear movements of the observer sitting face to face. Evidently the problem is essentially the same. In the one instance the action to be copied is carried out by a living person, in the other it is indicated pictorially. But both forms of test demand accurate silent formulation of the differentiating characteristics of the movements to be executed; both are affected more or less together and the degree to which they are disturbed depends rather on the severity than on the specific form of the aphasia.

Thus it is evident that the power of recognising the meaning of a picture suffers in a different way according to whether it implies a command or not. Most aphasics can understand a picture and appreciate its full significance, although they cannot translate into action some complex order it implies.

§ 2. DRAWING

The capacity to draw forms one of the most interesting means we possess for investigating the defects of function associated with these disorders of speech. But to be of any value the examination must be carried out systematically. To draw spontaneously, to copy a model, to produce the figure of an elephant to command, or to construct from memory a ground-plan of some familiar room are tests of a profoundly different order and must be investigated independently in each case of aphasia. For it is not the motor aspect of the act of delineation which is affected, but the power to translate some percept, image or idea into the symbolic terms of a drawing.

(a) *Drawing from a model and its reproduction from memory*

Most of my patients were delighted if asked to draw some simple object placed before them such as a jug, a glass or a candlestick. Many of them even reproduced in outline with considerable accuracy the complex structure of a glass spirit lamp. This is a severe test and demands considerable power of observation and intelligence; for the wick must be shown through the glass, not only as projecting above the brass collar but continued below it into the fluid contained in the body of the lamp.

I then remove the object from sight and, after an interval of five minutes or more, the patient is asked to draw it again from memory. Now it is a remarkable fact that the power of drawing from a model and reproduction from memory rise and fall together. The latter task, which is somewhat harder, tends to suffer first and to a more severe degree. But the same faults appear on both drawings and I shall therefore consider both aptitudes under the same heading.

Should the disturbance of symbolic formulation and expression be extremely severe or the aphasia associated with grave loss of intellectual capacity, all power of drawing from a model may be abolished. The patient moves the pencil aimlessly over the paper and fails to produce any semblance of the object before him.

But, whenever the disorder of speech is less massive and assumes some specific form, capacity to draw from a simple model is rarely destroyed completely. It may, however, be profoundly reduced if as with semantic aphasia the main defects depend on inability to appreciate the general meaning of a situation. Thus No. 10 failed to delineate a vase of simple form either from the model or from memory. Dr P. (No. 24) made a poor picture of a spirit lamp and failed altogether to reproduce it after it was removed from sight. In most instances of semantic aphasia the drawing is feeble, the lines uncertain and the patient complains that he has difficulty in knowing how to begin. A young Lieutenant (No. 8) had always been extremely fond of drawing and possessed a considerable reputation in his family for his sketches; but since he was wounded most of this facility had deserted him. He drew a poor representation of a wineglass from a model and repeated this drawing with all its faults almost exactly from memory. He complained

"I have difficulty in reasoning out how the lines go. I see but I can't get a clear impression in my mind how this (the stem) goes in and how the bottom comes." Miss S. (No. 25) had been taught to draw and to block out an object on paper; but the result of her attempt to draw a candlestick from a model was not up to her preparation or knowledge. She could not bring the figure within the limits of the sheet of paper, nor did she place it directly in the centre. Asked to draw it from memory, she made a bad reproduction of her previous drawing. "I can see the brass candlestick and know it wasn't fat in the middle like this (pointing to her sketch). If you ask me where the largest part was, I cannot tell you. I can see the square base. I can see the mass but I can't remember the detail to draw it."

Even the nominal aphasic, who suffers mainly from defective appreciation of the meaning of words and other symbols, may find some difficulty in drawing from the model and from memory provided the disturbance of function is sufficiently severe. Thus No. 7 made a poor outline drawing of a spirit lamp and did not attempt to represent the mechanism of the burner and wick; this drawing he reproduced from memory with all its faults. These defects were not due to permanent incapacity; for some years later he drew an excellent picture of the same lamp both before and after it was removed from sight. Moreover, even on the first examination shortly after he was wounded, he copied with complete accuracy a drawing made by me of the same object. No. 23, a congenital example of aphasia of this class, drew a spirit lamp fairly well from the model, but was much less successful in reproducing it from memory. On the whole, however, nominal aphasia does not materially diminish the power of drawing from a model unless the defects are severe, whilst drawing from memory tends to be more easily disturbed.

So long as the disorder of function consists mainly in want of capacity to formulate words and phrases, drawing is not affected. Thus all my verbal and syntactical aphasics carried out these tests with ease and remarkable accuracy.

(b) *Drawing to command*

To draw some definite figure to order without the aid of a model is a task of considerable intellectual difficulty and it is in consequence gravely affected in a large proportion of cases of aphasia. I am accustomed to test this loss of power by asking the patient to draw an elephant; this object was selected because the shape of the body is so characteristic and the trunk and tusks cannot be omitted even by the most unobservant normal individual. Fortunately many of my patients were familiar with this animal, not only from visits to the Zoological Gardens, but owing to military service in India, or voyages to that country and in one case to employment in the orchestra of a circus.

Massive loss of symbolic formulation and expression destroys all power of drawing an elephant to command. No. 21 had been employed as steward on board a boat travelling to India and had brought home some carved figures of elephants which stood on the mantle-piece of his sitting-room. Asked to draw an elephant, he answered, "Yes, I've been all over, seen lots." I enquired, "In India?" and he replied, "Yes, I've got some on my what you call it." But the drawing he produced was ridiculously insufficient.

Even when the aphasia assumes some specific form, all power of executing this task may be abolished. This is particularly the case with semantic defects. Several patients of this group scrawled aimlessly on the paper (No. 8 and No. 24) whilst No. 10 produced an outline which bore no relation to any known animal. He omitted the trunk and, when I enquired if he had left out anything, replied, "Elephant's nose; I'm not sure where the nose ought to be."

Miss S. (No. 25), a congenital example of this form of disorder, produced a picture distinctly resembling an elephant, except that she gave it a bushy tail and forgot the tusks. After she had finished she exclaimed, "I haven't put the tusks in. I can't remember where they come. They come from just below the eye I think; but I don't know, I believe they are teeth and should come out of the top of the jaw really." After making several attempts to argue the question out to herself, she asked, "May I do a diagrammatic picture according to what I know about tusks and teeth and noses and all that, on the assumption that the elephant is like every animal is?" She then produced the drawing on p. 385, Vol. II, carrying on a running commentary as each part was filled in. "This is a diagrammatic picture. It is made up of what I know about tusks and teeth and noses. I think what all animals have and then make it up. I made an open mouth; then I put in the teeth. I got rid of the nose by putting it like that (elevated). That's all I can do." Evidently her failure to draw an elephant's head to command was due to want of capacity to formulate and express by means of lines a general conception of its appearance; attempts to reason it out point by point led to less confusion.

Nominal aphasia is also associated with profound loss of power to execute this test. Any drawing the patient might be able to make was either absurdly unlike an elephant or lacked some characteristic feature. Capt. C. (No. 2), a Staff Officer, accustomed to draw both for business and pleasure, produced a figure which was devoid of a trunk and tusks and bore no resemblance to an elephant[1]. Yet, when attempting to describe the difficulties of transport in the East, he drew spontaneously a spirited picture of a camel[2]. With the gradual recovery of speech his power of drawing to command steadily improved and, two years and a half after the first examination, he drew an excellent representation of an elephant to order.

Syntactical disorders of speech do not materially affect the capacity to draw to command, unless the patient attempts to formulate aloud or to himself the various features he wishes to delineate. No. 15, who told me "I was good drawder...drawer...at school," was asked to draw an elephant. He replied, "Yes I seen them...up other end...India," but produced the figure in Vol. II, p. 232. When drawing he uttered the words aloud and instead of tusks said "irons, highons"; misled by the false nomenclature he added horns to the figure, but was finally able to explain his error by gestures. Even on subsequent occasions, when I persuaded him to remain silent, he produced an inadequate picture without trunk or tusks; yet he made an excellent drawing of a spirit lamp from the model and subsequently from memory. Another patient (No. 13), with clearly defined syntactical defects of a less severe order, was able to draw the figure of an elephant showing all its distinctive features.

The more closely the disorder of speech approximates to a specific defect of verbal formulation and expression, the less likely is it this test will be affected. All my aphasics of this group could draw an elephant to command and, even if the outline was crude and the lines were feeble, all the characteristic parts were represented[3].

In conclusion, the power to draw complicated figures of this kind to order is disturbed in two ways. Either the aphasia is extremely severe and massive, or the form it assumes is associated with more or less incapacity to appreciate the meaning of words and other symbols and to manipulate them for the purposes of representation.

But whatever the cause of these defects there is nothing specific about the records obtained with this test. Sometimes the patient scratches idly on the paper; at others he can draw a figure of some kind lacking one or more of the characteristic parts of an elephant. It would be impossible, however, to determine from the drawing alone to what class of aphasia

[1] Vol. II, p. 23.   [2] Vol. II, p. 22.
[3] Yet several of these patients were compelled to draw with the left hand.

the defects of speech belonged. This may be betrayed by the remarks of the patient, but not by the nature of the record on the paper.

(c) *Drawing a ground-plan*

At some period in the course of the examination the patient is asked to construct a ground-plan of his ward or of some other familiar room. This is a severe intellectual task and suffers gravely in many forms of aphasia.

Provided he could be transported from place to place, I have been accustomed to make most of my observations in some remote part of the hospital or at home, so as to avoid the noise and bustle of a great institution. Day after day the patient would come to my house and so grew familiar with the surroundings in which we worked. When this was the case, I asked him to look about him and to take especial notice of the position of the fireplace, windows and doors. He was then taken into another room and requested to make a simple plan of that in which we habitually sat.

As might have been expected most of those with semantic defects failed completely to carry out this test. Asked to draw a plan of his room in the hospital, No. 10 made no attempt even to put pencil to paper, saying, "I've all sorts of ideas, but I can't carry them out." But with his eyes closed he had no difficulty in pointing to the position which the window, fireplace and pieces of furniture would occupy in relation to himself as he lay in bed. When asked to say how the wash-hand stand stood in relation to the fireplace or the latter to the door, he entirely failed to do so; allowed, however, to say, "The fire is there and the door there," he pointed to their position with complete accuracy. He knew exactly where they were and was certain he could "see them in his mind," but was unable to express their relative position to one another in words or as a drawing.

On a subsequent occasion, after he had failed to draw from memory a ground-plan of the room in which we had so often worked, I modified my procedure as follows. I made him shut his eyes and point to the position of the various objects as I named them, which he did perfectly. His eyes were then opened and I put before him an outline plan representing the four walls only, on which he indicated with his finger the place of each piece of furniture in turn; this he carried out correctly in every instance. Finally, I asked him once again to draw a plan of the room in which we worked and he was now able to do so, at any rate as far as its main features were concerned. He said, "When you asked me to do this first, I couldn't do it. I couldn't get the starting-point. I knew where all the things were in the room, but I had difficulty in getting a starting-point, when it came to setting them down on a plan. You made me point out on the plan and it was quite easy because you had done it. After things were pointed out, I retained them in my memory and got them down on paper quite easily."

In the same way No. 5, after producing a completely inaccurate plan, complained, "I can see it all in my mind, but I can't put it down."

Miss S. (No. 25), who suffered with a slighter and congenital form of semantic aphasia, alone of this group succeeded in constructing a ground-plan. She explained her method as follows: "I put myself and then I went round the room putting in the fireplace and then the couch and so on. The way I got it was by putting in each thing as I remembered it. I made no general plan. I could see the things I put in quite clearly." It must be remembered that this patient is a woman of unusual intelligence, who has spent all her life in attempting to circumvent her disabilities.

Nominal aphasia is also associated with inability to construct from memory a ground-plan of some familiar room. Thus, from the time Capt. C. (No. 2) first came under my care, there was no doubt that he could recall the position of the various pieces of furniture in his room at the hospital. If I drew a foursided figure on paper to represent its shape in outline, he could point to the place of tables, chairs, cupboards and windows correctly. But as soon as he was asked to construct a ground-plan of the room, he failed entirely; he drew in elevation the table, the desk, the mirror on the wall and the electric light pendant from the ceiling. He could reproduce his visual images of these objects, but was unable to transpose them into terms of a ground-plan.

In the same way No. 11 failed to execute this test and drew the salient pieces of furniture in elevation. Asked to point to their position on a plan drawn by me, he did so without mistakes. I then handed him an identical outline sketch and on this occasion he was more successful in marking in the situation of the various objects; but he still tended to represent them in elevation, the door had a handle, the couch had four legs and the bookcase a projecting flap. He insisted that, when attempting to draw a ground-plan, he saw my room and the objects he was trying to indicate.

This tendency to represent the salient features of a room in elevation was present in all my patients who suffered from nominal aphasia. Evidently the power of recalling visual images at will was greater than with the semantic group, although there was difficulty in translating them into terms of a plan. The nominal aphasic therefore reproduced what he saw in his mind, just as he drew from the model or from memory; but he was unable to execute the more difficult act of translating them into a diagram.

Neither syntactical nor verbal aphasia disturbs the power of carrying out this test with accuracy, provided the patient is naturally intelligent and the loss of mental aptitude is not extremely severe. All my young officers (No. 1, No. 4 and No. 17), belonging to the group with verbal defects, showed unusual power of constructing a ground-plan, even though they were compelled by hemiplegia to draw with the left hand.

Records obtained by asking the patient to construct a ground-plan from memory obey the principles deduced from all other tests which demand formulation and expression in terms of drawing. Success or failure depends on the intellectual difficulty of the task and on the severity and specific form assumed by the loss of function. Semantic aphasia, which is associated with inability to formulate the general meaning or intention of an act, leads most readily to defective execution of this test. But the nominal aphasic also fails to carry it out perfectly and tends to fall back on representation of his memory images in elevation. These he can formulate with considerable accuracy, but he cannot translate them into the symbolic terms of a plan. On the other hand, the more nearly the disturbance corresponds to a want of verbal or syntactical formulation, the less is this test likely to be affected, unless the disease produces severe and wide-spread defects of function.

(d) *Drawing spontaneously*

It might have been assumed that, if a patient was unable to draw from a model or to command, he could not draw spontaneously; but this is not necessarily true. Should the disturbance of symbolic formulation and expression be extremely gross, all power of drawing may be abolished, especially if he is compelled in consequence of right hemiplegia to employ his left hand.

But so long as the aphasia assumes some specific form and the patient is intelligent, he can frequently draw spontaneously, although he is unable to do so to command. For instance Lieut. M. (No. 10) produced a feeble representation of a jug both from the model and from memory; a child could have done better. Asked to draw an elephant, he made a scrawl on the paper which bore no resemblance to any known animal; and yet, when told to draw anything that came into his mind, he made an excellent outline picture of a Dutch bee-hive, pointing out the high entrance which distinguishes it from the English form and indicated the bees on guard before the opening.

Capt. C. (No. 2) formed one of the most remarkable examples of the difference between drawing spontaneously and to command. Told to draw an elephant, he produced an absurd figure without trunk, tusks or ears; yet he was intimately familiar with this animal from his service in India. On one occasion, however, he was trying to describe the difficulties of transport in the East and, unable to express himself in words, drew a spirited rough picture of a camel.

A young man (No. 23) with nominal aphasia of congenital origin could draw a jug from a model, but reproduced it somewhat feebly from memory. He made a poor drawing of an elephant and explained his confusion as follows: "I can see it, but it keeps coming and going. It's more of a guess." But, when I asked him to draw anything he chose, he produced a remarkably detailed representation of the house in which he lived. He blackened over one of the windows with shading, saying, "That was a window, but they've closed it up; it's all blank." This, on questioning his sister, I found to be correct.

Sometimes, however, even though the disturbance of symbolic formulation and expression assumes a specific form, the power of drawing spontaneously may be diminished. This is particularly liable to occur with semantic defects. For example No. 8, failing to draw an elephant to command or to construct a ground-plan of the room in which we worked, asked to be allowed to draw a landscape. After making a few meaningless scrawls on the paper, he explained his difficulty as follows: "I want the thing in front of me. I don't know how to build it up, to build up the foreground. I can see it in my mind, but I can't put it down."

Verbal aphasia is not accompanied by any diminution of power to draw spontaneously, unless the lesion has produced considerable loss of intellectual capacity. Two young officers, No. 4 and No. 17, belonging to this group used to amuse themselves by drawing; both had been compelled in consequence of severe right hemiplegia to employ the left hand, but in spite of this disability No. 17 produced an excellent portrait of himself as seen in a mirror.

(e) *Summary*

Thus the power of drawing follows exactly the same principles as other forms of behaviour used as tests in these disorders of speech. When the loss of function is extremely grave, all acts of drawing may be affected and, even if the aphasia assumes some specific form, the amount of the disturbance depends on the severity of the task.

But in addition the capacity to draw depends on the extent to which the patient can appreciate the meaning of the act he is about to perform. He must be able to formulate to himself the manner in which to set about the task. Then he must be able to translate his sensations, images or ideas into the form of lines which possess indicative significance. A strong line is one which reveals the firm purpose and intention of the draftsman whilst a feeble one betrays his uncertainty.

Even defective appreciation of nominal significance may render the more severe tests impossible. For the patient has difficulty in formulating his mental processes precisely in linear symbols. He can, however, usually draw from a model, or in response to his own desires. When constructing a ground-plan, he is liable to fall back on a direct reproduction of his visual images and, unable to translate them into strictly diagrammatic terms, tends to draw the salient objects in elevation.

The more purely verbal forms of aphasia do not usually interfere with the power of drawing spontaneously or to command and the patient can construct a ground-plan with remarkable accuracy, even when compelled by right hemiplegia to employ his left hand. Want of capacity to evoke words and phrases seems to produce little or no effect on this form of behaviour.

Thus, it is not the motor act, even in its highest form, which is affected in association with these disorders of speech. For the power of drawing is least disturbed in those cases which approximate most closely to so-called "motor" aphasia. On the other hand, want of appreciation of general or verbal meaning is a potent cause of loss of capacity to formulate and express some process of thought in terms of drawing.

§ 3. VISUAL IMAGERY

In the past much stress has been laid on the important part played by loss of visual images in the phenomena of aphasia and kindred disorders of speech. These statements are uniformly based, not on actual observations, but on purely a priori assumption. It is in fact difficult, and perhaps impossible, to devise tests suitable for clinical application which are capable of revealing the condition of visual imagery in the same objective manner that we can record the capacity to read or to write.

I, at any rate, make no claim to have employed such tests. But in the course of the various methodical observations described in the two previous sections on the appreciation of pictures and the capacity to draw spontaneously, from the model or to command, most of the patients betrayed in conversation their powers of employing visual imagery. Such expressions as "I see it in my mind, but I can't put it down" occurred repeatedly and, although purely introspective, revealed a condition of the patient's mental processes worthy of closer consideration.

The fact that normal persons exist in whom visual imagery is apparently non-existent during waking life shows that such processes are not indispensable for thinking. But the large majority of the young men who formed the material of this research were obviously accustomed to visualise more or less strongly; some of them were conscious of this fact like No. 17, an ex-medical student, who said, "I always did visualise in my work." I am aware that the very existence of visual imagery has been called in question by some who are evidently devoid of this power. But to one whose most vivid mental life is closely bound up with such images this denial has no more value than the statements with regard to colour of a man blind from birth.

As far as the results of logical thinking are concerned, no obvious differences can be discerned between those whose memory consists mainly of visual images and those who depend on other methods for recalling what they have seen. The product of thought may be identical, although it has been reached by a different process. But when two such individuals are asked to describe from memory the appearance of some definite object, such as the breakfast table with its contents or the house in which they live, the difference between them is likely to be manifested in the expressions they employ. The man who depends on visual images tends to describe the objects as if he saw them in front of him and he usually mentions not only their colour but their relative position. If he is of a lively temperament, he points into empty space with the words "The teapot is there and the sugar basin there," adding "I can see the loaf of bread and the eggs and bacon." He begins his description of the house in which he lives by stating its shape, the number of stories and windows and the relative position of the front door. He tends to pass from the general to the particular, as if he was describing a picture; and in fact he frequently states that he sees it before him. To one who does not habitually employ this method, but depends on some other form of imagery or means of recall, these expressions are foreign and incomprehensible. He tends to build up his description step by step in detail, as if his attention was moving in order from point to point. In some of my cases a patient with a natural tendency to employ visual images was compelled by his disability to fall back on this method of logical reconstruction[1].

(a) *The power of forming visual images spontaneously*

If before the onset of the lesion visual images were habitually employed in the normal processes of thinking, their vividness may remain undiminished in spite of grave disorders of speech, even though the power of evoking them to order and manipulating them at will is profoundly affected. It will be well therefore to consider first of all what can be gleaned from my cases with regard to the behaviour of spontaneous visual images before dealing with the part they play in response to external prompting.

If the disorder of symbolic formulation and expression is extremely severe and is associated with much mental hebetude, visual imagery may suffer like any other psychical process. But it is remarkable how rarely it is affected so long as the disturbance of speech assumes a specific form.

Amongst my examples of verbal aphasia, No. 1 described from memory the exact position of his bed and the other objects in his ward, which was of an unusual and complicated shape. He recalled and distinguished accurately the colours of the uniforms worn by the Matron and her nurses and asserted that he had always had a strong visual memory. No. 17, who had been a medical student, showed a remarkable power of recalling visual impressions, describing exactly the colour of the curtains and walls of the ward; he volunteered the statement "I always did visualise in my work." Even No. 9, a severe example of verbal aphasia with hemianopsia and right hemiplegia, could recall the relative position of the beds, windows and table in his part of the ward and describe the colour of the curtains.

All three patients with syntactical aphasia showed evidence of possessing visual imagery, especially No. 15. After drawing an excellent picture of a spirit lamp from memory, he insisted that he could see the whole lamp and glass together with a "bit of string to light it" (the wick).

Nominal aphasia does not destroy the power of forming visual images, although they can no longer be manipulated with freedom and certainty

---

[1] See No. 25 and the drawing of an elephant's head (Vol. II, p. 385).

for the purpose of formulating and expressing ideas[1]. For instance, Capt. C. (No. 2) struggled with poor success to convey to me what he had gathered from the printed account of a famous prize-fight. As soon as I asked "Can you see the fight?" a profound change came over his narration. He said "Now I think about the fight I see the picture of Carpentier. I see Beckett falling...I see the Ref..Ref..what you call it... Referee...the last thing I can picture is Carpentier standing like this with both hands like this." He sprang from his bed and assumed an attitude, with both hands on his hips looking down towards the ground, in the position assumed by Carpentier in the photographs of the termination of the fight. The change in manner from the puzzled aspect of a man slowly recalling what he had read to the brisk smiling person describing what he saw was remarkable.

But, although he possessed the power of producing visual images, they were insufficient for consecutive and logical thinking. They formed isolated points, which would normally have been linked up by other symbolic processes of mental activity. On one occasion, wishing to tell me how he would walk from the hospital in Westminster to the War Office in Whitehall, he said, "Suppose I was going from the Army and Navy, that's what it is called, just round here (i.e. the Army and Navy Stores) I should then say some place to a hospital about a quarter of a mile away. I remember the hospital is on the way to the War Office, about half way. I believe it's the Abbey. No, it's near the Abbey on the way to the War Office." Later he added "I saw the hospital." I put the question "The Abbey?" and he replied as follows. "It's here and then it's gone again and I have to feel for it again. The only thing I can remember of it is the opening, the big opening, where everybody goes in. I can get that" (moving his hand to indicate a large arch). Since it was obvious that he was attempting to describe Westminster Hospital and Westminster Abbey, which are close to one another though on opposite sides of the road he would take, I asked, "Have the Hospital and Abbey anything to do with one another?" He replied, "Nothing except my focus, the place of them, the distance that is all." Later he added "You see, it's like this; with me it's all bits. I have to jump like this," marking a thick line between two points with a pencil, "Like a man who jumps from one thing to the next. I can see them, but I can't express. Really it is that I haven't enough names."

It is evident from this conversation that he was able to recall visual images of objects on his way from the hospital in Westminster to the

---

[1] Cf. No. 7, Vol. II, p. 106, No. 11, Vol. II, p. 195, No. 22, Vol. II, p. 335.

War Office. First of all he saw the Army and Navy Stores and then Westminster Hospital on the left, with the great door of Westminster Abbey on the right; but want of names prevented him from linking them up except by their position and he was forced to jump from one image to another without the cohesive bond of verbal formulation.

After No. 23 had drawn a jug placed before him, he described its shape and coloured pattern from memory in the following terms: "I can see it; it's white with a blue edging and crinkly all round the handle. There's a boy on one side and a woman on the other, green I think." All these details were correct. I showed him a wooden figure of a Venetian guitar player in a white mask, dark cloak and three-cornered hat. Five minutes after it had been withdrawn from his sight, he said "I see it. He's playing...I've been trying to think what they call those things. He's standing on a board. He's got a sluch (slouch) hat on. I can see the statue and then it's gone; it flies over, it comes up and then goes faint and then comes again." This fluctuating nature of visual images, when they cannot be fixed by some symbolic formula, is a frequent phenomenon in both nominal and semantic aphasia.

For instance No. 10, a striking example of the latter form of defective use of language, volunteered the following remarks a few days after I had tested his power of drawing in various ways. "I thought of what you asked me to do, drawing the glass. In bed I was trying to think about it. I was trying to see the glass bottle. I knew it was a bottle and I could describe the shape of it, and I remember making a drawing, and I could describe the drawing. But then, when it came to seeing it as a picture, I was more or less nonplussed. I often seemed to have got the picture, but it seemed to evade me. There is a photograph of my wife, which is hanging in the bedroom. I can see that; the expression in that photograph is very good, I can see that." He then added, "I can see the bee alighting on the alighting board. I see it quite clearly. Now, for instance, our hives are painted in two colours, one green, one white. I can see a bee alighting on the alighting board, say, for instance, yellow-coloured pollen. Yes I can see them quite clearly. The more I try to...to make them come, the more difficult is it to get in touch with them, as one may say."

Even so severe an example of semantic aphasia as Dr. P. (No. 24) un-doubtedly possessed some power of visual imagery. Thus, when I said to him "rose," he answered me he saw a red rose projected in space before him. He added "I can see your hall-door and your dining-room. I see your furniture, which is very pretty. I thought you had a taste, an appreciation of furniture. I saw the gentleman (my father's portrait), I saw his bearded face and I wondered was it your father or yourself. I noticed the antique mirror there. I can still see them all in my mind."

But as soon as he was told to describe some definite object, such as my front door which he had seen many times, he was liable to make absurd mistakes. He said the door was brown instead of green and thought the front of the house was grey instead of white; and yet he described the three bells on the door-post and placed my brass plate correctly. But he was obliged to reconstruct by formal argument the name it bore, saying, "I see the name in front of me now. I confused it first with Heath, then with an old friend of mine Heard, and now I have corrected it."

Thus none of the specific forms of aphasia interfere directly with the spontaneous recall of visual images. But both nominal and semantic defects limit the power to employ these mental processes for the purposes of consecutive and logical thinking.

(b) *Visual images and drawing from memory*

It is obviously possible to draw from memory without the aid of visual images; for otherwise no one devoid of this form of imagery would be able to delineate what he had seen or to recall detail sufficiently to construct a ground-plan. But most of my patients insisted during the performance of these tasks that they were representing on paper what they "saw" in their minds.

The various tests I have habitually employed are not, however, of the same order of difficulty. Once an object has been drawn from the model, it is easy to reproduce the drawing by recollecting the acts that have been performed, or with the help of an image of the original sketch. This was the method adopted by many of my patients, who made an exact reproduction of the picture drawn from the model with all its faults and omissions.

To draw an elephant to command or to construct a ground-plan of some familiar room from memory are tasks of much greater severity. Normally they can be executed with considerable accuracy; but, should they present any difficulty, the patient is liable to fall back on logical reconstruction, based on his knowledge of the characteristic features of the object he is attempting to represent. For instance, Miss S. (No. 25), after failing to draw the general outline of an elephant, begged me to let her make "a diagrammatic picture according to what I know about tusks and teeth and noses and all that, on the assumption that the elephant is like every other animal." As she filled in each detail, she carried on a running commentary. "This is my diagrammatic picture. It is made up of what I know about tusks and teeth and noses. I think what all animals have and then make it up." She drew from memory an excellent plan of the room in which we worked, saying, "I put myself and then I went round the room putting in the fireplace and then the couch and so on. The way I got it was by putting in each thing. I made no general plan"; and yet she asserted that she could "see the things" she indicated "quite clearly."

So long as the disturbance of speech consists mainly of inability to form words and phrases, the capacity to draw from memory is not materially affected. Even No. 9, a severe example of verbal aphasia with hemianopsia and right hemiplegia, not only made an excellent drawing of a spirit lamp from memory, but produced unprompted a sketch of a human face. But he became somewhat confused when asked to draw an elephant, and, although the principal pieces of furniture were indicated correctly on a ground-plan, he tended to represent them in elevation.

Should the defects of symbolic formulation and expression include want of power to discover adequate names or to appreciate the general meaning of the situation, visual images can no longer be employed freely for such acts as drawing from memory. Capt. C. (No. 2), who drew a spirited representation of a camel spontaneously, failed to depict an elephant to command, although he was equally familiar with the appearance of the two animals. No. 23 made a fairly accurate picture of a horse unprompted followed by a poor drawing of an elephant to command. But he asserted, "I can see what that is, same as I can see a horse what that is." Asked to draw anything he chose, he produced a remarkably detailed and accurate representation of the house in which he lived, saying, "If I put my mind on it I can see it clearly." But, when he attempted to reproduce from memory a jug he had previously drawn from a model, he was comparatively unsuccessful and complained, "It's not clear enough to put it down; I only guess it, then it goes. I can't see it always; I saw it all full and then it went. It always goes faint and I can't seem to get it when I want to." The fleeting character of visual images, unsupported by complete power of symbolic formulation, prevents their employment as an aid to expressive delineation carried out to command.

No. 18, a case of semantic aphasia, complained that he could not picture two objects in his mind together; "I can pass from one to the other, but as soon as I catch the other, it (the first) goes straight out of my mind. As soon as I attempt to think of the other before I seem to catch it in my mind, the first one has gone." This hampered him greatly, when he attempted to construct a ground-plan of my room and he omitted several of its salient details.

Sometimes semantic aphasia leads to so severe a loss of power to appreciate the full meaning and intention of an act to be performed that the patient cannot even draw from a model. In such circumstances, he is still less able to draw from memory or to command. He can evoke visual images spontaneously, but their fleeting nature, combined with the defective power of translating them into action, renders all expressive delineation difficult or impossible. Thus No. 8 complained, when drawing a wineglass from memory, "I have difficulty in reasoning out how the lines go. I see, but I can't get a clear impression in my mind how this (the stem) goes in and how the bottom comes." He produced a poor diagram of my room omitting the windows and doors, although he marked in such details as the typewriter and the ophthalmoscopic lamp.

(c) *Evocation of visual images in response to words*

When we are seeking a word in which to express our exact meaning, the presence of visual images may actually hinder its discovery by substituting a pictorial for a verbal symbol. We see the face and appearance of the person we are recalling so distinctly that there is no necessity for his name in order that we may think about him; a name is required only when we speak of him to others. I have no doubt that in some of my patients the appearance of visual images actually inhibited the discovery of names; but it is impossible to investigate such subtle difficulties clinically.

On the other hand, the patient not uncommonly complains that he cannot recall visual images with ease and certainty in response to words. In a normal person with active imagery, all external or internal verbalisation is associated with a cloud of relevant pictures, which add vividness and security to the expression of conceptual thinking. This association was undoubtedly weakened in many of my cases of aphasia.

For instance, when Capt. C. (No. 2) read aloud or repeated after me the simple phrases of the man, cat and dog tests, he complained, "I say them one after the other and I don't think. I don't have a picture; I say them like, what is the animal, the parrot, yes the parrot." On another occasion he said, "If you say dog to me, I can see the dog; but if you say the dog and the cat I think of the dog and can't think of anything else."

This lack of power to evoke an appropriate visual image in response to a word led to the following interesting phenomenon. Suppose Capt. C. was asked to choose some familiar object in response to a spoken or printed word, he passed his hand over the various articles on the table until he finally settled on the one which corresponded to the name presented to him. If, however, no duplicate lay before him, he was unable to grasp the meaning of the word. I handed him two cards, one bearing the word MATCHES, the other WATCH; he pointed to the match-box and, holding up the other card, said, "nothing here," which was correct. Asked what is the difference, he replied, "They are both written (printed); this one is here (pointing to the matches), the other there is nothing. I focus this one (matches) because it is here (pointing to the box). I can't focus this (the watch card) so well because it is not so clear." He then gazed round my room until, fixing his eyes on my clock, he said, "When I look at that big one, that helps me. I want to interpret the reading 'watch' into a picture or into that watch (pointing to the clock). If I think of a watch and don't have to read it, I see a picture of my own watch. If you say it to me the picture is alright; if you show it me like that (printed) I have to think. I don't get the picture easily[1]."

Thus, with nominal aphasia the word no longer recalls an appropriate visual image; this, in a man who habitually visualised strongly, is further evidence of loss of verbal meaning The significance of the word is not sufficiently potent to evoke a mental picture of the object. But, when once the meaning of the individual word has been elucidated by repetition and study, the total picture presented to the mind may be full and accurate. For instance, No. 23 had extreme difficulty in understanding a passage from Dickens describing a squint-eyed man in breeches and gaiters. But, after he had read it aloud and to himself, had written what he remembered and then listened to my rendering, he said, "I can see the man...I can see him with his leather gaiters and riding breeches and hat and swish...squint-eyed and a funny chin... There was something else...did you say he had a beard on his chin? No, not that; there was something else...I see someone with a black hat, black coat and waistcoat and yellow riding breeches and gaiters with boots and a switch...looking down he is with his squint eyes. I should see that for an hour or more. He'll keep coming on my mind." In this narration he was obviously describing what he saw and even deduced from his mental picture details that were not in the printed text.

But with semantic aphasia the difficulty consists in forming a complete picture from a series of words rather than in calling up an appropriate

[1] Cf. Lotmar [96].

image in response to a single name. Thus, at the close of a series of man, cat and dog tests, No. 10 volunteered the following statement: "I can see a man with his trousers cleanly cut. He is tall and straight; he has a hat on and is clean shaven." I said, "Tell me about the dog." He answered, "The dog has short legs like a terrier, roughish coated, may be a Scotch terrier." Asked about the cat, he replied "It's an ordinary cat; the whiskers are rather evident. She is sitting, not lying down. She's just sitting up on her haunches, that's the word I wanted[1]." Yet, although he had remarkable power of recalling detail, he had considerable difficulty in obtaining a clear mental picture from a consecutive series of spoken or printed words.

In the same way Miss S. (No. 25) could see the outlines, colour and lighting of visual images which recurred spontaneously, or in answer to command, "But I cannot see letters like I see you or the Tube Station, when I am away from you." Moreover, she had difficulty in evoking a complete mental picture of Landor's garden in Italy, until she had perused and heard the description many times in succession.

Thus, both nominal and semantic defects tend to disturb the power of forming visual images in response to spoken or printed words. But in the former variety of aphasia single words or phrases are not clearly understood and the visual image is therefore less easily evoked. With semantic aphasia the difficulty consists less in lack of verbal appreciation than in want of power to form a complete picture representing the total situation.

(d) *Summary*

I would gladly have investigated the effect of these disorders of speech on other kinds of imagery, especially the so-called "motor" or "kin-aesthetic" form. But I could discover no means of making this enquiry in pathological cases which did not run the risk of suggesting an answer, since even the most intelligent of my patients was ignorant of such mental processes. On the other hand, most of them volunteered much information with regard to their visual images. The tests with pictures and drawing aroused their attention to their lack of power and they were anxious to explain to me the nature of their difficulties.

The conclusions to which I have arrived in the previous pages may be summarised as follows:

Provided the lesion has not produced great mental hebetude, the vividness of spontaneous imagery may remain undiminished. But, in

[1] Slightly shortened, vide Vol. II, p. 172; also p. 178.

such circumstances, they form isolated moments in the act of thinking and are not linked up effectively by coherent bonds of verbal formulation. They cannot be evoked with certainty to command, nor translated at will into some other form of symbolic representation. But they are never destroyed completely in those who have been accustomed to employ them in an active form before the injury; they come and go and fluctuate involuntarily. In such circumstances, the greater the effort expended by the patient, the more difficult is it "to get in touch" with the appropriate visual images. Should this be the case, they cannot be evoked with certainty in response to a spoken or written word, phrase, or narrative.

Though not in themselves conceptual, visual images take part amongst the other activities of the mind which result in symbolic formulation and expression. In this way they come to be affected in certain forms of aphasia. Images may appear spontaneously, or be evoked voluntarily, but their relation to one another cannot be expressed as a logical deduction, a formal statement, or a diagrammatic representation.

So long as the disturbance in the use of language consists of defects of verbal or phrasal formulation and expression, visual imagery is little if at all affected. But the closer the disorder approximates to a want of appreciation of either the details or general meaning of a situation, the less easily can appropriate visual images be evoked at will.

Visual imagery adds to the vividness and certainty of conceptual thinking, like a series of pictures illustrating a printed text which is comprehensible without them. It helps to elucidate the meaning of words in whatever form they may have been presented to the mind. Should the power of finding the appropriate name or appreciating verbal significance be diminished, the word is no longer sufficiently potent to call up the appropriate mental image and it may be impossible to recognise its meaning, unless the object indicated is actually visible at the moment. In nominal aphasia this increases the difficulty in understanding both spoken and written symbols of every kind.

Semantic defects, on the other hand, are accompanied by inability to evoke a complete picture corresponding to the total meaning of the situation. Visual images may appear freely in response to detail, but some essential aspect is frequently wanting in the general mental picture.

Thus, it would seem as if the visual images called up by words and isolated phrases tended to be uncertain and fluctuating in nominal aphasia, whilst in the semantic form these defects were more manifest in the total picture than in its separate details. But, although it may be possible to suspect the existence of such differences from the statements and behaviour of the patient, there is nothing in the actual records to betray them with certainty. It is only by watching his method of action and by listening to his explanations that we can recognise these specific differences between nominal and semantic aphasia.

§ 4. MUSIC

Most of the soldiers who came under my care had been accustomed to sing the popular songs of the day by ear, although few possessed any knowledge of music. In no case was the power of singing these simple airs in time and tune abolished, provided no attempt was made to say the words. It was usually necessary for someone to sing or play on the piano the first bars of the melody and the patient then picked it up and continued it to the end.

But as soon as he tried to say the words, he usually broke down. No. 7 had been on the music hall stage as a singer of serious and sentimental songs before he joined the army. He had never been able to read musical notation easily and had been accustomed to learn mainly by ear. If he was given the opening notes of a song he had known before the injury deprived him of speech, he sang it through accurately without words. Time, tune and modulation were perfect and his voice had the full volume of a powerful high baritone. But, when he made any attempt to pronounce the words, he was unable to sing at all. He steadily regained his power of speech and four years and nine months after he was wounded might have passed on superficial examination for a normal man. He still sang well without words; his voice had its full volume and showed no unsteadiness. But as soon as he attempted to add the words he fell out of tune, the volume of his voice decreased and a bad tremolo made its appearance. Evidently the words hindered him, and he complained, "It's the words that worry me...better without words." He had returned to his occupation as a music hall singer, but lost his engagement because of these defects.

In the same way No. 23 could recall a melody provided he did not utter the words. He insisted, "I can get the tune better than what I can the words. Same as when they are playing the violin or piano, I can tell them if they go wrong. I hear the sounds alright, what they ought to go."

Capt. C. (No. 2) could sing several songs through without words, provided his sister played the melody and accompaniment on the piano. When first admitted to the hospital, he could not whistle unprompted and said, "I did not seem to know where to get the tune from." But ten months after the injury, when on a walking tour, he passed a mill and asked his sister what it was. On her replying that it was a mill, he began to whistle "She was a miller's daughter" and continued in perfect tune to the end.

When about this time his sister began to teach him music, she told him that the scale consisted of three tones, a half tone, two tones and another half tone. This puzzled him completely, even when she demonstrated it on the piano. But as soon as she drew a diagram where each horizontal line represented a tone and each short vertical one a half tone, he understood and from that date never forgot it[1].

Major X. (No. 14), although a profound example of syntactical aphasia, had not lost his power of playing the piano and comprehending musical notation. He played for me Chopin's Largo (Op. 20) very slowly, reading the notes and giving the change of key correctly. The right hand was clumsy in consequence of incoordination; but he succeeded in bringing his fingers on to the right notes of the chord and, if he was wrong, immediately corrected his error. Keeping his eyes on the paper he recognised by ear that he had struck a false note and that it did not correspond to the text of the music. Thus it is evident that even a severe degree of syntactical aphasia does not diminish the power of appreciating musical sounds, although it is usually attributed to defects of "auditory images."

No. 22, an example of nominal aphasia, was a professional performer on the double bass and the cornet. He lost the power of understanding not only printed words, but also musical notation and became entirely unable to play either instrument. He said, "I can't read music; I can't tell an a from a b. It affects me the same as reading this," pointing to words in print.

Thus, it would seem that these defects of speech do not directly disturb the power of singing or whistling a melody. It may be necessary to start the patient with the first notes of a tune, or the first words of a song; once the act is initiated in this way, he can continue perfectly.

But any aphasia which interferes with verbal formulation and expression, especially the nominal variety, destroys the power of singing if any attempt is made to utter the words. Nominal aphasia also interferes with the comprehension of musical notation and so destroys the capacity to perform on an instrument.

[1] Vol. II, p. 33.

CHAPTER VIII

SUMMARY STATEMENT OF THE RESULTS OF CLINICAL EXAMINATION

§ 1. PRINCIPLES UNDERLYING THE TESTS EMPLOYED

WE are now in a position to sum up the results to which we have arrived in the previous chapters and to state categorically the nature of the clinical manifestations in aphasia. First of all it is important to remember that my observations were made with the help of new tests, which not only yield more complete information than those in common use, but are also designed to avoid certain fallacies inherent in the ordinary means of examination. No criticism of my results is valid unless the patient's condition has been explored by similar or more perfect and extensive methods.

Our researches on sensation had taught us that a remarkable want of constancy in response was one of the most striking defects produced by injuries of the cortex. A series of stimuli, identical in strength and character, might be appreciated at one time, whilst at another they remained unnoticed. Moreover, a graduated increase was not of necessity followed by an equivalent improvement in the certainty and accuracy of response. The answers frequently varied so profoundly, that it was impossible to say whether a particular stimulus could be appreciated or not, and the patient seemed to be untrustworthy. This tendency for attention to fluctuate occurs in healthy persons, especially under the influence of fatigue; but, as the result of a cortical lesion, it may reach proportions far in excess of any normal variation.

Since this was true of sensory defects, it was obviously useless to judge of the powers of an aphasic by a single answer to some task set before him. Every test must consist as far as possible of an orderly series of observations in which the same problem recurs on several occasions. Sometimes the patient responds correctly, at others he gives a wrong answer or fails to reply at all, and it is often impossible to say whether he can or cannot execute a particular task. But this is in itself evidence that his capacity to carry it out is diminished, provided the test is not abnormally severe.

Thus, when investigating the power to make a choice in response to oral or printed commands, the name of each familiar object or colour is repeated twice or more in the series. If the aphasia is severe, the same order is at one time executed accurately and with ease, whilst on other occasions the patient fails altogether or experiences great difficulty in choosing correctly. The same irregular responses appear throughout all the serial tests; they are equally apparent whatever the nature of the task.

The tests I have employed in this research embody a second principle new to the study of aphasia; for an attempt has been made to graduate them according to the severity of the intellectual problem they present. When investigating defects in spacial sensibility due to cortical lesions, we had already found that tests which depended on recognition of movement in three dimensions, suffered first and most severely; then followed those based on discrimination in two dimensions and last, to a still smaller degree, "spot-finding" or simple localisation.

In the same way an oral or a printed command can be graded in severity according to the number of possible alternatives it presents. Thus, when told to touch the nose, to put out the tongue or to shut the eyes, the patient has to appreciate an order necessitating a single action only and to execute it correctly. Next we combine two of these forms of behaviour and finally raise the task to the full complication of the hand, eye and ear tests, where the difficulty is enhanced by the constant necessity of choosing between right and left. Somewhere along this line of graduated tasks the patient with aphasia may falter or break down according to the nature and gravity of his defects of speech.

The arithmetical tests, as I usually set them, illustrate the same principles. The first consists in adding together two numbers each of which is composed of three figures, so chosen that the sum of any pair of them does not exceed ten; no carrying over from one column to another is necessary. The second exercise in addition demands that the operation of carrying over should be performed once, the third twice, in order to arrive at a correct answer. The three problems in subtraction are graduated in the same manner and the severity of the task is found to rise with the number of times it is necessary to carry over. It must be remembered, however, that subtraction is throughout somewhat more difficult than addition.

Such tests illustrate the importance of graduating the difficulty of the task set to the patient, if we are to arrive at any definite conclusion with regard to his powers of symbolic formulation and expression. For not uncommonly he can solve the first addition correctly and perhaps even the easiest problem in subtraction, although he may fail entirely with all the others. Now if he had been set a test of the first order of difficulty only, the records would have shown that he possessed the power to manipulate numbers. Had the observer chosen one of the more severe tasks in subtraction, or even in addition, he would have concluded that the patient was unable to solve even simple problems in arithmetic. But if the observations are carried out according to the graduated method, we learn the extent to which this power has been affected in any particular case of aphasia, whether slight or severe.

Another rule which runs through all these serial tests is to employ the same sequence whatever the nature of the behaviour required. Thus, with familiar objects or colours, the order in which they follow one another remains the same whether they are named aloud and in writing or are chosen to oral and printed commands. In the same way the patient's power of writing is tested by showing him two pictures of the man, cat and dog tests and asking him to put down on paper the combination he has seen. Then these simple phrases are dictated in exactly the same order and finally he is asked to copy them from print in cursive script. When he is set the far more difficult task of conveying in writing the contents of some paragraph he has read to himself silently, he is also asked to write exactly the same words to dictation, and finally to copy them from print. He is not set to write one sentence spontaneously, another to dictation and to copy a third completely different group of words and phrases.

Moreover, in all these serial methods of examination certain tests are interspersed which do not demand symbolic formulation and expression; these are not affected in uncomplicated cases of aphasia and form a useful guide to the patient's mental capacity. Thus he is asked to choose an object or colour corresponding to one he has just seen, or some article of definite shape is placed in his hand and he selects its duplicate from amongst a set lying before him on the table. These are simple acts of matching, which are not affected in pure aphasic conditions, and the fact that they can be carried out with ease frequently serves to encourage a patient who is depressed or angry at his repeated failures.

But apart from these tests which can be executed with uniform ease, unless the aphasia is complicated by a general loss of intellectual capacity, I have habitually included others so simple that they remain unaffected in the majority of cases. Thus, it is a difficult matter even for normal persons to reproduce exactly movements made when examiner and patient sit face to face; but the task becomes an easy one if the movements to be copied are reflected in a mirror. For it is no longer necessary to choose between right and left; provided the patient understands what he is expected to do, the act becomes one of direct imitation. This is also true when a diagram representing such movements is reflected in a mirror; whereas, if the picture is held in front of the patient, the task becomes difficult because of the necessary translation into right or left. But all these forms of behaviour, however simple they may be under normal conditions, may suffer if he fails to comprehend exactly the aim and intention of the command; then he is puzzled, even by the significance of the reflection, and attempts to reason out what he is expected to do, instead of imitating directly what he sees in the mirror.

Sometimes every answer to a particular series of tests may be given correctly and yet it is obvious from the slowness or number of corrections, that in this respect the power of symbolic formulation and expression is defective. The importance of speed and promptness of response has not been sufficiently recognised in the clinical study of aphasia. Usually it is amply sufficient to record that a particular reply was given slowly or after one or more corrective efforts; but in many cases I have timed the period between question and answer with a stop watch. For, long after all the formal tests can be carried out correctly, those which were originally affected are still distinguished by the slowness or uncertainty of response[1].

With lesions of the brain, especially those affecting the cortex, the patient is still aware of some abnormality of function, when no changes can be detected by the finest methods of clinical examination. Thus, if the sensibility of one hand has been affected, he may complain that the fingers "feel different," although it is impossible to discover any measurable sensory defect. Introspectively the loss of function is always more persistent and severe than the changes to be found experimentally. This is still more evident with disorders of speech; for, although the patient may respond to all the tests correctly, he is conscious that he lacks freedom and ease. It is therefore of the greatest importance to record fully his own statements as to the difficulties he encounters and any conceptions he may have formed, however crude, of the nature of his behaviour. In this way it is often possible to discover profound differences between two series of tests both of which were executed without mistakes.

Bearing these principles in mind I gradually evolved the methods of examination described in Chapter I. These I applied to such patients with aphasia as came my way in civilian practice and by the middle of

---

[1] Cf. Lotmar [96].

1914, after many tentative observations, these new tests had assumed a practicable form. Then came the war and the young men who were under my care with gun-shot wounds of the head gave me unexpected opportunities for testing the validity of these methods and for utilising them clinically.

§ 2. FORMS OF BEHAVIOUR WHICH ARE NOT AFFECTED IN THESE DISORDERS OF SPEECH

It soon became evident, as in truth I had previously recognised, that the manifestations of disordered speech could not be brought under any categories so far recognised; they could only be described in terms of the act which was affected and not in those pertaining to some other form of behaviour. When my tests were applied systematically in suitable examples of aphasia and amnesia, the results did not correspond with any known classification and showed that these affections of speech belonged to an order different from any previously described.

Moreover, in those cases which threw most light on the nature of the disorder, the loss of power was relative and not absolute. A man who was entirely unable to read or write under certain conditions, might be able to do so if the task was presented to him in some other form; the response to any particular test depended not only on the intrinsic nature of the action demanded, but also on the intellectual difficulty which it presented.

These conclusions were to a great extent adumbrated in the writings of Hughlings Jackson and the morbid manifestations are in the main explicable on the general views he enunciated. Yet, although he showed that such disorders in the use of language were due essentially to lack of power to "propositionise," he did not apply this explanation in detail to actual instances of aphasia. But the systematic employment of the tests I have described exposed the fundamental characteristics of these abnormal reactions and showed how they could be differentiated from other mental processes, which remained at the same time unaffected.

It has been universally recognised that a person who is usually speechless may utter words or even phrases under the influence of emotion. Many who can scarcely employ "yes" and "no" correctly can swear; and one of my patients in this condition, who had been to India, when asked to draw an elephant, exclaimed "Yes, I've been all over, seen lots," and "Yes, I've got some on my what you call it," alluding to the figures of elephants on his mantle-piece. But even the longest of such exclamatory or automatic phrases does not convey a complete logical statement of some propositional act of thought. In Jackson's phraseology "a speech-less patient is not wordless, but he does not possess words for voluntary use." This truth is so well established that it needs no further amplification.

Systematic use, in suitable cases, of the methods I have employed enables us to lay down a further rule for distinguishing the mental processes which suffer in aphasia from those which remain relatively intact. The more closely a task set to the patient approximates to a simple act of matching, the less likely is it to be affected, whilst on the other hand the higher the degree of symbolic formulation and expression it demands, the grosser will be the disturbance of function. Thus, for example, a patient who has difficulty in imitating movements made by the observer when they are reflected in a mirror, may be unable to write down what he sees without making many mistakes in right and left.

In uncomplicated cases of aphasia the patient can always pick out from amongst a set of familiar articles or colours the one which cor-responds to that which he has just seen. This is a simple act of matching; a certain object on the table corresponds in its essential characters with the memory of his previous visual impressions and recognition of this similarity is immediate.

But, suppose he is shown two objects at the same time and is told to choose their duplicates, he may fail; for he now attempts to retain them in his memory by formulating the two names[1]. The necessity for even so simple a symbolic representation is liable to disturb the act of selection.

If, instead of allowing the patient to see the object to be selected, some article of familiar use or a wooden block of distinctive geometrical shape is placed in his hand out of sight, he can choose without fail its duplicate from amongst a set of objects of the same class. This apprecia-tion of likeness and difference is based on his tactile impressions. No symbol intervenes between the results produced by his manual sensations and immediate recognition that the object in his hand corresponds with one of those he sees before him and differs in some essential particular from all the others.

Should he disobey the instructions and attempt to name the object he holds in his hand instead of executing the task silently, he may cease to make a choice of any kind. The intervention of a word between the im-pressions he receives from his hand and the act of recognition destroys the power of selection. If, however, the necessity for silent and im-mediate choice of a duplicate is again impressed upon him, he can

[1] No. I, Vol. II, p. 6.

perform the desired action perfectly; but as a rule he does not of his own accord revert to the easier method of carrying out the task. Having shot his bolt and failed to attain his end, he neglects the simpler and more direct means which is within his grasp.

To set the hands of one clock in imitation of another is for the normal individual a direct act of matching and can be executed with ease by most aphasics. But it is in essence somewhat less simple than selecting an object corresponding to one held in the hand. For the long and short hands of the clock have not the same significance and are not inter-changeable; however exactly one hand may be set opposite some point on the clock face, it is important that it should be the right one. This necessity for appreciating a difference in symbolic meaning may render this otherwise simple task difficult in certain forms of aphasia.

We can sometimes notice another defect, when a patient of this kind is asked to match one clock with another. Supposing he has just set 8.50 correctly and is then shown a clock marking 7.45, he may move the hands all the way round the face to the new position without recog-nising that he has only to shift them back five minutes. He fails to adopt the shortest way of reaching the goal.

Some forms of behaviour, which at first sight appear to be purely imitative, demand for their perfect performance more or less symbolic formulation. In order that one person seated opposite another may copy certain movements exactly without saying anything aloud, there must be some expressed recognition of the crossed relation of the hand to be employed to touch either eye or ear. This may be so gross that the subject says to himself with each test, "That is his right hand touching his left eye," or he may adopt the general formula, "It's always the opposite." But in some symbolic form or another the inverse nature of the act to be performed must be present in consciousness before it can be carried out correctly. Consequently this test tends to be affected in all forms. of aphasia and amnesia, if sufficiently severe.

When the movements to be imitated are reflected in a mirror, the task is much easier. No deliberate thought is, as a rule, necessary; the subject has simply to copy what he sees and, with most varieties of disordered speech, is able to do so correctly. But in semantic aphasia there is profound lack of power to appreciate the intention of an act to be performed and, asked to imitate these movements from reflections in a mirror, the patient begins to argue silently with regard to the nature of the task. He thinks, "It's a looking glass and so it must be opposite," thus misleading himself and confusing his conception of what he is asked to do.

25—2

Exactly similar results are obtained if the orders to carry out these movements are conveyed in the form of a picture. When the card is held facing the patient, he makes many mistakes; whilst if it is reflected in a mirror every movement may be performed correctly and with ease. But here again, with the semantic form of aphasia, confusion is liable to arise from attempts to argue out the nature of the act to be performed instead of immediately copying the reflected diagram.

Thus, provided he understands the intention of what he is told to do, a patient with these disorders of speech can imitate movements, if they are not translated into words or do not require the intervention of some symbolic formula. This explanation of the clinical facts is supported by the following experiment. Suppose the patient is told to write down what he sees in a mirror, he may fail grossly although for other purposes his writing is little affected. He can imitate the reflected movements perfectly, but makes many mistakes when he is compelled to translate them into written symbols.

Many of these patients are profoundly puzzled by right and left and adopt all sorts of expedients before they can decide which hand to move in response to a command. Thus No. 2 said, "I can't remember which is my right hand; but I know, if I was going to fight, I'd go like this," throwing himself into the correct boxing attitude with the left hand in front. Then he added, "Now I know, this is the right, this is the one I would use to do this," making the movements of writing. Yet he undoubtedly retained the conception of right and left, although he was unable to formulate the idea in symbolic terms. For he not only appreciated, but was able to convey to me by gestures, that in England the traffic of the streets moved to the left, whilst in every other country it kept to the right side of the roadway; and yet he could not employ the terms right and left correctly to express this idea, although he had words in plenty at his disposal for the purpose.

To copy printed capitals exactly is little more than a form of imitative drawing and can usually be carried out without mistakes; but many patients find extreme difficulty in transcribing them in ordinary hand-writing. This is not due to actual inability to write; for if the copy is set in cursive script it can be reproduced without difficulty. Failure or success in completing the task is not determined primarily by the actual form of the letters, but by whether some act of symbolic formulation intervenes of necessity between appreciation of the model and the kind of writing in which it is copied.

The power to produce a drawing from a simple model is not as a rule disturbed in uncomplicated cases of aphasia. One of my favourite means of testing an intelligent patient is to place before him a glass spirit lamp, with the request that he will draw it in outline; amongst other points, his representation of the way in which the wick passes through the brass collar to reappear in the globe below is a valuable indication of his intellectual capacity. Some semantic patients, it is true, unable to obtain a general conception of how to set to work, move the pencil slowly from point to point and may fail to complete the outline; but even they can copy a rough sketch of the same object made for them by the observer.

If the model is removed and the patient is asked to reproduce it from memory, his drawing usually resembles, both in its faults and excellencies, the one he made when the object was in sight. In most cases it is evidently constructed by retracing an action recently performed and not by an independent formulation of the task.

But, although an aphasic can draw from a model and subsequently from memory, he may have profound difficulty in doing so to order. Even those who are familiar with the form of an elephant produce an absurd drawing of this animal devoid of trunk, tusks, ears or any of its distinctive parts. They are unable to formulate and express with ease its salient features and so cannot transfer them to paper. But if I drew the body and legs of an elephant, leaving blank spaces for the forgotten parts, the patient could frequently fill them in correctly; for the shape on the paper suggested the additions necessary to make it complete.

Many of these patients, who were unable to draw to order, could represent spontaneously some object that was in their thoughts. Thus No. 10, wishing to describe to me the sort of hive he was using for his bees, drew an outline of the one he employed, indicating the metal cover to keep off the rain; and yet he was unable to draw a single object to command. On one occasion, when trying to describe the difficulties of transport in the East, No. 2 produced spontaneously a spirited rough sketch of a camel. Told to draw an elephant, a familiar object to him during his service in India, he drew an absurd figure without trunk, tusks or ears; asked what he had left out, he added a tail and marks on the forehead evidently intended for horns, but was completely unable to produce anything corresponding approximately to an elephant.

None of these disorders of speech in an uncomplicated form disturbs the power to appreciate the details of a picture, provided it does not carry a definite command to action. Thus all my patients who possessed sufficient words at their disposal could show that they recognised the various objects in a picture, even if they were unable to coordinate them as a whole and extract their general significance. But, whenever the picture contained an order, as with the pictorial commands of the hand, eye and ear tests, the failure was as great as if the movement to be performed had been suggested by any other means. The necessity of translating the picture into a formula preparatory to action led to apparent lack of power to comprehend its significance.

The existence of persons of high intellectual capacity, who are devoid of visual and auditory images, shows that they are not essential for the processes of logical thought. But the larger number of the inhabitants of this country depend to a greater or less extent on visual images as a factor in their normal mental activity. Throughout the explanations offered by the vast majority of my patients, drawn from every social class, some such expression as "I see it in my mind" occurs repeatedly. That this is no metaphorical mode of speech will be granted at once by anyone endowed with strong visual imagery, and is supported by the detailed and vivid description given by intelligent patients of their mental difficulties.

Now the power of evoking visual images as such is not affected by the disorders of speech, which are the main theme of this work. But, whenever they form an integral part of an act of symbolic formulation and expression, they are liable to suffer exactly in the same way as any other mental function involved in the process.

Thus, most patients, having made an outline drawing of some object in sight, can reproduce it from memory after removal of the model. This is undoubtedly due in part to a repetition of the movements made on the first occasion; but the various details recalled with accuracy and expressed in speech during the execution of this task show that in many instances a visual image has been invoked to reinforce the memory. Whilst repeating his drawing of a spirit lamp after removal of the model, one of my patients said that he "could see the whole lamp and glass and the bit of string to light it" (i.e. the wick). Several gave an accurate description from memory of the coloured pattern on the jug, although they could not represent it in a drawing. Many could remember and distinguish the colours of the uniform of Nurses and Sisters, the appearance of their fellow patients in the ward, the pictures in my room and the appearance and shape of its furniture. These descriptions were prefaced and accompanied by verbal expressions and gestures which could have no meaning unless they were associated with the evocation of visual images. To those of us, who possess strong visual imagery, the whole procedure is familiar in every detail.

But in many instances of aphasia these images cannot be employed for propositional thought; they cannot be evoked to command or translated at will into some other form of symbolic representation. Thus, a man who has made an excellent reproduction of a spirit lamp from memory after drawing it from the model, may be unable to draw an elephant to order; he complains that he cannot recall "What it looks like" or that "I can see the elephant, but I can't seem to draw it." Another patient expressed his difficulty in drawing to order as follows: "I want the thing in front of me, I don't know how to build it up; I can see it in my mind, but I can't put it down."

The difficulties experienced in translating a visual image into a drawing are greatly accentuated, when the patient attempts to write down in words what he has seen. Even if visual images can be evoked spontaneously or in response to a word said by the observer they cannot be employed with certainty as symbolic formulae. Asked to describe the appearance of some familiar house, he asserts that he can see it plainly "but I can't put it properly into words"; or "I often seem to have got the picture, but it evades me; the more I seem to make them come the more difficult it is to get into touch with them," and yet this man described to me accurately the form and colours of the hives he employed and visualised the bees alighting laden with yellow pollen.

The description by No. 2 of how he would walk from the Empire Hospital to the War Office in Whitehall is a splendid example of the maintenance of visual images without power to use them in constructive thought. He recalled that on the way he first passed the Army and Navy Stores and then on the left a hospital (Westminster Hospital). He added "I saw the hospital" and indicated that it was close to the Abbey (Westminster Abbey). When I asked about the latter, he replied, "It's here, but then it's gone again and I have to feel for it again; the only thing I can remember of it is the opening, the big opening where everybody goes in; I can get that," moving his hand in the form of a large arch. After further description, he concluded "With me it's all in bits; I have to jump like a man who jumps from one thing to the next; I can see them, but I can't express; really it is that I haven't enough names, I've got practically no names." It was evident from this conversation that he could recall visual images of objects seen on his walk, first the big Stores, then Westminster Hospital on the left with the great door of the Abbey on the right. But want of names prevented him from connecting them in a logical sequence and he was forced to jump from one image to another without the coherent links of verbal formulation.

Thus, visual images may remain unaffected in these disorders of speech, although they cannot be employed in continued processes of symbolic formulation and expression or evoked in response to words and other symbols. Mental pictures remain, but the means of converting them into the materials for logical thought have been disturbed or grossly diminished.

Many of the tests I have employed depend on capacity to choose some familiar article or colour, shown to the patient or named by the examiner orally and in print. After a few observations, most persons rapidly learn the order in which the objects lie on the table and do not waste time by passing the finger along the whole series in search for the one they want; they pounce on it at once, showing that they recognise, not only its characteristic differences, but its position in space. An intelligent aphasic, asked to indicate what he has seen or has held in his hand, soon shows that he has learnt where to look for its duplicate amongst the articles lying on the table. If they are hidden from his sight by a piece of cardboard and it is not removed with sufficient rapidity, he may place his finger over the very spot on the screen, which lies above the object he is seeking. All such forms of choice are acts of matching and remain unaffected in uncomplicated aphasia.

But as soon as the selection to be made by the patient depends on the name of an object or colour presented to him orally or in print and he finds difficulty in appreciating its significance, his finger wanders up and down the series of objects on the table, until he finds the one he wants. If he is asked to state the position in which they lie, he may fail to do so, although he still acts as if he knew the exact position of each of them, when indicating the one he has seen or held in his hand.

Thus relative position in a series is as much part of the characteristic features of an object as its shape and colour. So long as an aphasic is not required to formulate these characters, but makes his choice directly by an act of matching, he behaves as if he knew its position in the series. But further investigation shows that, although he may remember the exact spot it occupies, he cannot reproduce at will its relation to the others. For, whenever he has difficulty in recognising the meaning of a verbal symbol presented to him in any form, he loses the power to recognise the relative position of the object he is seeking, although he may ultimately make his choice correctly. He is not only uncertain about such qualities as its shape and colour, but also with regard to its spacial relationships.

This want of prompt and immediate movement in the right direction is found only in patients who have difficulty in recognising the exact significance of verbal symbols. As recovery progresses and the power to appreciate names increases, this uncertainty as to relative position passes away and the finger no longer wanders up and down the whole series of objects before making a correct choice.

When testing the patient's memory of his surroundings, we encounter the same capacity to state the position of an object directly, associated with inability to formulate its relation to others of a series. Thus if he is asked to recall some familiar room, such as that in which we habitually worked together, he can indicate the position of its salient features one after the other. He says, "The fire is here, the window there and this is where the door would be." But, asked to describe the position of the fire compared with that of the window or the door, he may fail completely; he can indicate the position of each in turn, but is unable to express their relation to one another.

This becomes still more evident, if he is told to construct from memory a ground-plan of some room he knows well. In many cases he cannot represent its main structural features or the position of the furniture correctly. But, if a quadrilateral figure, representing its boundaries, is drawn for him and a mark is made within it to indicate his habitual seat, he can point to the position of each surrounding object correctly provided he is asked in turn "Where is the fire, the window, the door, etc." He remembers the locality of each of these objects as he saw them, but he cannot construct a plan to express their relation to one another and to the confines of the room.

In the same way an intelligent aphasic can usually recall an actual occurrence, although he may be unable to relate it to other facts of experience and to draw the obvious deduction. Thus he remembers that, when he placed two shillings on the counter and asked for two ounces of tobacco, he received three pence in change; and yet he is totally unable to tell the cost of an ounce of tobacco[1]. Whenever No. 2 came from his home to my house by train, he handed in five shillings and expected the booking clerk to give him two-pence halfpenny; but he could not say, without laborious calculation on paper, how much the journey cost him.

Thus in conclusion, any task which depends solely on direct matching and does not imply some other formulated relation, can be carried out successfully in uncomplicated cases of aphasia and amnesia. Memory as a whole is not affected; the patient can recall actual facts of experience,

[1] No. 10, Vol. II, p. 169.

although he may not be able to use them for purposes of deduction. Images continue to appear spontaneously or in response to some external suggestion; but they cannot be evoked at will to take part as essential factors in logical thought. The mind retains vividly all forms of activity which do not demand the use of certain symbols or the formulated and expressed relation between two or more facts of experience.

§ 3. FORMS OF BEHAVIOUR WHICH SUFFER IN THESE DISORDERS OF SPEECH

Aphasia and kindred disorders of language consist essentially of a want of power to carry out with ease acts connected with articulated speech and the comprehension of spoken words. Man acquired the capacity to utter his thoughts and to understand what was said by his fellows long before he could formulate and express a relation between two events in any other manner. This power he developed and enlarged, adding one means of symbolic representation after another, until he was not only able to record his verbal formulations in writing, but could manipulate symbols for profound deductions of logical thought. No one is born ready equipped with these powers; every individual is compelled to acquire, during his life-time, the primitive art of speaking and understanding what is said by others.

Many methods of thought are possible without words and remain unaffected in uncomplicated cases of aphasia. But words and other symbols bind together and give permanence to non-verbal processes of thought, that would otherwise be fleeting. The most diverse activities of the mind become accreted into a coherent whole and, should they participate in acts of language, are liable to suffer with disorders of speech. Thus, visual images may still be available for spontaneous thought, although they cannot be employed in a normal manner for registering relations.

Aphasic disorders alter behaviour in a specific manner; an action can be performed in one way, not in another. The lesion does not of necessity destroy the power to think, but one method by which thought is carried into action is disturbed. The patient is robbed of certain forms of effective symbolic representation and has lost the normal means of communicating with his fellows.

Let us imagine that he has been deprived of articulated speech, the comprehension of spoken words and all the complex activities derived from them, such as reading, writing and the use of numbers. He may still possess the power of matching familiar objects or colours and of indicating the duplicate of something held in his hand out of sight. He can imitate some simple action performed by the observer, such as touching his nose or protruding his tongue, although he is unable to carry out these movements to any form of order, spoken, written or pictorial. Capital letters in print are laboriously copied, but cannot be written spontaneously or to dictation, nor can they be translated into cursive script. Counting is impossible, except perhaps for the first three or four numerals, and the patient can carry out none of the alphabetical tests successfully. He has no means of expressing the relative value of coins and is not even able to pile up, from those laid on the table, the equivalent value of a single piece of money placed before him.

An individual reduced to this condition of impotence would appear at first sight to be demented. But closer observation shows that he still possesses the power to think, often in an extremely intelligent manner, although he is deprived of all formal means of communicating and registering his thoughts.

Fortunately few aphasics show such profound loss of the functions connected with speech, although vascular lesions in elderly men frequently produce a condition which approaches it more or less closely [e.g. No. 26]. The patient cannot utter spontaneously or repeat a single intelligible word and responds solely by modifications of some meaningless sound (such as "lowla"). He carries out simple oral or printed commands with some difficulty, but fails completely to execute more complex tasks; thus, he can choose a common object correctly, although he is unable to set the hands of a clock or to execute the hand, eye and ear tests to orders, given by word of mouth or in print. He may be able to copy exactly words or letters placed before him, but he cannot transcribe printed words into ordinary handwriting. All power of spontaneous writing is abolished, except that he can perhaps write his surname. Arithmetic is impossible owing to his want of power to employ numbers and he cannot express the relation of two coins to one another by any means.

No. 21 was a somewhat less severe example of this type of aphasia. He employed "yes" and "no" correctly and could utter a few ejaculatory phrases, such as "don't know," "can't get it," "I know what it is," "I can't say what it says," "thank you" and the like; yet he was unable to repeat a single one of these to order. He appeared to understand all that was said to him and chose common objects or colours easily to oral commands; to print he was somewhat less accurate. But, with the more complex clock tests and the movements of the hand to eye or ear, he failed whatever form the order assumed. Although he seemed at first sight to be totally unable to read a printed phrase, he selected a card bearing the legend which corresponded to any two pictures of the man, cat and dog tests shown to him. All power of writing was not abolished and he succeeded in reproducing his name imperfectly spelt, but he could not append his address. He was unable to write the simple words of the man, cat and dog tests spontaneously, from pictures, or to dictation; he could not even copy the printed phrases in cursive script. Counting was defective and arithmetical exercises were carried out badly; but he was able to express in a most ingenious manner on his fingers the relative value of two coins shown to him simultaneously.

In spite of the extreme severity of the loss of speech, both these patients retained some elementary power of symbolic formulation and expression and in neither case was there any failure of general intelligence, apart from the defective use of language. Moreover, in both instances the loss of function was relative and not absolute; certain simple tasks were successfully performed, whilst more complex tests of the same order could not be carried out correctly.

This dependence of the manifest defects on the intellectual difficulty of the act to be performed is one of the most important factors in the problem of aphasia. For it is obvious that any disturbance of symbolic formulation and expression must be looked for, and can be discovered soonest, in those tasks which require the greatest expenditure of mental effort in this direction. Thus, since it is harder to carry out a test which offers three possibilities of an erroneous answer, than one which demands a single choice, the former is the first to suffer and is most severely affected throughout the course of the disorder.

The patient tends therefore to adopt every means in his power to simplify the task. Asked to imitate the movements of the examiner, when face to face, he may give up all attempt to employ the right or left hand correctly and consistently select the one that is opposite. Power to carry out this test accurately is acquired between the ages of nine and twelve, and the aphasic reverts to the simpler method of response habitual in childhood. In the same way, when adding two numbers together, he counts from one to the other and may even use his fingers to do so; for instance, instead of stating "six and three is nine," he says "six, seven, eight, nine."

To describe an object or to indicate its use is easier than to name it directly and many patients adopt this method, even if they succeed ultimately in finding the correct word. To explain "that is the thing you cut with" often facilitates the final answer "scissors." In the same way the name of an object can be embodied in a sentence, although it could not be formulated immediately as a single word. Shown an ink-pot it is easier to say "that's a pot for holding ink" than to answer "ink" without any preliminary; "that's what I should call a cedar pencil" comes more readily from the tongue than "pencil" only. Such apparently complicated methods of expression are in reality simpler than mono-verbal designation.

Apparently meaningless ejaculations such as "you know," "it's like this," "what you call it" or even the familiar "er, er" of the unpractised speaker, serve the same purpose. They are "taking off" words; just as it is easier to jump successfully after a run than from a standing position, so a word can often be discovered more readily by uttering irrelevant sounds than by sitting silently in front of a problem until the answer emerges fully formed.

The more abstract the name the greater difficulty does it present to most aphasics. Such words as "knife," "penny," "pencil," designate objects of definite shape and appearance, with a multitude of distinctive characters. But colours are more abstract; red, for instance, is a quality we discover in many different objects that have nothing else in common. Now it is a remarkable fact that this difference appears in the records obtained in many cases of disordered speech; the patient may be able to name and choose correctly articles of familiar use, although he fails to do so with a set of simple colours. He succeeds with the more concrete intellectual task, but not with one that is more abstract.

It is always easier to employ descriptive or metaphorical terms. A Staff Officer (No. 2), though unable to name colours, was in no sense colour-blind; if he was permitted to say "what you do for the dead" for black, "what the Staff wear" for red, and to employ other equally significant terms, he could designate all the colours correctly. Moreover, with practice he went so far as to employ the single word "dead" in place of black, the name he could not apply correctly; the metaphorical term was easier than the more abstract designation.

A most intelligent house painter (No. 22), who could not name colours with certainty, indicated exactly how they could be composed from the crude materials he used in his trade. Thus violet was "blue and black with a small portion of red"; when shown orange, he replied "It's easy enough to make it, if I'd the stuff, a bit of red, a bit of yellow and a bit of white lead."

If there is any difficulty in deciphering the printed name of some familiar article, the patient may be greatly aided by seeing the object on the table before him. I showed No. 2 a card bearing the word KEY, and he replied, "I'm not quite sure of that; I was not certain if it was a key or a knife. I have to spell it K E Y and I say 'key' and look on the table and then I know that's the key. I still puzzle what K E Y means; if I see that (pointing to the key) then I don't have to worry, I know K E Y is that...is a key." I then handed him two cards, one bearing the word MATCHES, the other WATCH; he pointed to the match-box and holding up the latter card said "nothing here," which was correct. Asked "What is the difference?" he replied "They are both written (printed); this one is here (pointing to the matches), the other there is nothing. I focus this one (matches) because it is here. I can't focus this (the card bearing the word WATCH) so well because it is not so clear." He then moved his eyes round my room, as if seeking something, and added "When I look at that big one (my consulting room clock), that helps me. I want to interpret the reading WATCH into a picture or into that (pointing to the clock) watch." Later he added "Suppose you had shown me looking glass, written like this (printed), I should have had to think a long time. But if I looked up and saw that looking glass (pointing to the one on the wall) I should have known it at once."

Here again to render a task less concrete increases its difficulty. It is easier to appreciate the meaning of a printed name, when the appropriate object is present to sight, than if the word must be deciphered in response to the verbal pattern on the paper only.

It is always easier to solve a problem by progression than by a direct propositional act. Suppose for instance that a patient fails to appreciate the significance of "Thursday the twenty-fifth of March," he may arrive at a correct conception by saying the days of the week up to "Thursday," counting up to "twenty-five" and then repeating "January, February, March." In order to recognise a particular letter he may be compelled to say the alphabet, in part at any rate, up to the point where it stands in the sequence. Such tricks are familiar to those who are imperfectly acquainted with some foreign language; in French, for instance, many persons do not appreciate the significance of "quatre-vingt-treize" until they have formulated to themselves "eighty and thirteen is ninety-three."

When setting the hands of a clock, many an aphasic can carry out an oral or printed command in railway time more readily than if it is given in the ordinary nomenclature. Told to set "5.40," he places the hour hand opposite the figure 5 and then swings the long hand round the face until it reaches a position corresponding to 40 minutes. But "twenty minutes to six" puzzles him; he wants to set the short hand at 6 and is in doubt as to whether the other one should be placed at "twenty past" or "twenty to" the hour. This is not due to any greater facility in employing numbers rather than words; for, if he attempts to tell the time aloud, he has equal difficulty in formulating and expressing it by either method.

Habitual acts, which have become almost automatic, cease to be possible if they are started in some unfamiliar manner. Thus, a patient may be able to write his name and address, but not that of his mother with whom he lives. The unusual beginning "Mrs." destroys his fluency and he can no longer transfer to paper the remaining words, which he otherwise writes with ease. An officer, who in signing his name usually appends his rank and regiment, may be unable to write these words if he is not allowed to precede them by his name. An oft-repeated action can only be carried out successfully, if it is started in the accustomed manner.

Many aphasics cannot draw a ground-plan of some familiar room; they may perhaps begin by outlining a quadrilateral figure, but the salient features are indicated in elevation. The chair has a back and legs, the windows are shown with their panes and the electric light is suspended from the ceiling. Evidently the patient recalls his visual image of the room and transfers it directly on to the paper, incapable of expressing the relation to one another of its contents in the more abstract form of a ground-plan.

Symbolic formulation and expression is no more than an empirical term invented to designate those forms of behaviour which are disturbed in aphasia. They consist essentially of capacity to speak and to understand spoken words; these powers are gradually extended at a later stage of man's career, both individual and racial, until they comprise not only reading and writing, but also the higher operations of logical thought.

Speech and the use of language, in its widest forms, require the exact performance and interaction of a series of processes of great complexity. Acquired during the life of the individual, these are perfected by voluntary effort and finally come to consist of the orderly exercise of functions conscious, subconscious and wholly automatic, all working together in harmony.

Once a child has learnt to say a few intelligible words and to understand the significance of what he hears, he has started to develop an aptitude, which may ramify widely and reach a high degree of perfection.

If the facility is disturbed by a structural lesion, the essential disorder of function appears as defects of verbal form and meaning. But it must not be supposed that the clinical manifestations of aphasia can be classified strictly into two mutually exclusive groups according to these categories. In every case the patient has some difficulty in finding words and phrases in which to express his thoughts, associated with more or less want of comprehension of their exact meaning. But it is to these two primitive aptitudes, verbalisation and understanding of verbal symbols, that we must look for distinctive and specific disorders in the use of language.

The diverse meaning given to the expression "internal speech" has been one of the greatest obstacles to comprehension of the phenomena of aphasia. In no language has the term been used consistently; it is habitually employed in three different senses. Firstly, it is limited to silent articulation, as, for instance, when we move the lips or vocal apparatus during the process of writing; secondly it is made to comprise that formulation in words which precedes their utterance and, lastly, it is used for the general processes of thought which result in propositions, spoken or unspoken.

Speech is not simply the utterance of words, but consists of the formulation and expression of propositions. In this respect external and internal speech do not differ from one another; they differ solely in that the one leads to some act of articulation, even though the lips alone move silently, whilst the other is not expressed, unless perhaps in writing[1]. Speech is a mental process which we may or may not exteriorise; an aphasic is not only deprived of power to speak aloud, but he has also lost the capacity to formulate his thoughts to himself in certain symbolic terms. As Jackson says, "We speak not only to tell other people what we think, but to tell ourselves what we think."

Throughout I have followed Jackson's use of the term "internal speech" to signify the formulation of some proposition or relation in symbols, which are not necessarily expressed in vocal movements. The measure of the capacity for internal speech in any one case is given by the content, as opposed to the mechanical act, of writing; for in most aphasics writing betrays the same sort of defects in verbal form and meaning, that are evident in articulated words and phrases. The only difference lies in the fact that ability to write, an art more recently acquired, is liable to suffer to a greater extent than vocal speech.

[1] Jackson [81], pp. 15-16.

External speech suffers in the most diverse ways, ranging from defects in verbal form to want of power to express the ultimate intention of some process of thought or action. The patient may have profound difficulty in discovering the word he requires, and yet he can show that he recognises the name of an object or colour by selecting correctly the card upon which it is printed. Moreover, in his struggle for expression, he utters sounds which bear some definite resemblance however remote to the word he is seeking. Even repetition may be difficult or impossible if the disturbance is severe. But such a disorder of speech is not a purely articulatory change; for internal speech also suffers from the same defects. The patient is puzzled when he attempts to formulate what he has been told or has read to himself, and his writing shows the same kind of defects in verbal structure that are manifest in what he says aloud. In all such cases speech is slow, deliberate, hesitating and words of more than one syllable may be divided by a more or less prolonged pause.

When balance and rhythm are mainly affected, the patient talks rapidly in phrases which are syntactically defective. Sometimes the pronunciation of the individual words may be so grossly disturbed that speech becomes incomprehensible gibberish. But usually, if the test demands an answer in a single word only, this may be given correctly and the patient shows that he is familiar with names and relative characteristics of common objects. Internal speech suffers less than articulation and writing is often called in to supplement the defects of external speech. But closer study shows that even the silent formulation of thought tends to suffer from the same sort of errors; this is especially evident if the patient attempts to repeat to himself what he has been told or has gathered from conversation and reading.

So far we have considered those difficulties of expression, which are due mainly to defective structural formation of words and phrases. But, when the disorder of speech depends on inability to find names and other nominal terms, the patient may possess words in plenty, although he cannot discover the one which satisfies the meaning of the situation. His want of fluency is due to lack of power to select the particular expression, which exactly fits his conceptual wants. In the attempt to name an object or a colour he tries one word after another, all of them bearing some significant relation to their usual nomenclature. An excellent instance was the voluble lady called "Blanche," who when asked her name replied "Yes it's not Mount Everest, Mont Blanc, blancmange, almonds to put in water...you know, you be clever and tell me." Complex tasks in naming are reduced to simpler terms. For instance, orange is called "yellow" or "red" and violet "blue," or in the case of a house painter are described according to the colours which, when mixed, would produce them.

Words are wrongly employed because their meaning is not accurately distinguished. The patient confuses right and left, high and low, up and down, to and past the hour, especially if they are offered to him as alternatives in the same phrase.

Internal speech shows exactly the same defects. The patient writes wrong words and muddles himself in his repeated attempts to find the right expression. He obviously knows what he wants to say, but cannot discover suitable terms in which to express his thought to himself or to others. Verbal form suffers both in external speech and writing, because he no longer has at his disposal an accurate nomenclature.

Sometimes the main defect in speech consists in want of power to formulate exactly in words the intention of some mental process. This produces no material effect on verbalisation, but the patient is liable to lose the thread of what he is saying, either aloud or to himself, and his conversation or writing tails away without reaching its natural end. The words are well formed, syntax is not disturbed, and yet the sentences are incomplete, confused or logically inconclusive. In such cases any defects in form are due solely to want of power to appreciate and manipulate with ease the ultimate or general meaning of symbols.

When we turn to the second primal aspect of speech, comprehension of spoken words, we find a similar diversity in the manifestations of aphasia. Should the main faults lie in verbal formation, the patient frequently appreciates what is said to him and can carry out oral commands with ease; but, if the disturbance is extremely severe, even these acts may be affected, although they suffer to a less degree and are restored at an earlier period of recovery than the more formal aspects of language. Uncertainty in the use of words for internal speech is liable to reduce the capacity to recall what has been said, or to formulate thought for the purposes of memory. Thus, full and exact comprehension of spoken words tends to be diminished even in the most definite verbal aphasia, provided it is sufficiently severe.

If rhythm and balance are disturbed, the comprehension of spoken words may suffer because, when the patient attempts to formulate what he has heard, he is puzzled by his own internal jargon. Simple, direct oral commands are executed correctly; but, any attempt to recall the order silently before acting upon it, is liable to lead to confusion. For the same reason there is often difficulty in picking up a conversation, even if the theme has been started by the patient himself, and his spontaneous mental processes are disturbed by the defective symbolic forms in which they are conceived.

Nominal aphasia, on the other hand, is characterised by a definite want of comprehension of verbal meaning. Even single words are misunderstood and oral commands are badly executed. This has a profoundly disturbing effect upon memory. So long as the patient does not attempt to embody his thoughts in symbolic forms, his actions are coherent and exactly suited to the occasion. But he is liable to fail, when forced to employ terms of definite significance, especially if they are contrasted with one another, such as right and left, up and down, to and past the hour, etc.

The gravest disturbance of meaning is associated with what I have called semantic defects. The patient has lost the power of grasping the general aim of some proposition, whether arising spontaneously or in response to external suggestion. He can no more use verbal symbols with certainty to express the ultimate intention of his thoughts than he can construct a piece of furniture, or assemble the necessary utensils for a meal.

Verbal form and verbal meaning are complementary aspects of elementary acts of speech; so long as any power of symbolic formulation and expression is retained, the defects fall more heavily on one side than on the other. But disorders of speech cannot be separated into two sharply defined groups, one of which consists solely of abnormalities in verbal structure and syntax, whilst the other depends on want of comprehension of spoken words or phrases. For, although one form of behaviour may be disturbed to a preponderating degree, both tend to suffer provided the aphasia is sufficiently severe. Ultimately defects in verbal formation will confuse the comprehension of words and phrases, whilst want of recognition of verbal meaning creates difficulties in finding the terms necessary for exact expression. We cannot therefore class the clinical phenomena as motor or sensory, aphasia or amnesia, apraxia or agnosia. These disorders are the manifestations of a general response on the part of the patient to a situation created by the defective mechanism of speech. He attempts to express himself, to understand what is said to him and to formulate his thoughts, in spite of verbal difficulties which hamper both the structure and meaning of language.

When we pass to more recently acquired and complicated methods of symbolic representation, such as reading and writing, the defects assume a graver form and persist longer in the course of the disorder. For to write with ease and certainty demands the translation of words into arbitrary symbols, which must be reconverted into verbal forms, before we can interpret them even to ourselves. To perform the acts of reading and writing in perfection it is necessary not only to possess the capacity of manipulating words, but to understand and to shape correctly those conventional signs, which stand for them. Although we do not habitually spell out each word letter by letter, the pattern on the paper must be endowed with some symbolic meaning, before it can be appreciated for the purpose of thought or action. In the same way, when writing, we do not linger over the details of the process, which as the result of long practice have become almost automatic; but any obstacle to its perfect performance is liable to destroy the power of writing down even propositional statements, which can otherwise be expressed freely in verbal symbols.

To read to oneself and to carry out silently a command given in print is not the pure exercise in verbal meaning it might appear at first sight. For most persons, when reading, carry out a certain amount of verbalisation; some even move the lips or whisper. The highly educated may snatch the significance from a page of print without paying anxious attention to the structure of the words; but any obscurity in the text at once leads to definite acts of internal speech.

Thus, although the majority of patients with verbal aphasia can carry out simple printed commands correctly, most of them confess that they read a book with difficulty, even when recovery is far advanced. A young officer (No. 17) complained that he could not read with pleasure "because I'm bothered when I say the words to myself; I can get the meaning of a sentence if it's an isolated sentence, but I can't get all the words." In the same way any defect of syntax or internal jargon is liable to cause confusion, if the patient attempts to formulate to himself silently what he has gathered from print. But direct appreciation of its meaning is little affected; books or the newspaper can be read with understanding and printed orders carried out correctly.

In both these varieties of disordered speech, the main difficulty centres round the formation of words and phrases, even for internal use. Consequently reading aloud suffers profoundly and shows the same gross defects as spontaneous speech. But, provided the patient can talk comprehensibly, he usually retains some power of reading aloud and the defective sounds he produces bear a distinct relation to the words and phrases he is striving to utter.

Such defects of external and internal verbalisation do not entirely destroy the capacity to extract the meaning from printed words. Many verbal aphasics can choose an object with ease to printed commands, although they find great difficulty in reading the name aloud. When No. 1 attempted to read aloud the name of a colour and to select the appropriate one from those lying on the table, he made his choice with great rapidity; but he did not utter the word on the card until long after he had indicated the colour correctly. The response to the printed command was immediate and did not necessitate complete verbalisation. Even No. 21, who was unable to say the simple words "man," "cat" or "dog," could pick out correctly a printed card which corresponded exactly to the combination shown to him. Evidently the words conveyed their appropriate meaning, although he was unable to express them in articulated sounds.

Patients, who cannot read aloud a single word of this test from print, may be able to evoke the words in response to pictures. For the pictorial representation of such familiar objects as a man, a cat or a dog recalls the verbal designation more readily than the name displayed in printed characters. Thus, with all such faults of formal expression, it is easier to find words for pictures than to read aloud from print.

Inability to recognise verbal meaning leads to grave want of capacity to understand printed matter read silently. Simple commands are badly executed, the patient cannot read a newspaper and is scarcely able to decipher a letter. Should the defects lie mainly in comprehending the general significance of some group of statements or a complex order, the ultimate conception, or the method of carrying out the act demanded, is liable to suffer. Commands, given in a single word or short phrase, are executed correctly. The patient can read to himself, but is puzzled with regard to the ultimate meaning of what he has read. He may comprehend the details, although he cannot combine them into a logical and consecutive whole.

Whenever the disorder of speech affects mainly the meaning of words and phrases, reading aloud is a distinct help to understanding. A patient with nominal aphasia can not uncommonly carry out a printed order, if he is allowed to utter the words of which it is composed, although he fails when he reads silently. For, in such circumstances, he reinforces what he gathers from the printed characters by a self-given oral command, and this is of assistance because verbal formulation is less affected than the appreciation of meaning. If the defects in comprehension are more general and less detailed, it makes comparatively little difference whether the words are read aloud or not; the patient tends to fall into the same kind of mistaken ideas with regard to the ultimate significance of the printed matter.

To copy exactly line by line printed letters or single words is little more than imitative drawing and is within the capacity of any aphasic who can be made to understand what is required of him; but to translate print into cursive handwriting necessitates some power of symbolic formulation and expression. It is, however, the simplest of all written tasks and demands no more than transformation of the printed letters of the copy into script, familiar from childhood and employed for the purposes of daily intercourse. This test, therefore, reveals in its purest form the way in which the acquired act of writing is affected and modified in association with disorders of speech. Freedom and ease of execution are diminished; writing becomes laborious. The letters are poorly formed and there is difficulty in recapturing the exact shape of the cursive symbols, which correspond to the printed characters. This is not due to want of ability to execute the movements of writing; for if the copy is set in cursive script, it can be reproduced correctly. There is no "motor" or "apraxic" defect; the capacity to transform print into cursive forms is at fault and not the mechanical actions of the hand in writing.

Writing to dictation is as a rule a somewhat more difficult task; for the words spoken by the examiner must first be appreciated before the patient can translate them into written signs. Any loss of facility in this direction is liable to be associated with calligraphic errors of all kinds, to an even greater degree than when print is copied in cursive script.

But in addition to these faults in the art of writing, each variety of aphasia tends to affect in some particular manner the capacity to record dictated words and phrases. With verbal defects the patient has lost the power to form the words correctly and cannot remember those he has heard long enough to place them on paper. Disorders of syntax reappear in the structure of the dictated phrases and want of balance frequently adds to the difficulty in writing the longer words. Loss of nominal power and want of recognition of verbal significance causes confusion and difficulty in reproducing exactly what has been said. Finally, semantic aphasia is associated with a tendency for portions of the dictated matter to be omitted or misunderstood.

All these defects become apparent to an even greater degree, when the patient attempts to reproduce his own thoughts in writing. For the words must be formulated as an exact expression of the writer's meaning and then transformed into adequate verbal symbols. The same sort of faults are obvious, if the patient attempts to convey in writing the substance of what he has been told or has read to himself. Strictly speaking this is not a spontaneous act of writing; but, although he is not compelled to originate all the words in which he expresses what he has heard or read, he combines them into a personal narrative and does not reproduce them mechanically.

All the varieties of spontaneous writing are consequently defective both in structure and intellectual content. Anything which hampers free exercise of the art is liable to lead to calligraphic errors, common to all forms of aphasia, if sufficiently severe. Letters are malformed, capitals are employed unnecessarily or omitted where they are required, stops are badly placed and spelling is uncertain.

But such acts of writing also reveal the condition of internal speech. Examination of the written text shows the presence of faults in structure and meaning corresponding to those found in other manifestations of disordered speech. Sometimes it is mainly the form of words and phrases which is defective; at others the writing suffers from want of nominal expressions and faulty appreciation of verbal or general meaning. These specific differences will be treated more fully, when we consider the various forms which can be assumed by an aphasia.

The tests with the alphabet form an excellent illustration of the principles just enunciated. For, when a patient attempts to say the alphabet spontaneously or to arrange the block letters in order, he depends on perfect evocation of a rhythmic sequence, either expressed aloud or silently. This habitual act can be disturbed indifferently by any loss of symbolic formulation and expression, provided it is sufficiently severe. To write the alphabet is an even more complicated act; for the letters must not only be formulated in their proper order without external help, but also translated into adequate written symbols. Here again owing to the complexity of the task the loss of aptitude is more or less general and does not exhibit those specific differences which characterise the various forms of aphasia. These become apparent in the simpler tests only, such as repeating the alphabet aloud after the examiner or in copying the printed letters in cursive handwriting.

The perfect use of numbers is closely dependent on verbal formulation, external or internal, and on the comprehension of symbolic meaning. It tends, therefore, in its simplest aspects, to suffer in a more or less distinctive manner according to the form assumed by the aphasia. But, when as with arithmetic the tasks set demand the exercise of higher propositional powers, this is no longer the case. Any severe degree of aphasia may disturb the solution of simple problems in addition and subtraction; and yet it is impossible by examining the crude records of these tests alone to determine the specific form of the disorder of speech. We can only conclude that the patient is suffering from some loss of symbolic formulation and expression, which affects the use of numbers for arithmetical purposes.

To name the various coins as they are exhibited one by one, or to choose them correctly to oral or printed commands, differs little from similar tests carried out with other objects of common use. But to express the relative value of two pieces of money to one another is an intellectual task of a different order; it is essentially a high-grade problem in formulated meaning and suffers gravely in many forms of aphasia. In the same way a patient may remember that, when he placed two shillings on the counter, he received two ounces of tobacco and three pence in change, without being able to calculate the price of an ounce. He can even build up a pile of coins which exactly equals some one of high value laid before him, although he cannot state the relation of any two of them with certainty. One piece of money can be added to another until the sum total equals the value of the single coin; the difficulty lies in expressing this fact in propositional form.

Pictures always convey some meaning, so far at least as their simple details are concerned. But the power of weaving them into a coherent whole, exhibiting their general significance, may suffer in certain varieties of aphasia; in such circumstances jokes and humorous allusions conveyed in pictorial form are not completely apprehended. Moreover, the full meaning of a picture is frequently missed, if it can only be gathered by combining the pictorial representation with the legend printed beneath it.

When a picture is made the vehicle of an order of any kind, this suffers like any other suggestion to behave in some particular manner. The extent to which oral, printed and pictorial commands are affected relatively to one another varies with the different forms of aphasia; but a patient who has no difficulty in appreciating the direct significance of a picture may fail to execute some order presented to him pictorially.

Capacity to draw from a model is not as a rule disturbed, unless the aphasia is extremely severe. Some patients can draw such images as arise spontaneously in the mind, although they cannot do so to order; thus, the majority are unable to reproduce to command such a figure as that of an elephant. There is, however, nothing distinctive in the form assumed by such a failure, except that it is more likely to accompany loss of symbolic meaning than defective verbalisation.

So long as the disorders of speech are concerned mainly with the formation of words and phrases, spacial orientation is entirely unaffected. The nominal aphasic can usually go about unaided, if he is allowed to take his bearings with the help of familiar landmarks in sight; but he may have difficulty in planning his path, or in describing beforehand how he would find his way from one place to another. But gross want of orientation is a prominent feature of that lack of aim and intention, which characterises semantic aphasia. The patient cannot take his bearings, wanders without guidance from point to point, misled by false resemblances and absurd conclusions and fails entirely to follow a direction given in such terms as "take the second on the right."

To construct a plan of some familiar room or other well known place, demands the power of calling up relations in space and their subsequent translation into a highly abstract form. This is not materially disturbed in verbal and syntactical aphasia, but suffers more or less severely, whenever there is any want of appreciation of verbal or general meaning.

Musical capacity, in the strict sense of the word, does not suffer in association with these disorders of speech; for it has no functional relation to word-formation or verbal understanding. The patient can still recall a melody and sing in time and tune. Before he joined the army No. 7 was a professional singer, accustomed to learn mainly by ear. Given the opening notes of a song previously known to him, he sang it through accurately without words; time, tune and modulation were perfect and his voice had the full volume of a high baritone. He could not, however, sing any song, if he attempted to pronounce the words. In the same way, No. 23 was able to remember a melody, but was hampered by the words; when members of his family played the violin or piano, he could tell if they struck a wrong note or were out of tune, and he insisted that he "heard the sounds alright." No. 22, who performed professionally on the cornet and double bass, was entirely dependent on musical notation and never played by ear. From the time of his stroke he ceased to be able to read the notes and in consequence lost all power of execution.

On the other hand No. 14, a pronounced example of syntactical aphasia, played for me a Largo of Chopin, reading the notes and giving the change of key correctly. His right hand was clumsy, owing to in-coordination produced by the cerebral injury; but he succeeded in bringing his fingers on to the right notes of the chord and, if he went wrong, immediately corrected his error. Keeping his eyes on the music, he recognised by ear that he had struck a note, which did not correspond with the text.

Direct imitation of some simple movement is an easy task demanding little or no symbolic formulation; but, as soon as right or left are in question, its intellectual difficulty is greatly increased. Any aphasic, who can be made to understand what is required of him, is able to protrude his tongue, shut his eyes or lift his hand in imitation of similar actions carried out before him. Even the most intelligent patient, however, is liable to make mistakes if asked to imitate exactly movements of the right or left hand made by the examiner sitting face to face. In such circumstances the natural tendency is to reverse the action, employing for instance the left hand to touch the right eye instead of vice versa. For, in order to execute a test of this kind, some sort of symbolic formulation and expression is required; the patient is compelled to say to himself "it's the right hand and the left eye," or this may be shortened to the general formula "it's always the opposite." Gordon[1] has shown that ability to carry out such movements correctly is not acquired by normal children until between the age of nine and twelve; some adults never learn to perform them perfectly. It is not remarkable, therefore, that the hand, eye and ear tests show gross defects in most forms of aphasia, if sufficiently severe. The commonest fault consists of a systematic reversal of right and left, a return to the simpler mode of response customary in childhood; but the errors assume most variable forms, and eye or ear may even be mistaken the one for the other.

It is interesting to find that exactly similar defects appear, when the movements to be copied are represented diagrammatically. The picture of a figure, carrying out the action demanded, is given into the patient's hand and he attempts to imitate it exactly. In most forms of aphasia he fails grossly; here again the commonest fault is a tendency to direct reversal, although every variety of mistake may be present at one time or another.

The character of these erroneous responses does not differ materially according to the type of aphasia. The more formal disorders of speech tend on the whole to produce less disturbance than those which interfere with the comprehension of symbolic meaning. The profoundest lack of capacity to carry out a task of this kind is associated with semantic defects, whilst the milder degrees of verbal aphasia produce little or no change; but it would be impossible to determine the specific form assumed by the loss of speech from the records of these two varieties of the hand, eye and ear tests alone.

The difficulties in carrying out a task of this kind are based on defects

[1] Cf. Gordon, Hugh [61].

of internal verbalisation and are not due to want of power to initiate the acts required. For, if either the movements of the examiner or the diagrams are reflected in a mirror, most patients can give a perfect series of responses, except where the intention of the command is in doubt. Thus, an aphasic, who gives grossly erroneous responses, when attempting to imitate movements sitting face to face with the examiner or when holding a picture in his hand, may reply throughout correctly, if they are reflected in a mirror. This is an almost purely imitative act and little or no symbolic formulation is necessary for its perfect performance. The only difficulty arises should the patient fail to grasp the intention of the action he is asked to carry out.

It is impossible to find any single term to include logically all those forms of behaviour, which suffer in association with the manifestations of aphasia and amnesia. Any process is peculiarly liable to be affected, which demands a formulated proposition, some general recognition of relations, or conveyance of an abstract idea in words and other conventional signs. But, in order that these acts may become possible, certain definite symbols must be evoked with ease and at the same time convey their exact and appropriate meaning. A man must be able not only to speak to his fellows or to himself, but he must interpret the sounds he hears in mental terms.

If these powers are enfeebled, the patient loses the capacity to retain words and phrases in his mind correctly. At the same time he cannot think with clearness and precision; he may arrive at some preliminary conclusion, but, failing to register it, is unable to pass on to the next step in reasoning. His memory is weakened and he complains that he cannot read to himself or write down accurately what he has gathered from conversation or reading.

I have therefore chosen the empirical term "symbolic formulation and expression," for the forms of behaviour which are affected with these disorders of speech, to indicate that the effects of the lesion are manifested most often and to a profound degree in the use of words, numbers and other analogous symbols.

§4. CLINICAL VARIETIES OF APHASIA

This group of functions is rarely if ever uniformly disturbed and cases of aphasia differ profoundly in their manifestations. The majority, especially in the earlier stages, show evidence of wide-spread defects in the use of language; the more acute and severe the lesion, the graver and more extensive is the disorder it produces. Many of these abnormal reactions disappear rapidly and sometimes the patient recovers his powers of speech entirely; but more often certain aspects of symbolic formulation and expression remain affected and the aphasia consequently assumes some particular form.

Analysis of these clinical varieties seems to show that the various forms of behaviour, included under the term "symbolic formulation and expression," can be disturbed in different ways in consequence of organic injury. These diverse defects of speech do not reveal the elements out of which the use of language is built up; on the contrary, they show the way in which a highly complex series of acts can be disturbed by lesions of certain portions of the brain. No two examples exactly resemble one another; for the form assumed by the disorders of speech depends not only on the site, severity and nature of the lesion, but also on the intelligence and degree of education of the patient. The clinical phenomena represent the mode of response of an individual to an abnormal situation, produced by some disturbance of structure or function.

But broadly speaking cases of aphasia can be gathered together into definite clinical groups. To each of these varieties I have given a name chosen to signify the most salient defect in the management and comprehension of words or phrases. These names are purely indicative and are not intended in any way to define a specific set of psychical functions or aptitudes.

(a) *Verbal Defects*

In severe forms of this disorder the patient's utterance may be reduced to "yes" and "no" and even these words cannot always be evoked for voluntary use. As speech returns his vocabulary increases, but his enunciation is slow and halting. Any word he is able to recall can, however, be used for naming an object. It may be so badly pronounced as to be scarcely recognisable, but it is applied correctly. When the patient attempts to repeat what has been said to him, the articulatory sounds are imperfect, although he can usually repeat more words than he can pronounce spontaneously. It is characteristic of this form of aphasia that words are evoked with difficulty and tend to be abnormal in structure.

At first the comprehension of verbal significance may be somewhat impaired. But, after the stage of neural shock has passed away, the power of understanding the meaning of words is rapidly restored; these patients can not only choose an object to oral or printed commands, but even complex orders may be executed correctly.

The power of reading to themselves with enjoyment is spoilt by difficulty in remembering a series of words accurately; they are frequently compelled to look back to the beginning of a long sentence in order to obtain its full meaning. On the other hand, reading aloud is hampered by the same defects as articulatory speech.

As the spoken vocabulary increases, the power of writing is regained, although throughout it tends to show the same errors as articulatory speech. These patients cannot spell and find difficulty in remembering the order of the letters, even in simple words. They write more easily to dictation, but are unable to carry in the memory a string of words or a long phrase. Ability to translate printed words into cursive script, though at first diminished, is as a rule rapidly recovered.

The verbal aspect of numerals is affected and not their significance. Thus, when looking up the page of a book or scoring at cards, the patient may utter the wrong number, but acts as if he had said the right one. Simple arithmetical operations can be carried out correctly, except in severe cases; then it is not the process of addition and subtraction which is forgotten, but the act fails because of the difficulty in remembering accurately the requisite figures.

These patients can draw, play card games and enjoy jokes set out in print or pictures. In fact, the disorder from which they suffer affects mainly verbal structure and words as integral parts of a phrase; their nominal value and significance are perfect, except for the disturbance produced by articulatory abnormalities which affect both external and internal speech.

(b) *Syntactical Defects*

This is an easy form to distinguish, because the patient tends to talk jargon. Not only is articulation of the words ill-balanced, but the rhythm of the phrase is defective, and there is want of grammatical coherence. The power of naming objects may be retained in spite of the gross defects by which speech is hampered. Not infrequently, when the patient cannot utter a name, or when the sound emitted is incomprehensible to his auditor, he writes it correctly, proving that he is familiar with the usual designation of the object.

Comprehension of the meaning of words is always in excess of their use in conversation. These patients can choose common objects or colours without fail to oral commands in the form of a single word; if, however, the order is conveyed in a spoken phrase, it may not be understood correctly. In daily intercourse they suffer from inability to recall with certainty what they have been told; not only is phrasal utterance defective, but phrasal memory is transitory. This makes consecutive conversation difficult or impossible, and leads to an apparent slowness of apprehension.

Such patients can understand what they read to themselves, provided they are not compelled to reproduce the meaning in words, either silently or aloud; for their internal speech is also disturbed by jargon.

Single words may be written correctly; but any attempt to convey a formulated statement in writing is liable to end in confusion. Patients suffering from the more severe degrees of this affection cannot write a letter; but in slighter cases writing is easier than articulatory speech and all of them can copy correctly, transcribing print into cursive hand-writing.

Counting and the use of numbers is not materially affected, except that the pronunciation of the actual numerals is liable to be defective. There is no difficulty with the manipulation of money, or in giving the names and relative value of coins.

These patients can understand the full meaning of pictures, but they are greatly hampered by their jargon, if they attempt to convey to others or silently to themselves what they have gathered. They are able to draw, unless misled by defective verbalisation, and can often produce an accurate ground-plan of some familiar room.

This disorder is essentially one of balance and rhythm in symbolic expression, and syntax suffers greatly. The patient has plenty of words, but their production is ataxic and they are strung together without the usual connecting links. This leads to jargon and renders difficult even internal formulation of words and their meaning.

(c) *Nominal Defects*

This is essentially a loss of power to use names and want of compre-hension of the nominal value or meaning of words and other symbols. Not only does the patient fail to name objects placed in front of him, but, when asked to point to one of them named aloud or in print, the choice, even if correct, is made slowly and with effort.

There is no lack of words and, if the patient is intelligent, he evokes one after another all more or less aptly associated with the name or ex-pression he is trying to discover. He frequently employs some des-criptive statement, such as "what you cut with" for scissors, or in the case of a colour, may indicate how it is composed or the circumstances under which it is used. Verbal structure may suffer during the struggle to find the right word, but repetition is not materially affected; provided they are presented in articulated form the sounds can be reproduced correctly. The essential defect is inability to fit a name to an object or an object to a name, to recognise the difference between words of contrasted significance and to execute promptly oral and printed commands. This disorder is mainly due to defective appreciation of meaning and inability to evoke a desired name; both internal and external speech suffer as a secondary result.

Such patients read with extreme difficulty both to themselves and aloud, especially if they attempt to spell out the words. Single letters, even if correctly enunciated, frequently fail to convey their full nominal significance. Printed orders are badly executed; but to read them aloud is a decided aid to their correct performance.

Both the act of writing and the power of conveying the intellectual content of ideas, evoked spontaneously or in response to something heard or read, are greatly affected. Writing to dictation shows the same calligraphic faults, although the subject matter is somewhat better reproduced, and, in the severe forms, these patients slavishly copy printed or cursive letters, but cannot consistently translate print into ordinary handwriting.

They can usually count, but suffer from defective appreciation of the meaning of single numbers. This interferes with the power to carry out simple arithmetical operations, and capacity to formulate the relative value of two coins, or to calculate change, is usually more or less affected. Games, such as cards, which demand rapid and correct recognition of names and power to register a score, are impossible. On the other hand chess, draughts and dominoes may be played correctly.

Drawing from a model, or from memory after the object has been removed from sight, is easily performed. But, when the patient is asked to draw some such figure as that of an elephant from imagination, the result is extremely unsatisfactory; all the distinctive features are usually omitted.

He can usually find his way from place to place so long as distinctive landmarks are in sight; but he may have considerable difficulty in planning his route beforehand, or in describing the salient objects he would meet on his journey. One of the most instructive forms assumed by the loss of function in these cases is the want of ability to draw a ground-plan of some familiar room. Asked "where is the table?" or "where is the window?" he can point to the situation of each correctly;

but he cannot express their relative position in the abstract form of a ground-plan. Moreover, he tends to slip into an attempt to express the principal pieces of furniture in elevation, evidently reproducing his concrete visual images.

(d) *Semantic Defects*

This form of aphasia is characterised by want of recognition of the ultimate significance and intention of words and phrases, apart from their direct meaning. But other functions suffer that have no immediate bearing on verbalisation; for in this form of disordered speech there is loss of power to appreciate or to formulate the general conclusion of a connected train of thought. The patient may understand a word or short phrase and can appreciate the various details of a picture, but the significance of the whole escapes him. Thus, although he comprehends the meaning of "summer" and "time," and knows that "summer-time" has something to do with the "Daylight Saving Act," he is unable to say if the clocks are put forward or back, when it begins. He can carry out a manoeuvre where each action suggests the next, but fails to do so if he is compelled to formulate it to himself as a whole and is unable to bear in mind with certainty the final goal towards which his efforts are directed.

He has no difficulty in forming words and can repeat what is said to him. But in general conversation his sentences tend to tail away aimlessly, as if he had forgotten what he intended to say. If he is told some simple story and asked to reproduce it by word of mouth or in writing, many essential elements may be omitted; this occurs to an even greater degree after reading it to himself silently[1]. He cannot retain the total conception of its meaning, which is necessary for perfect narration. He may be able to enumerate the details one by one correctly, provided he is allowed to mention them in any order as they may happen to recur to his memory; but his knowledge is episodic and is not coordinated by a general, logically expressed formula.

The clock tests reveal the nature of this disorder in a striking manner. The patient confuses the two hands, does not know how to approach the task of setting them to oral or printed commands, and forgets the meaning of "past" and "to" the hour. Even direct imitation on one clock of the time shown on another may lead to confusion; for, whatever

---

[1] This is an exaggerated form of a phenomenon familiar from psychological experiments on normal persons.

the form assumed by the test, the patient is liable to misunderstand the intention of what he is asked to do. On the other hand, except in the gravest cases he has no difficulty in telling the time, provided he is allowed to keep the clock in sight until he has given his answer.

Such patients can write, but the result tends to be inaccurate and confused. Although spelling may be careless and the letters imperfectly formed, semantic defects are more liable to disturb the intellectual content and logical sequence of what is written than its verbal form. Not infrequently the written account of a set of ideas arising spontaneously, or suggested by something the patient has heard or read, tails away aimlessly just like the spoken narration of the same subject. The power of reproducing a logical and orderly sequence suffers more severely than the direct act of writing.

Counting is possible and the actual value of numbers and coins may be recognised correctly. But the patient becomes confused if he is asked to state the relative value of two pieces of money; in daily life he finds profound difficulty in calculating the price of an article he has purchased, although he remembers how much he has expended. Arithmetical operations, such as addition and subtraction, are carried out uncertainly and with difficulty, because the nature of such mathematical processes is incomprehensible.

Such patients fail to understand jokes which demand complete comprehension of printed words or pictures. They cannot play card-games, draughts or dominoes; nor can they put together puzzles, which confuse them greatly.

Drawing, even from a model, shows considerable loss of general constructive power. These patients do not as a rule block out the drawing, but tend to begin at some one point and follow round the outline of the object detail by detail; this weakness of design is also evident when they try to reproduce it from memory. Attempts to draw an elephant to command usually end in confusion and occasionally the marks on the paper do not correspond to a coherent figure of any kind.

None of this group could draw a plan spontaneously of a room with which he was familiar; unimportant details might be filled in though salient features, such as the windows and doors, were omitted. This is not due to lack of memory of details, but to want of power to unite them into a coherent whole. For if I drew an outline plan and indicated upon it the position of each object as the patient pointed it out to me, he could subsequently reproduce this plan without fail. No. 10 complained that he "had difficulty in getting a starting point," but "after things were pointed out I retained them in my memory and got them down on paper quite easily."

These patients are completely unable to find their way alone; they do not take their bearings and fail to recognise landmarks, or to appreciate that they are passing over ground that should be familiar. They do not know which way to turn and, if they chance to cross to the opposite side of the road, become confused, ignorant in which direction to walk.

Semantic disorders interfere seriously with the activities of daily life. The patient finds difficulty in collecting the objects required to set the table for a meal, in adjusting the complexities of a military belt, or in putting together the different parts of a piece of furniture he has constructed. Such defects render him useless for any but the simplest employment; yet his memory and intelligence may remain on a relatively high plane. He does not forget people and places and his power of remembering detail is sometimes remarkable. He can recall spontaneously events both recent and remote and may be able to furnish valuable information with regard to his disabilities. It is not "memory" that is affected, but the power to coordinate details into a general formula for internal or external statement.

The tendency to confusion and want of comprehension of what is going on around them leads these patients to seek solitude and to shun their fellows. In some instances this produces an odd form of behaviour or even a definite psychosis.

§ 5. GENERAL MENTAL CAPACITY

All these processes which suffer in aphasia are essentially psychical and, in so far as they are defective, the capacity of the mind is restricted. Yet it is not "memory" and "general intelligence" which are primarily affected, but the mechanism by which certain aspects of mental activity are brought into play. In proportion as these forms of behaviour are necessary for the perfect exercise of psychical aptitudes, "general intelligence" undoubtedly suffers. For a man who is unable to express his thoughts or comprehend the full significance of words and phrases, cannot move freely in the field of general ideas. Moreover, defects of internal speech make it difficult for him to arrange and formulate his deductions, even when they are drawn from correct observation. If in addition he cannot manipulate numbers with ease, or find his way from one place to another, he will certainly be less capable than his fellows of carrying out intellectual acts successfully.

Let us consider the condition of a patient suffering from an extremely severe form of aphasia, in which the power of symbolic formulation and expression has been profoundly affected. Speech is reduced to "yes" and "no" and even these words are not always used correctly. He may perhaps be capable of uttering automatic expressions, such as "Oh! dear me," but is unable to employ them at will or repeat the words when they are said to him. He can imitate a simple action, such as touching his nose, closing his eyes or putting out his tongue, although he is unable to do so to command. He matches an object or colour shown him with one lying on the table, but fails to make a correct choice to orders given orally or in print. Reading is impossible; he may pick out his own name from others written on paper and yet is unable to recognise that of his wife under similar conditions. He can copy capital letters line by line, a purely imitative act, but is unable to translate them into cursive script, or put together in writing even the simplest word or phrase. Given a coin, such as a two-shilling piece, he selects another which exactly resembles it; but he can neither express its relative value nor pile up its equivalent from the various coins laid before him. All arithmetical operations are impossible and this prevents him from carrying out even simple business transactions. Such a patient shows by his response to tests, which do not require symbolic formulation and expression, that he is not demented; he can carry out certain mental processes, but not others. For the purpose of daily life his intellectual capacity is profoundly diminished. He resembles a prisoner in solitary confinement, whose sole communication with the outer world is by means of a defective telephone; he can neither comprehend exactly what is said to him nor make others understand his wishes.

Moreover, the intellectual life of civilised man is so dependent on speaking, reading and writing that any restriction of these powers throws him back upon himself; he shuns company and cannot occupy himself with the newspaper or social intercourse. The working man no longer goes daily to his employment and, if he is an ex-soldier, vegetates on a pension. This life without occupation or interests inevitably leads to a diminished field of thought and many aphasics gradually deteriorate in mental capacity. Yet closer observation shows that this lack of intelligence may be secondary to defects in some distinctive form of behaviour.

But it must not be forgotten that the large majority of these disorders of speech are due to some wide-spread destructive lesion of the brain, such as a haemorrhage deep in its substance, which interferes with a multitude of converging and diverging paths. Many gun-shot wounds of the head, which produced aphasia, were so gross that, even if they had not been accompanied by defects of speech, they would have lowered the patient's mental capacity.

Moreover, the larger number of those in whom the lesion is the result of cerebral haemorrhage, suffer from wide-spread disease of the vessels. They have long lived up to the limit of their mental capacity and the stroke plunges them into a state of profound psychical insufficiency. This is greatly aggravated by the disorder of speech and many a patient of this kind has been supposed to be demented.

Most of the aphasics encountered in civilian practice are enfeebled by age and easily become fatigued by effort. Any severe or exacting test is liable to result in a state of mental incapacity far in excess of that which could be attributed to the disorder of speech alone. The methods of examination I have adopted are intended for young and vigorous persons in full bodily health and must be shortened and adapted to the capacity of older and more easily exhausted individuals.

Anxiety and worry are liable to reduce profoundly the power to carry out these tests; a patient, who has shown obvious signs of improvement, may regress to a previous condition and appear to be degenerating mentally. This loss of capacity can be shown on examination to be due to the recurrence of specific defects of function, which were present at an earlier stage; if it is possible to remove the disturbing psychical factors, the patient may rapidly recover the powers he has lost.

In a highly intelligent and sensitive patient disappointment at failure to perform the tasks set him, or any emotional disturbance, may produce a want of power, which makes further testing impossible. He loses heart and no longer tries to solve the problems placed before him; he appears to be unusually stupid, for he may cease to execute even those tests which are not as a rule affected in uncomplicated aphasia.

For this reason I have laid particular stress on the results obtained from the examination of young men with limited gun-shot wounds of the head. The majority are buoyed up by obvious improvement in their physical condition and powers of speech. They are on the up-grade and day by day acquire increasing capacity, whilst most patients with non-traumatic lesions progress more or less steadily towards dissolution, or at best remain stationary. Active and full of hope, the young aphasic shows an intense desire to do well and to recover; he works, he exerts his will, he seeks out every expedient to make himself understood and triumphs in his success. His behaviour forms an extreme contrast to the conduct of an elderly patient with diminished intelligence and lack of mental vigour.

The results obtained with the tests I have employed also depend greatly on the state of the patient's education. If for example the power to manipulate numbers is affected, the extent to which he can solve problems in arithmetic depends on the ease with which he could do so before the injury. Thus an intelligent private soldier, who had left school at thirteen, failed to bring out an answer to the last simple addition and to all three subtraction sums. But two young officers, also suffering from verbal aphasia, carried out all these tests successfully; one of them had been a student of medicine and the other a clerk in a bank, accustomed to deal with figures.

One of the most characteristic features in cases of nominal aphasia is the close parallel between the results usually obtained in response to oral and to printed commands. No. 22, however, showed much greater difficulty in executing the latter, probably in consequence of his defective education. For, although he was an unusually intelligent house painter and musician, he had had little schooling and reading was always a somewhat laborious process.

The effects of general education on the answers to specific tests was particularly evident in the two congenital cases. These patients acquired the art of reading and writing in spite of disabilities which had apparently existed from birth. Thus, No. 25 gave the following instructive account of her difficulty in learning. She always knew she was not like other people. She had always been extraordinarily alive to all matters of experience and speculative questioning, but did not learn to read until she was thirteen years of age. She attended no school, being taught at home by governesses and having no regular lessons after twelve; for it seemed a hopeless task to teach her reading, writing and arithmetic. Her father, a school inspector, who took endless trouble with her education, always said, "The way to your mind is by all sorts of roundabout paths, through hedges and over ditches." After all organised lessons had ceased, she learnt to read "with a rush"; but she first read intelligently some years later, when she stopped in a house where there was a copy of the Encyclopaedia Britannica. She read with avidity one article after another and this awakened her desire for theoretical knowledge.

On examination this patient evidently suffered from a moderate degree of semantic aphasia; but her powers of reading and writing were unusually bad, considering her outstanding intelligence and ability.

In the same way, No. 23 was unable to learn like other boys and at the age of thirteen had reached the second standard only at an elementary school. When I first saw him, he was a remarkably intelligent young man, but reading and writing were grossly defective owing to his con-genital disabilities. A clever school mistress, recognising that he was abnormal, definitely concentrated her efforts on teaching him to tell the time and, in consequence, the results I obtained with the clock tests were consistently above what might have been otherwise expected.

It must not be forgotten that the erroneous responses, which result from specific defects of symbolic formulation and expression, are in themselves liable to produce mental confusion. Even a highly intelligent aphasic may be misled by wrong words, said to himself silently or aloud. Thus, should he say "horns" instead of "tusks," when drawing an elephant, he is liable to add these appendages to the forehead of the figure. We are familiar with the difficulty produced by inadvertently saying the wrong number to ourselves when telephoning; in the same way a patient suffering from syntactical defects of speech is liable to be confused by his own internal jargon. One of the most characteristic features of semantic aphasia is want of power to appreciate the ultimate aim or intention of some mode of behaviour, initiated either spontaneously or to command. When these defects are sufficiently severe, the patient may act in some foolish and apparently inexplicable manner.

Moreover, this fundamental want of comprehension of general meaning and consequent mental confusion sometimes leads to a mild psychosis. Thus, two of my patients with semantic aphasia of traumatic origin became somewhat mentally affected. But this is in no sense universally the rule; for in no other instance of this form of defective speech was there any sign of mental instability.

Even limited defects of symbolic formulation and expression are liable to reduce the patient's mode of behaviour to a lower level of efficiency. Should he be unable to carry out the task in a normal manner, he falls back on a simpler and more childish method of solving the problem. He counts with the aid of his fingers instead of adding or subtracting, he states the amount of change he has actually received in place of the cost of the article he has purchased, and describes the use of an object before mentioning its name. But, as with many children who are supposed to be mentally deficient, this loss of intellectual capacity is specific and not general[1].

Another simplified but insufficient mode of response, common in the more severe degrees of aphasia, is liable to be attributed to want of general understanding. When, for example, the patient is asked to read

[1] Cf. Fildes, Lucy G. [47].

aloud and to execute some printed command, he utters the words correctly but does nothing further; the second half of the order fails to take effect, although he can execute it without fail if the same words are said to him by the examiner. Having performed the action of reading aloud, he has no impulsion to follow it up by another, even though it is implied in the phrase he has just enunciated. Shown an object and told to write down its name, he may say the word correctly but writes nothing. If, however, he can be persuaded not to utter the word, he writes it with ease. When one action has been performed, all desire is satisfied and a second command is required to elicit a further response; there is no compulsion to follow one action by another, although both are implied in the order.

Thus every patient suffering from aphasia is liable to exhibit in his conduct more or less evidence of intellectual insufficiency. This may arise solely from his defective use of language or from a general lack of mental capacity induced by the severity of the lesion or coincident disease of the brain and its vessels. At the same time it must not be forgotten that the mental enfeeblement and readily induced fatigue, consequent on advancing age, gravely affect the character of the answers to the more severe tests. Even in aphasics who have shown considerable signs of recovery, worry and anxiety may cause regression to a previous condition and the reappearance of abnormal responses.

§ 6. CONCLUSION

No single term can be discovered to include logically all those forms of behaviour which are affected in aphasia and kindred disorders of speech. Symbolic formulation and expression is a purely descriptive designation, chosen to signify that the principal disturbance is to be found in the use of symbols, such as words and numbers. In the same way, the names I have given to the different clinical varieties of the disorder are intended merely to indicate the characteristic defects in verbal form and meaning; they are in fact purely grammatical designations.

All such terms are labels applied to phenomena observed experimentally; they must not be employed as definitions. Because it cannot be deduced logically from the name applied to the disorder of speech, there is no reason why a particular form of abnormal conduct should not appear with some variety of aphasia. The constituents of each clinical group must be determined by observation and designated empirically by some more or less indicative appellation.

Such empirical use of technical terms is entirely new to the study of aphasia. All previous observers have assumed that the various defects of speech reveal the elements out of which the use of language is composed, exactly in the same way as a salt is split up into an acid and a base by chemical analysis. On this fallacious supposition names were applied to the different forms of disordered speech to express definitely the elementary function which was responsible for the morbid manifestations. From a priori considerations speech seemed to be dependent on integrated movements of the articulatory apparatus and on visual or auditory images. Aphasia, which was supposed to reveal these elementary processes, was therefore divided into "motor" and "sensory," "auditory" or "visual."

Closer clinical investigation showed that this was not the case. No one who examined his patients with due care and an open mind, was able to discover an example of pure "motor," "auditory" or "visual" aphasia. In every instance some forms of behaviour were affected, which by the definition should have remained intact, whilst other functions escaped in an apparently inexplicable manner. To anyone who was not obsessed by the idea that the clinical manifestations revealed the elements out of which speech was composed, it was obvious that these categories were inapplicable to the phenomena actually observed.

These morbid states express the manner in which the organism meets a novel situation with all the means at its disposal. Each abnormal act of speech is the response of an individual to some interference with the mechanism necessary for the perfect use of language, and is governed by the conditions of the moment.

But with the aid of systematic tests it is possible to show that these pathological responses tend to assume certain distinctive forms. Regarded simply as abnormal acts of speech in its widest sense, the clinical varieties of aphasia fall naturally into certain groups. Each class exhibits different defects in the use of language, which in no way represent the analytical elements out of which this process is composed from a physiological or psychological point of view.

Thus symbolic formulation and expression does not correspond to a human "faculty," which, having once been discovered, can be accurately defined and treated as a predetermined form of intellectual capacity. It is the name given to a system of aptitudes, which have been gradually acquired in conjunction with acts of verbal formation and comprehension. It does not correspond to any single psychical or physiological process. Nor is there any unitary function underlying verbal, syntactical, nominal

or semantic aphasia. All these terms designate abnormal modes of behaviour, discovered by observation and grouped together experimentally
in cases where the disorder of speech is due to some cerebral lesion.

Although aphasia does not reveal the psychical or physiological elements of speech, the forms it assumes are determined to a considerable
degree by the manner in which the use of language has been acquired.
This has its own history, peculiar to each individual, but with certain
common features in men of the same race and cultured affinities.

The earliest and most primitive acts of speech, apart from emotional
manifestations, consist of the employment of certain articulated sounds
to convey a distinct meaning to others. This power may be developed to
a high degree, but the majority of human beings advance no further in
symbolic formulation and expression. Civilised man, however, enormously widens his intellectual capacity by converting these verbal
formulae into written symbols, which in turn can be retranslated into
articulated words by anyone conversant with their conventional significance. This places at his disposal the recorded thoughts of those distant
from him in space and time, and his capacity for logical generalisation
is enlarged to a corresponding degree. Once he has learnt to read and
write his propositional powers may continue to increase in range and
amplitude until their development is terminated by death alone.

In the same way a child learns to count on his fingers and can advance
a considerable distance in the use of numbers without the help of reading
and writing. Once he has acquired these arts the most complicated
mathematical calculations become possible. So, in the history of the
race, man originally recorded number by a series of strokes or notches;
as soon as a single sign was invented to express a group of units, the first
step was taken in symbolic formulation and expression of numerical
relations. The value of an object was at first determined by the amount
of some other commodity for which it could be exchanged; but, when
a conventional significance was given to certain pieces of metal, barter
was replaced by the use of money.

Thus in time the more primitive acts of speaking and comprehension
of spoken words became associated with many other aptitudes, linked to
them for the purposes of human inter-communication. The nature and
extent of the morbid manifestations which accompany disorders of
speech increased profoundly with the growth of man's intellectual
attainments, and in any individual instance depend to a considerable
degree on the patient's education.

It is a universal law that those aptitudes suffer first and in the severest manner which are most difficult to carry into action or have been recently acquired. This rule is illustrated throughout by the phenomena of aphasia; for the patient tends to fail altogether in the execution of tests based on the higher developments of symbolic formulation and expression. On the other hand, tasks approximating closely to acts of verbal formation and comprehension show defects, which are less massive and more distinctive. Thus the abnormalities in counting and understanding of numbers vary in character according to the form assumed by the aphasia, whilst it would be impossible to determine from the crude records of arithmetical tests alone to what group the patient belonged.

Analysis of results yielded by tests, based on the simpler and more primitive aptitudes of speech, shows that the morbid manifestations consist mainly of defects in verbal form and meaning. Whilst the principal disturbance in verbal aphasia is found in the structure and formation of words for external or internal use, nominal aphasia is based on defective appreciation of their meaning and inability to employ them correctly as names. In the same way syntactical aphasia destroys the rhythmic balance of words and phrases and interferes with the grammatical structure of the sentence; on the other hand semantic aphasia is mainly characterised by inability to comprehend the general intention and significance of a series of logically consecutive statements.

But here again it is a profound error to classify the clinical phenomena in two mutually antagonistic groups, such as "aphasia" and "amnesia," "apraxia" and "agnosia." For such terms postulate that every example of disordered speech can be analysed into a disturbance of verbal form or verbal meaning, and depends on lack of some distinct and accurately definable set of functions.

In fact, however, there is no disorder of verbal formation, which, if sufficiently severe, does not involve some want of power to appreciate the meaning of words and phrases. Even in the slighter forms of verbal aphasia, the patient complains that he cannot always grasp the meaning of what he reads to himself, because he tends to forget the words before he reaches the end of the sentence. On the other hand, even the purest form of semantic aphasia may affect the structure of written words or even the letters of which they are composed; the patient forgets how to set to work to produce them, just as he fails with other operations demanding constructive aptitudes.

The defective responses, however closely they may approximate to the formative or significant aspects of speech, are a disturbance of the use of language as a whole. Defective capacity to find words and phrases is associated with some lack of appreciation of their meaning; on the other hand, forms of aphasia, due mainly to want of power to understand their significance, tend to be associated with some disturbance of verbal or phrasal structure. The use of language cannot be separated into two sharply defined categories, structure and meaning. In each group of aphasia one aspect tends to be affected to a preponderating degree, and to this it owes its characteristic features. But any attempt at rigid and definable classification on these lines serves only to obscure the nature of the phenomena. The more strictly drawn and logical a definition, the more remote does it become from reality and the less does it correspond to the actual events we set out to describe.

To attempt to collate these conclusions with older views on the nature of aphasia and kindred disorders of speech is to pour new wine into old bottles. Most previous theories were based on certain assumptions, which I believe to be erroneous. The clinical phenomena cannot be classed as isolated affections of speaking, reading or writing; the effects of the lesion do not analyse speech into its constituent elements and the various disorders in the use of language cannot be strictly divided into defects of verbal formulation (aphasia or apraxia) and want of appreciation of meaning (amnesia or agnosia).

I have attempted to show that all these disorders of function are manifestations of the reaction of the individual as a whole to an abnormal situation. Each response can only be described as an act of speech in the widest sense and not in terms of some elementary process, of which it is presumed to be composed under normal conditions.

Summary

(1) Speech and the use of language in its widest forms require the perfect performance and interaction of a series of processes of great complexity. Acquired during the life of the individual, these are perfected by voluntary effort, and finally come to consist of the orderly exercise of functions, conscious, subconscious and wholly automatic, all working together in harmony.

(2) Once acquired, this form of behaviour can be disturbed by anything which interrupts the orderly precision of the physiological processes on which it depends.

(3) The resulting loss of function is expressed in terms of the complete act, and does not reveal the "elements" out of which it is composed or developed.

(4) To the group of functions, which suffer in these high-grade disorders of speech, I have applied the term "symbolic formulation and expression." This is a purely empirical designation, chosen to signify that the power to manipulate such symbols as words and numbers is of all most profoundly affected.

(5) Acts of symbolic formulation and expression are integrated on a level superior to that of motion, and are of a higher order than sight or hearing. Consequently, the clinical manifestations cannot be classified as "motor," "visual" or "auditory" defects of speech.

(6) Moreover, the clinical facts entirely fail to bear out the contention, that the various forms assumed by these disorders in the use of language can be classified in distinct categories as faults of speaking, reading or writing. These are purely linguistic terms for diverse human actions, and do not correspond even to specific groups of psychical functions.

(7) The group of functions, classed as symbolic formulation and expression, is not uniformly disturbed in every instance and cases of aphasia differ profoundly in their clinical manifestations. Each one represents the response of an individual patient to an abnormal situation. But analysis of the various forms assumed by these disorders of speech shows that they can be classed roughly into groups possessing certain common characteristics. To each I have given a name chosen from the most salient defect in the use of words. These terms are purely indicative and are not intended to define any specific set of psychical functions.

(8) Verbal aphasia consists of a difficulty in forming words for external or internal speech. The patient may be reduced to almost complete dumbness and cannot even repeat what has been said to him. His comprehension of the meaning of words is greatly in excess of his power of uttering them and he understands most that he hears. Silent reading is hampered by difficulty in remembering a series of words and writing shows the same sort of errors as articulated speech. The verbal aspect of numerals is affected, but not their significance; except in severe cases arithmetical operations can be carried out accurately. The disorder affects mainly verbal structure and words as integral parts of a phrase; their nominal value and significance remain comparatively intact.

Syntactical aphasia is essentially a disorder of balance and rhythm; syntax suffers greatly. The patient has plenty of words, but their arrangement into coordinated phrases is defective; this leads him to talk jargon and renders even internal verbalisation difficult. But the power of writing is in excess of that of articulated speech. He understands most of what is said to him, but in daily intercourse suffers from inability to recall with certainty things he has been told or has gathered from reading; not only is phrasal utterance difficult, but phrasal memory is transitory and consecutive conversation becomes difficult or impossible. Comprehension of the meaning of words, however, is always in excess of power to employ them in daily intercourse.

Nominal aphasia comprises loss of power to use names and want of comprehension of the significant value of words and other symbols. Not only does the patient fail to give names to objects placed before him, but, when asked by word of mouth or in print to point to one of them, the choice, even if correct, is made slowly and with effort. Such patients read with extreme difficulty, writing is grossly affected and they suffer from defective appreciation of single numbers or letters. Games, such as cards, which demand rapid recognition of names and power to register a score are impossible, though draughts and dominoes may be played correctly.

Semantic aphasia consists in a want of recognition of the full significance of words and phrases apart from their direct verbal meaning. Other functions suffer, which have nothing to do with verbalisation. The patient may understand a word or a short phrase, but its ultimate significance escapes him and he fails to comprehend the final intention of some command imposed upon him orally or in print. He cannot formulate, either to himself or others, a general conception of what he has been told, has read to himself, or has seen in a picture. Such patients can read and write, but the results tend to be inaccurate and confused. Counting is possible and the significance of numbers and coins may be recognised; but arithmetical operations are disturbed by defective appreciation of the procedure required. There is a wide-spread lack of constructive power both for processes of logical thought and orderly manipulations.

(9) The harder the intellectual task set by any test for symbolic formulation and expression the more readily and profoundly will it be affected.

(10) The degree and form assumed by the disturbance of any particular aptitude depends on the stage at which it was acquired. Recently adopted forms of behaviour are liable to suffer more severely and in a less specific manner than those developed at an earlier date in the life-history of the individual. Thus, articulated speech and the comprehension of spoken words exhibit specific defects with the various forms of aphasia, whilst writing and arithmetical calculations suffer in a less distinctive manner.

(11) Each specific form of aphasia depends on a predominant disturbance of certain aspects of symbolic formulation and expression. As recovery advances, those functions are restored first which have suffered least. Thus, by watching the gradual improvement of the patient's powers, we gain a further insight into the essential nature of each variety of disordered speech. Moreover, the records obtained at various stages of recovery enable us to understand those "partial" cases, where the defects of speech are slight from the beginning.

(12) On the other hand, should the powers of speech again deteriorate, those tests suffer first which were originally affected most severely. Regression retraces the lines along which recovery has advanced.

Apart from any increase in the structural lesion, epileptiform attacks, fatigue or worry are potent causes of regression.

(13) The direct use of visual images may remain intact, although they cannot be employed readily in acts of symbolic formulation and expression, or evoked with ease in response to words and other symbols. Mental pictures remain to those who originally possessed this form of memory; but the capacity for converting them into materials of logical thought has been destroyed or greatly diminished.

PART III

CHAPTER I

WHAT IS MEANT BY LOCALISATION OF FUNCTION

No one doubts that speech in its highest forms can be disturbed by destruction of the tissues of the brain, or that the manifestations differ according to the situation of the lesion. These crude facts have been habitually cited to prove the existence of "centres" for the various aspects of speech and an enormous literature has grown up around their supposed anatomical localisation. But before it is possible to talk of "centres" for speech, we must first determine the nature of the functions that we believe to be "localised" in these particular areas of the brain, and consider what we understand by this expression.

Now the views as to the nature of these "centres" vary profoundly. According to a prevalent conception they consist of specially restricted depositions of cells which initiate and carry out those motor, auditory, or visual activities of which speech in its widest sense is composed. The surface of the brain is thought to be starred with a number of minute areas, each of which is responsible for initiating a specific act of motion or sensation; these are combined synthetically to form groups of functions of varying complexity. Each such "centre" has a definite position and function; like the push of an electric bell, it is fixed at one spot and produces a constant and predetermined effect.

§ 1. "MOTOR CENTRES" AND EXCITATION OF THE CORTEX

These mechanical ideas were based mainly on the results of electrical excitation of the cortex, particularly over the "motor" area. But they no longer appeal to more thoughtful experimenters, and the work of Sherrington and his colleagues on the anthropoid apes has shown how little such an interpretation is justified, even by the positive effects of stimulation. For the response from any one cortical point is not constant; it varies both in the nature of the movement evoked and in the part of the body thrown into action. The reaction depends not only on the site of excitation, but on the character of the events by which it has been preceded.

Successive stimulations of one and the same spot at short intervals of time usually produce definite facilitation and an increase in the amplitude of the response. Sometimes, however, the nature of the reaction changes; thus, a point, which began by yielding primary extension, may come to yield flexion in the latter part of a series of stimuli. This reversal, when it occurs, may appear slowly or, in some cases, develop with great rapidity; it may consist only of relaxation of the muscle, which was originally thrown into contraction from the particular cortical points; or there may be simultaneous contraction of its antagonist, previously the site of inhibition[1]. Repeated or strong excitation of a flexor point often temporarily diminishes or suppresses the subsequent response of an extensor point; a similar increased resistance to flexion can also be produced, though less easily, from an extensor point. Even stimulation applied to the afferent fibres of a peripheral nerve, such as the ulnar, may have a profound effect upon the nature of the response subsequently obtained from a definite cortical area.

Graham Brown and Sherrington sum up as follows[2]: "What we desire to stress in regard to the reaction of the cortical point on the antagonistic muscle-pair is the influence of shortly pre-current excitations, both of itself and of other points, and of afferent channels. And in this respect the functional instability of some cortical points seems to be greater than that of others. The instability is great enough to be easily demonstrable under narcosis as in our experiments. It may well be even greater in normal conditions without narcosis. Indeed, the frequency of reversal as a phenomenon attaching to the reactions of points in the motor cortex suggests that one of the functions of the cortex may be performance of reversals, and that the greater predominance of reversal under cortical than in purely spinal or decerebrate reflexes is because reversal is one of the specific offices of the cortex cerebri."

These ideas were developed still further in the remarkable paper of Sherrington and Leyton, published in 1917[3]. Cortical motor points are functionally unstable and, during systematic exploration, three phenomena are liable to appear, all closely akin, "facilitation," "reversal" and "deviation" of response. For example, the whole anterior border of the motor field can be made to extend further forward by facilitation, and the area from which some particular movement can be obtained may be considerably enlarged. On the other hand, the nature of the response

---

[1] Brown, T. Graham, and Sherrington, C. S. [30], p. 254.
[2] [30], p. 277.
[3] Leyton, A. S. F. and Sherrington, C. S. [85].

can be reversed either by repeated excitation of the same point, or by a previous stimulus applied to some part, which normally yields an opposite reaction. Deviation was exemplified by the following experiment, which I quote verbatim[1]:

"The examination of the motor area had in this experiment been begun at the top limit of the arm area in shoulder region, and proceeded systematically from point to point in the downward direction. Followed in this manner elbow flexion soon became the leading (primary) movement, and continued so very nearly or even quite down to the inferior genu of sulcus centralis. Beyond a certain point, which was minutely and precisely marked on the map made, elbow flexion disappeared abruptly, and facial movements appeared in the form of closure of opposite eyelids. The lower margin of arm area having thus evidently been reached, we turned to the delimitation of the face area. The examination of this area we started at the lower (Sylvian) end of sulcus centralis, and thence proceeded point by point upward along the precentral gyrus not far in front of sulcus centralis. In due course the point yielding closure of opposite eye was again reached, and it was found that then on proceeding farther upward to the point that had previously yielded elbow flexion as its primary movement, that point now yielded adduction of the thumb as its primary movement, and, a little farther upward, movement of index, chiefly extension, was added to that of thumb; and movements of thumb and index continued to be primary movements right up through the region which previously had given elbow flexion as primary response, and thumb and index movements as primary responses trespassed actually into the area that had previously yielded shoulder movements." Here "deviation of response" affected a series of points forming a considerable fraction of the whole arm area.

But this "deviation" could be produced in a still more remarkable manner. An electrical stimulus, applied to the post-central convolution, evoked no direct response in the anthropoid apes; yet it might profoundly influence the nature of a subsequent discharge from the motor cortex[2]. Not only could it facilitate the response from adjacent precentral points, but even the form of movement evoked might be fundamentally changed by antecedent stimulation of an apparently "silent" area.

They conclude that phenomena such as facilitation, reversal and deviation of response, evidence of the functional instability of cortical

---

[1] [85], p. 141.
[2] Cf. Brown, T. Graham [29]. See also [28] and [30].

motor points, are indicative of the enormous wealth of mutual associations existing between portions of the motor cortex. "The acquirement
of skilled movements, though certainly a process involving far wider
areas (cf. v. Monakow) of the cortex than the excitable zone itself, may
be presumed to find in the motor cortex an organ whose synthetic
properties are part of the physiological basis, which renders that acquirement possible." They add, "Such synthesis involves time adjustments
as well as spacial adjustments." In fact, in the words of Franz, "the
motor cortex is a labile organ."

These luminous experiments show the fallacy of conceiving the
motor cortex as the seat of strictly limited "centres" of preordained
function. Cortical activity, even when aroused by electrical stimulation,
is revealed as a march of events with a definite temporal relation. The
response obtained from any one point, at a particular moment, depends
on what has happened before. Excitation of a spot, which caused
flexion of the elbow, may provoke the opposite effect if it follows some
event, motor or sensory, favourable to extension. In the same way an
area, associated at one time with contraction of the face, may yield
movements of the elbow if approached from above downwards on the
precentral gyrus. The past plays a predominant effect in the response
obtained at any one moment, and this in turn helps to determine in
advance the form of the future reaction.

These facts show that the "motor" centres cannot be the sole and
primary foci from which movements are initiated. They form rather the
means by which we are enabled at will to interfere with otherwise automatic acts. A series of high-grade movements are associated together
in the acquirement of some aptitude, which, though at first learnt
wittingly, ultimately becomes automatic. Cortical activity can then
interfere with this series of actions and modify them in accordance with
our voluntary requirements.

§2. THE EFFECT OF CORTICAL ABLATION OR INJURY

Even complete ablation of one of these "centres" produces a transitory loss of function only, provided the injury does not extend deeply
into the substance of the brain. Sherrington and Leyton[1] removed
the whole area from which movements of the hand could be evoked by
electrical stimulation. After recovery from the transient loss of power,
the site of the injury was again exposed and stimulated without effect;

---

[1] [85], p. 188.

the cortical tissues were then excised over a still wider area without producing any permanent or material change in the condition of the hand. Evidently the restoration of function was not due to the residue of a limited "hand area," which had escaped removal; nor was it the result of some vicarious activity on the part of neighbouring "centres." But, after neural shock had passed off, the animal still possessed the power of re-learning an action which had been disturbed by the anatomical destruction.

Any change that may result permanently from the ablation of limited areas of the cortex is too subtle to be betrayed under experimental conditions by destruction of the so-called "motor centres," even in the anthropoid apes. But the afferent activities of the cortex stand in closer relation to consciousness than movement, and the condition of sensibility in man, after local injury to the surface of the brain, forms a better indicator of the nature of the functional disturbance.

We were able to show that the cerebral cortex is the organ by which we can focus attention upon the changes evoked by sensory impulses. A pure cortical lesion, which is not advancing or causing periodic discharges, may change the sensibility of the affected parts in such a way that the patient's answers appear to be untrustworthy. Such diminished power of attention makes estimation of a threshold impossible in many cases; uncertainty of response destroys all power of comparing one set of impressions with another and so prevents discrimination.

But in addition to its function as an organ of local attention, the "sensory" cortex registers and retains the physiological dispositions produced by past events. These profoundly modify all subsequent actions. They may be manifest in the form assumed by sensations or images, but more often, as in the case of spacial impressions, remain outside consciousness. Here they form organised models of ourselves, which we termed "schemata." Such schemata, although they may act solely on the physiological level, are essential for all accurate spacial recognition; for they modify the impressions produced by incoming sensory impulses in such a way that the final sensations are charged with a relation to something that has happened before.

The part played by the cortex in sensation is concerned with those physiological processes which underlie projection and discrimination. The loss of function appears in three forms, as inability to appreciate spacial relationships, defective reactions to stimuli of graduated intensity, and failure to recognise similarity or difference in objects of various shapes and weights. The crude qualitative aspects of touch, pain, heat and cold are not affected by a superficial lesion of the brain; they are functions of a subservient organ, the optic thalamus.

We saw reason to believe that these three aspects of sensibility were not always affected uniformly, or in any constant relation to one another by a cortical injury. Sometimes one group of tests, sometimes another, revealed a disturbance of greatest severity and widest extent. Such variation proves that the physiological processes, necessary for the due appearance of these different aspects of sensation, can be thrown into disorder more or less independently by lesions situated at different positions on the surface of the brain.

Moreover, I was able to show that the various portions of the body were not equally affected by injuries of the "sensory" cortex; those closely connected with the performance of conscious acts, variable at will, showed the most intense loss of function and could be disturbed from a wider extent of surface on the brain. Such parts as the hand, which are endowed with the greatest power of discriminative sensibility, suffered most severely; for the fingers and thumb of man are little more than mobile sense-organs. Next in order came the sole of the foot, which habitually exerts discriminative activity in walking. The trunk is less likely to be affected, for the movements in which it is employed are mainly carried out automatically.

All cerebral activity consists of a march of events performed in part consciously, but to a greater extent unwittingly. On the physiological level the cortex undoubtedly plays a rôle in many automatic acts; but it also permits us to intervene to alter a sequence or to initiate some variation in accordance with circumstances. Thus, we are enabled to acquire with ease new aptitudes and facilities; once fully learnt, these in turn become more or less automatic. The deeper and wider therefore the injury to the cortex and underlying structures, the graver and more permanent is likely to be the loss of function; but we must never forget that it has disturbed a highly organised act and has not removed a strictly definable anatomical "centre."

§ 3. A LOCAL LESION OF THE BRAIN PRODUCES SOME DISTINCTIVE LOSS OF FUNCTION

It is a primary fact of both clinical and experimental observation that localised destruction within the limits of the precentral gyrus, if sufficiently severe, produces loss of voluntary movement in some definite part of the opposite half of the body. This may be transitory, although the lesion is permanent. Moreover, the various portions of the limb affected cannot be associated with rigidly definable areas of the cortex. But, roughly speaking, the higher the site of the injury on the pre-central gyrus and the closer it approaches the vertex, the more likely is it that the motor power of the lower extremity will suffer. Conversely, the lower it is placed, the greater the disturbance in the face and tongue. Destruction of tissue somewhere between these two situations will probably affect the hand and upper extremity.

Thus, in spite of the transient nature of the disturbance of function and the indefinite limits of the areas on the cortex from which it can be evoked, we are justified in associating topographically destruction of certain regions of the brain with defects of movement in portions of the opposite half of the body.

The same principles hold good for sensation. The area of the cortex within which destruction of tissue causes an alteration in sensibility extends at least from the central fissure back to the parietal region and below reaches the Sylvian fissure. A lesion within these limits tends to affect the leg or the arm of the opposite side, according as it is situated higher or lower on the surface of the hemisphere.

Thus, after taking into account their indefinite limits, we are justified in asserting that these areas of the cortex are associated topo-graphically with the motor and sensory functions of the opposite half of the body. At first sight this would not seem to be true of the so-called "visual centre." But I think a little consideration shows that vision also comes under a similar law. The total visual field stands in definite relation to projected bodily space; it consists of a right and left half and each of these again is divisible into an upper and a lower quadrant. A lesion, within a certain portion of the occipital lobe of one hemisphere, produces defects of vision confined to the opposite half of the field. The lower quadrants are similarly associated with the upper parts of this region of the cortex and vice versa. It must not be forgotten, however, that the fibres of the optic radiations lie extremely close to the surface and rare must be the lesion which does not destroy both cortical and sub-cortical tissues. This would tend to make the loss of function topographically more definite than if the lesion were strictly confined to the substance of the cortex.

But, in spite of this complication, we may conclude that local destruction within a certain area of the occipital lobe is associated with defects of vision in equivalent portions of the spacially projected field. This loss of function is not represented in defective movements of some part of the body, nor can it be delimited on its surface like the changes in sensibility; but the loss of vision, produced by local destruction of the brain, can only be expressed in terms relative to the projection of the body in space, and are strictly confined to parts of the field opposed to the site of the lesion.

Thus, all these primitive functions, motion, sensation and vision, can not only be affected independently from different parts of the surface of the brain, but the situation of the functional disturbance is associated topographically with the position of the lesion within any one of these areas.

Disorders of speech, or defects of similar high-grade functions, due to local destruction of the brain, differ from those of motion, somatic sensation or vision in that there is no such relation to parts of the body or its projection in space. Moreover, the lesion to be effective must be situated in one definite hemisphere. With the majority of right-handed persons this is the left, whilst conversely in the only left-handed man who came under my care with aphasia the injury was confined to the right half of the brain.

On this high level the problem of "cerebral localisation" acquires a somewhat different aspect and is greatly increased in complexity. We no longer have the comparatively simple task of associating some focus of destruction in the brain with loss of function in a definite part of the body or visual field, but are compelled to ask ourselves the much more difficult question, What form does it assume in accordance with the site of the lesion? We must first distinguish categorically the various defects in the use of language and then attempt as far as possible to determine their relation to the locality of the lesion in the left hemisphere.

Such questions as to the exact nature assumed by the specific loss of function also arise on the level of motion and sensation. But this aspect of the problem is usually neglected for the more diagnostic and easily determined relation between the site of the lesion and the part of the body or visual field affected. Yet, from the strictly scientific stand-point, voluntary movements, or those excited by stimulating the pre-central cortex, are not "motor" in the sense that this term is applicable to the response obtained from a motor nerve. For the cortical response is a highly coordinated movement, which depends to a considerable degree on the events which preceded it; in form it is mobile and variable according to circumstances other than the nature and strength of the stimulus. A muscular contraction, on the other hand, is definite, predetermined and inevitable. The term "motor" can only be applied to these two phenomena with a clear recognition of their fundamental difference; the one is a highly integrated movement, the other a muscular act.

In the same way a disturbance of sensation produced by a lesion within the limits of the so-called "sensory cortex" produces defects which differ fundamentally in character from those which follow injury to the spinal cord or afferent nerve. The more discriminative aspects of sensibility are alone disturbed; the loss of function appears as want of accurate appreciation of posture, of differences in intensity and of relations in size, shape, weight and texture of various test-objects. The cruder and more qualitative forms of sensory appreciation remain on the whole unaffected. Here a local lesion of the brain disturbs a psychophysical process and the consequences are expressed in terms of the act itself and not in those of touch, pain, heat and cold, which are categories of a lower functional order[1].

Study of defects in sensation produced by various injuries of the brain showed that there was no absolute criterion by which a cortical could be distinguished from a sub-cortical lesion. When the afferent impulses are interrupted before they reach the grey matter, the disturbance of function is usually graver and more definite than if the surface of the brain was alone affected. The closer the lesion lies to the internal capsule the grosser is the loss of sensation and the more certainly does it assume a hemiplegic disturbance.

Secondly, the loss of sensation is extremely severe compared with that which follows more superficial injuries. The patient frequently fails entirely to recognise the position into which his limb has been moved passively; when he wakes at night he has no idea where to find

---

[1] There is some evidence that the disorders of vision produced by cortical injuries tend to differ in character from the grosser forms of blindness due to lesions of the optic radiations or more peripheral portions of the visual apparatus. Supposing one half of the field is affected, the patient may recognise a moving object within it, although he fails to do so when it is stationary. Moreover, in certain cases, if two exactly similar objects are exposed simultaneously at identical points to the right and left of the middle line, he may fail to appreciate the one which falls in the defective half of the field; yet, if it is exposed alone in the same position, he can undoubtedly see it and indicates its shape correctly. (Cf. Case 8, Vol. II, pp. 109–110 and p. 117.) These changes have not been completely investigated; but, like other forms of sensation, vision tends to become inconstant and fluctuating under the influence of a cortical lesion. There is also some evidence to show that the power of spacial projection may be affected apart from appreciation of form and colour. (Cf. Holmes, Gordon, and Horrax, G. [77], and Riddoch, G. [118].)

the affected limb, although he is still conscious of the existence of his hand or foot. Contact may be appreciated, but contains no element of oneness or twoness; every application of the compass points is "just a touch." Spot-finding is gravely affected and touches are thought to be situated in some part of the limb remote from the site of stimulation. All power of appreciating weight, form, size and texture may be abolished. There may be some want of recognition of differences between warmth and coolness, though hot and cold can be recognised. Even the threshold for pricking may be appreciably raised.

All these defects are more definite and easier to determine than when the injury is confined to the superficial structures of the hemisphere. The effect of a sub-cortical lesion on sensation is shown by straightforward raising of the threshold for the affected aspects of sensation rather than by inconsequent and uncertain responses. Moreover, the deeper the lesion the more permanent are its effects; not only is the loss of function graver and more widely distributed, but it is also less transient.

Now in all my war-cases of defective speech, with the exception of No. 19, both the surface and deeper structures of the brain were more or less affected. On the other hand, most of the examples of aphasia met with in civil practice are instances of purely sub-cortical destruction. It is therefore impossible from such material to determine any absolute difference between the results of isolated destruction of the cortex or of the deeper structures of the hemisphere only.

But I think there can be little doubt that the effects produced by lesions of the surface are more transient and less severe than those of deeper parts. Thus the most definite and straightforward example of verbal aphasia was No. 19, who was thrown from a motor bicycle and evidently injured the base of his brain; there was no wound on the surface of his skull and at first he was both hemiplegic and aphasic. Three years and nine months after the accident his defects of speech were well defined and extremely gross.

On the other hand, in No. 20, who also suffered from verbal aphasia, the defects were more transitory and fluctuated within wide limits. Her loss of speech was consequent on the removal of a small extra-cerebral tumour and the sub-cortical destruction must have been comparatively slight.

All high-grade aptitudes acquired by conscious effort, such as the use of language, are carried out with practice more and more unwittingly; the functional processes upon which they depend become gradually engulfed in the automatic activities of the central nervous system. Thus a complete act of speech comes to be a wide-spread response of the organism to each fresh situation; this employs conscious, subconscious, automatic and purely physiological processes. The deeper the lesion the grosser and more definite the disorder. On the other hand, since the cortex is a more flexible organ with less rigid and preordained reactions, the disturbance of function due to injury of the surface is not so severe and permanent and is less easily determined.

These are differences in degree and are not categorically distinctive. All attempts shortly to differentiate a cortical from a sub-cortical aphasia are bound to fail. In both cases the defects in the use of language can only be described in terms of the act itself and not in those of anatomy.

That lesions situated in different localities of one hemisphere can produce specific changes in the power to employ language is one of the most remarkable facts which emerge from the study of aphasia. The material at my disposal is in no way sufficient to determine this relation with precision. Moreover, in all attempts to correlate the site of structural changes with defects of function it must never be forgotten that the severity and acuteness of the lesion exert an overwhelming effect on the manifestations.

But, in spite of these deficiencies, I think we are justified in drawing the following conclusions from the cases cited in this work. The more definitely the injury destroys the lower portion of the pre- and post-central convolutions and the parts which lie beneath them, the more likely are the defects of speech to assume a "verbal" form. A lesion in the neighbourhood of the upper convolutions of the temporal lobe tend to produce "syntactical" disorders. Destruction round about the region of the supra-marginal gyrus causes defects in the use of language which I have called "semantic"; whilst a lesion situated somewhat more posteriorly seems to disturb the power to discover and to understand names or other "nominal" expressions.

THE ANATOMICAL SITE OF THE LESION IN SOME TRAUMATIC CASES OF APHASIA

SUCH are the views to which I have been led by the study of selected cases of aphasia and kindred disorders of speech. It now remains to discover what relation the site of the lesion, when it can be determined, bears to the clinical manifestations. An ideal example for this purpose would be a chronic aphasic in the prime of life, who, after thorough examination at frequent intervals, had died from some cause unconnected with the central nervous system. One such example came under my notice, but unfortunately an autopsy was refused.

We must therefore be content for the present with the less satisfactory material provided by gun-shot wounds and the removal of non-malignant tumours. From an anatomical point of view these injuries are of less localising value than cases in which a complete microscopical examination could be carried out. But, on the other hand, such patients as I have used in this research are of infinitely greater scientific interest for determining the exact nature of the phenomena during life, than those broken-down wrecks in whom disease was terminated by death. These young men with gun-shot wounds of the head were in the prime of youth and their defects of speech and other symptoms were on the mend; they could be exposed to long continued observations, which would have been impossible in the case of an ordinary aphasic suffering from the diffuse effects of organic disease.

Moreover, in all attempts to associate a lesion of the brain with some form of loss of function, we must always bear in mind the effects of diaschisis. A small area of destruction of tissue can produce profound and wide-spread defects, if the lesion is acute or progressive. On the other hand a much larger loss of substance may cause a comparatively trivial disturbance, provided it is of old standing, slow onset and has occurred in an otherwise healthy brain.

Many gun-shot injuries, which produced clinical manifestations of great interest, were too diffuse to throw any light on the relation between the site of the lesion and the nature of the disturbance of speech. But amongst my cases were a small number which seemed to bear on this question and these I shall consider in closer detail in the following pages.

§1. METHODS EMPLOYED FOR DETERMINING THE POSITION OF THE CEREBRAL INJURY

In every instance of an injury to the head which came under my care during the war, the relative extent and shape of the wound were recorded on a set of diagrams showing the head from different aspects. An X-ray photograph was taken from the front and from the side, and in many cases stereoscopically, especially where we desired to localise the position of some foreign body in the substance of the brain.

Measurements were made according to the following plan. The distance from the root of the nose to the external occipital protuberance along the middle of the scalp was recorded in centimetres and the point determined at which it was cut by the interaural line. Then the position of the wound was mapped out, its diameters measured and the distance of its various parts determined in relation to the nasion-inion line and the middle of the scalp.

After the wound had healed, the head was subjected to another complete examination, to determine the extent to which bone had been lost and the condition of the parts that covered the opening in the skull.

If an operation was performed, I was invariably present to record its nature, the parts removed, and any indications that could be used for cerebral localisation. Such autopsies in the living often furnish evidence of the greatest value.

In order to determine the exact site of these brain injuries, I attempted to reconstruct them on the cadaver. For this purpose I applied for help to Professor Elliot Smith, who not only placed all the resources of his Anatomical Institute at my disposal, but poured out for me his unique knowledge and experience of cerebral topography. I cannot sufficiently thank him and his assistants, Dr Shellshear, Dr Tudor Jones and the late Dr John Hunter for the enthusiastic manner in which they helped and guided me in my difficult and laborious task.

The method we adopted was as follows. The head of a male body was selected, which corresponded as nearly as possible in its measurements to that of the patient, whose wound we intended to localise. The exact extent of the loss of bone was marked out on the scalp and holes were drilled through the skull to mark its dimensions. Through these a coloured fluid was passed with a small brush to fix the relation of the bony opening to the surface of the brain. Then the skull-cap was removed and a cast taken of its inner surface. This gave us a solid reproduction of the brain, covered by its membranes, on which were indicated the limits of the external wound. The situation and course of the principal fissures were determined by careful dissection and drawn on the cast. Thus we finally obtained a record of the area occupied by the wound on the surface of the brain, together with its extent in relation to the main landmarks of cerebral topography.

Fortunately the size of the head in these patients fell into a comparatively small number of groups; by selecting cases where the wounds were far apart, and by employing both halves of the brain in each cadaver, we were able to reduce the expenditure of bodies within reasonable limits. But none the less I cannot sufficiently express my thanks to Professor Elliot Smith for his open-handed generosity.

§ 2. THE SITE OF THE LESION IN VARIOUS FORMS OF APHASIA DUE TO GUN-SHOT INJURIES OF THE SKULL

(a) *Verbal Defects*

No. 6[1] (see Fig. 7) formed an excellent case for our methods of anatomical localisation. For the wound was an almost vertical cut in the left temporal region, 5 cm. in length, penetrating all the tissues, including the bone. The dura mater was laid bare in its deepest part, but the brain substance was not exposed. There was no wide-spread fracture of the skull and healing was complete in thirty days. No operation was performed at any time.

The upper end of this linear incision was 5·5 cm. from the middle of the scalp and 14 cm. behind the root of the nose; it lay 0·5 cm. anterior to the interaural line, whilst its extreme lowest point was 3 cm. in front. The whole nasion-inion measurement was 34·5 cm. and this was intersected at 14·5 cm. by the interaural line.

When this wound was plotted on the brain of a skull with approximately the same measurements, it was found to lie over the anterior portion of the precentral gyrus, extending downwards on to the inferior frontal convolution.

On admission to the London Hospital four days after he was wounded this patient was speechless, but he soon began to make articulate noises, which seemed at first to bear no relation to the words he was striving to pronounce. He could neither say his name spontaneously nor repeat it after me. His power of finding words rapidly improved during the first month, although throughout it was verbal structure and not nomenclature that formed his main difficulty.

---

[1] Fully reported, Vol. II, p. 76 et seq.

He could understand what was said to him and commands exacting a single choice were carried out accurately; but, as soon as two of these orders were combined, his response became slow and hesitating. Comprehension of printed phrases was obviously defective. He wrote his name and address correctly, but not that of his mother with whom he lived. When he attempted to record the names of objects he saw from the window, the words showed the same kind of structural faults as his

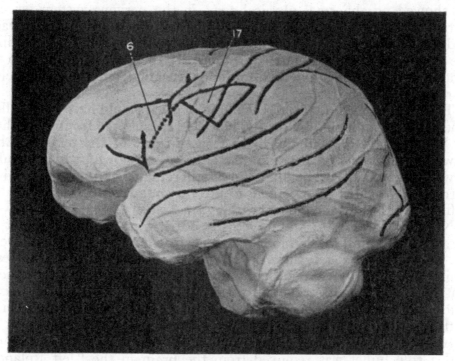

Fig. 7. To show the site of injury to the brain in No. 6 (dotted line) and in No. 17, cases of Verbal Aphasia.

articulation. Simple phrases were badly written to dictation, but he could transcribe print into cursive handwriting. He counted with extreme difficulty, although he wrote the numbers up to 21 correctly.

When examined more closely, five months after the injury, he still had great difficulty in verbalisation. The words were badly formed and evoked with difficulty, although they corresponded in nominal significance to what he wanted to say. He did not employ wrong words and his power of naming was perfectly preserved.

He understood what was said to him and carried out oral commands slowly, but on the whole correctly.

His power of comprehending the meaning of what he read to himself was undoubtedly good, and he carried out printed commands with several corrections, though few actual errors. As soon as he was permitted to read them aloud, his responses became perfect, for the sound of the words formed a self-given oral command.

Associated with these disorders of verbal formulation and expression he showed no abnormal physical signs in the nervous system, except a transitory weakness of the right half of the lower portion of the face and some deviation of the tongue to the right. All the reflexes, including the abdominals and plantars, were normal; there was no affection of motion, no incoordination, no disorder of sensation, and the visual fields were not diminished.

This man formed a splendid example of what would have been called true "motor" aphasia. Evidently, however, he suffered from more than an "anarthria," even in the highest significance of the term, for his powers of internal verbalisation were affected, as shown by his difficulty in writing and faults of spelling. But he still retained his power of naming correctly, provided he was able to utter a sound which corresponded sufficiently to the name he was seeking.

No. 17[1] (see Fig. 7) was much less satisfactory from the point of view of anatomical localisation; for the extraction of a rifle bullet from the substance of the brain was followed by formation of an abscess, which undoubtedly caused a considerable amount of deep destruction. But he was a superb example of defective verbal formation and, as a student of medicine, was able to give valuable introspective information with regard to his symptoms.

About ten days after he was wounded he was trephined in France, and a rifle bullet was removed from the brain in the "left Rolandic region." When he came under my care five months later, the wound was represented by a sinus from which issued a considerable quantity of pus. This opening was situated 16 cm. backwards along the nasion-inion line, in the centre of an irregular area, from which bone had been removed; this measured 4·5 cm. vertically, and 6 cm. horizontally, and extended between two points 13 cm. to 19 cm. posterior to the root of the nose. The upper border of the bony opening lay 6 cm. from the middle line of the scalp.

After removal of some fragments of bone from the substance of the

---

[1] Reported in full, Vol. II, p. 248 et seq.

brain and efficient drainage of an abscess cavity, the wound finally healed within eight months from the injury.

When the extent of this bony opening, which corresponded to those parts denuded of dura mater, was plotted on the surface of the brain, it was found to occupy an area extending between the inferior precentral and the lower third of the post-central fissures (Fig. 7). It corresponded in front with the upper part of the incision in No. 6, but did not extend so low. On the other hand, the destruction was not only superficial, but extended deeply into sub-cortical regions of the brain.

He showed characteristic difficulty in finding words to express his thoughts, and said, "At first I don't think I had more than a twenty-word vocabulary." Words were uttered singly or in short groups, isolated by pauses of varying length, and a single word of many syllables was liable to be slurred. Even a year after the injury he could not say the alphabet perfectly, and had much difficulty in counting. He was able to repeat the content of what was said to him correctly, but had the same difficulty in word-formation as during spontaneous speech.

He seemed to understand completely what he heard, and oral commands were executed quickly and with accuracy. But he confessed that, for the first fortnight after he was wounded, he had difficulty in understanding things said to him, unless they were "very simple and said very slow."

He carried out printed commands correctly, but could not read to himself with comfort, nor could he be certain that in the long run he understood exactly what was in the book before him. "I can get the meaning of a sentence, if it's an isolated sentence, but I can't get all the words." When he read aloud, his articulation showed the faults evident during voluntary speech, though to a less degree.

He wrote slowly and with great effort; his spelling was preposterous considering his education, and the form of the words showed the same defects that were manifested in voluntary speech. He complained, "I have to spell out every word, even the little ones; I have to say 'of'— I know it's a preposition, but then I have to think is it 'to' or 'from' or 'of.'" So much was this a matter of defective verbal formulation, that in writing a simple word like "help" he found it difficult to remember if the l or the p came last. A word such as "manager" was spelt "man-ger" exactly as it was pronounced, even when writing silently.

He showed remarkable powers of arithmetic and checked his own bank-book, in spite of his difficulty in counting. When he uttered a wrong number, as for instance whilst scoring at bridge, or looking up the page in a reference book, the false number did not mislead him; if he said twenty-eight instead of forty-one he scored it as forty-one. "I do the sum right, but get the figures wrong."

As might have been expected from the nature of the lesion, these defects of speech were accompanied by signs of profound injury to the nervous system. For a time he suffered with Jacksonian convulsions, which began in the right hand; these, however, passed off gradually, but were always accompanied by some increased loss of verbal capacity. He showed the characteristic signs of a spastic hemiplegia; isolated movements of the right hand were impossible, and although he possessed considerable power at the elbow and shoulder, the movements were clumsy and the whole limb was hypertonic. The right leg was in a state of extensor rigidity accompanied by loss of power of dorsiflexion at the ankle. The lower portion of the right half of the face was some-what affected and the tongue was protruded to this side of the middle line. Gross sensory changes of the cerebral type were present in both arm and leg of the affected half of the body. All the deep reflexes were greatly exaggerated on the hemiplegic side, the plantar gave a characteristic upward response and the abdominals were absent. Vision was unaffected and the fields were of normal extent.

This is another excellent example of so-called "motor" aphasia. He recovered to such an extent that the last traces of his disorder of speech were manifested solely as slight defects of word-formation. But these were evident not only on articulation and in his writing, but also when he attempted to formulate a word to himself for the use of internal speech. The power of naming was unaffected throughout, from the moment when it could be definitely tested.

(b) *Syntactical Defects*

Pick[1] has always contended that "agrammatism," as he defined it, was produced by lesions of the temporal lobe; and, in so far as it is included under "syntactical defects," my experience exactly bears out his contention. It is important, however, to remember that not all forms of jargon belong to this group of disorders of speech.

No. 15[2] (see Figs. 8 and 9) was a typical example of this condition. A rifle bullet had entered just to the left of the inner canthus of the right eye, destroyed the left eye, and had made its exit directly above the

---

[1] See Part I, pp. 126, 127.   [2] Reported in full, Vol. II, p. 227 et seq.

insertion of the left ear. A month later the wound of entry was represented by a minute perfectly healed white scar. On the other hand, the
exit consisted of an irregular opening in the bone and tissues of the scalp,
through which protruded a small pulsating hernia cerebri. Bone had
been removed over an irregularly quadrilateral area about 3 cm. in
vertical and horizontal extent; below, this opening reached the level of
the insertion of the ear and above it was about 13 cm. from the middle

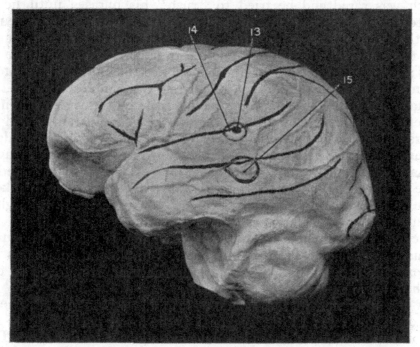

Fig. 8. To show the site of the injury to the brain in No. 13, No. 14 and
No. 15, cases of Syntactical Aphasia.

line of the scalp, corresponding anteriorly to a point on the nasion-inion
line 13 cm. from the root of the nose. The total distance from the
nasion to the external occipital protuberance was 35 cm.

Thus, the track of the bullet passed back through the left temporal
lobe, entering its substance in front close to the tip and passing out at
the level of the insertion of the left ear (Fig. 9). When plotted on the
surface of the brain, the exit wound lay over the middle of the second
temporal convolution, but must have produced some destruction both
above and below the superior temporal fissure (Fig. 8). In its course it
injured the extreme lower fibres of the optic radiations and so produced

the upper quadrantic hemianopsia described by Cushing[1] as characteristic of lesions within the temporal lobe. This wound healed completely in eighteen weeks.

His speech was a perfect example of that form of jargon which is
due to disturbance of rhythm and defective syntax. He did not use
wrong words and, if the subject under discussion was known, it was
not difficult to gather the sense of what he said. Once started, his
speech was rapid and he tried to "rush" his phrases until he was
arrested by the utterance of pure jargon. It was extremely difficult to
hear the prepositions, conjunctions or articles, and these parts of speech
were frequently omitted. The same errors marred his attempts to read
aloud; even when reading to himself, he became confused by internal
jargon and lost the significance of all but the simplest phrases. His
spontaneous writing was poor and he had little power of reproducing in
written words the contents of a paragraph he had apparently read with
understanding. His defective power of orderly symbolic formulation
and expression led to a curious error when he was asked to draw an
elephant; he said "irons," "highons" for tusks, and so provided the
figure with horns, although he was able to correct his mistake by
suitable gestures. His power of naming was preserved, although his
nomenclature was sometimes unusual, and he could tell the time
correctly. On the whole he understood what was said to him, unless
he was compelled to repeat it to himself. Simple oral commands were
well executed, but he hesitated and made several errors over the complex hand, eye and ear tests.

On his admission to the London Hospital, a fortnight after he was
wounded, there was a little weakness of the lower portion of the right
half of the face and the tongue deviated slightly to the right. There
was no loss of motion or sensation in body or limbs. The deep reflexes
were somewhat greater on the right than on the left side; the right
plantar reflex gave an upward response and that from the right half of
the abdomen was diminished. All these abnormal signs passed away
entirely within five months from the date of the wound, leaving only
the upper quadrantic hemianopsia, so far as such a condition could be
observed in the one remaining eye.

This was a perfect case for our methods of localisation. Beyond a
transitory affection of the reflexes and slight defect in the movements
of face and tongue, there was nothing to point to any morbid condition
beyond the limits of the temporal lobe. Moreover, the form of the

[1] [33].

visual field, so far as it could be determined from the one remaining eye, together with the curious attacks of "smells" accompanied by "dizziness," were characteristic of a lesion in this part of the brain.

Number 13[1] (Fig. 8) would have been equally valuable from the point of view of localisation, had it not been for the uncertainty introduced by the operation, carried out at the Front.

He was struck by a shell-fragment in the left temporal region, but did not become unconscious. When he came under my care about three weeks later, he brought no records of any kind. It was obvious that some operation had been performed; for there was a long, linear, surgical scar extending from the fronto-temporal to the parietal region on the left side of the head. This incision had closed, except for a small granulatory area in front, which healed rapidly and was of no importance. Farther back was a pouting sinus, which exuded pus; it was level with a point 16 cm. along the nasion-inion line and lay 8 to 9 cm. from the middle of the scalp. An X-ray photograph showed that bone had been removed over an irregular oval area, which lay exactly under this suppurating opening and was bisected by the surgical incision. On plotting out this area on the surface of the brain it was found to lie just behind the central (Rolandic) fissure.

But exactly below this area, 11 cm. to the left of the middle line, lay another fungating sinus passing down to and apparently penetrating the bone, from which exuded a considerable quantity of pus. The skull had not been trephined in this region, and yet the probe passed through

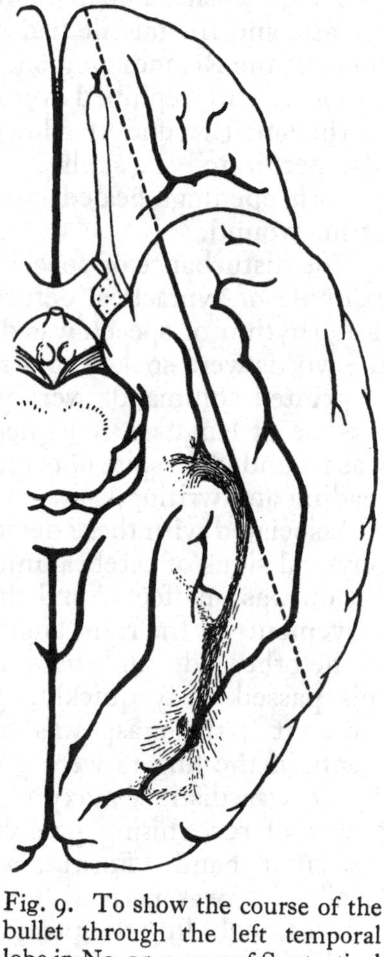

Fig. 9. To show the course of the bullet through the left temporal lobe in No. 15, a case of Syntactical Aphasia.

an opening into the cranial cavity. Moreover, the orifice in the scalp was at a distance from the surgical incision and had not been subjected to operative treatment of any kind. It undoubtedly represented one of

[1] Reported in full, Vol. II, p. 198 et seq.

the original wounds, and, when plotted on the surface of the brain, lay over the upper portion of the first temporal gyrus and the Sylvian fissure, on a level vertically with the foot of the post-central fissure (Fig. 8).

I should like to suggest that this was the lesion responsible for his loss of speech. The patient, on receipt of the wound, was obviously aphasic and the missile had possibly injured the skull in the neighbourhood of the Rolandic region. The surgeon therefore performed a linear exposure and trephined over the central fissure: but he paid no attention to the small wound at a lower level over the temporal lobe, which had also perforated the skull.

Both openings healed completely within eight weeks from the date of his wound.

The disturbance of speech produced by this injury formed a beautiful example of syntactical defects of symbolic formulation and expression. The rhythm of speech was disturbed and syntax was defective, whether the words were spoken or written. Naming, and comprehension of oral or printed commands were perfect. The character of these disorders in the use of language remained essentially unchanged five years after he was wounded, in spite of profound improvement in his power of speaking, reading and writing.

Associated with these defects of speech, he showed very few abnormal physical signs of cerebral injury. He had no fits or seizures of any kind. Vision was unaffected and the fields were of normal extent. At first the movements of the right angle of the mouth were slightly less than those of the other side, and the tongue was protruded a little to the right; but this passed away quickly. He complained that the right hand "felt different"; the grasp was comparatively feeble, but individual movements of the fingers were possible and they were somewhat hypotonic. There was distinct ataxy of the fingers with the eyes closed, and the power of recognising passive movement and posture was defective in the right hand. Form and weight were correctly appreciated and localisation was perfect. The lower extremity was unaffected. All the reflexes, including the plantars and abdominals, were normal.

The lesion responsible for these changes lay over the middle of the first temporal gyrus; but the slight disturbance of the higher aspects of sensation in the right hand during the earlier stages pointed to some affection of the post-central convolution.

No. 14[1] (Fig. 8) suffered from a much more severe injury, which lay,

[1] Reported in full, Vol. II, p. 215 et seq.

however, exactly over the same situation as what I have presumed to be the effective wound in No. 13.

He was hit by a fragment of shell casing or by shrapnel just above the insertion of the left ear. When I first saw him seventeen days later, the wound was represented by a granulating surface of 2 cm. by 1·5 cm. situated 11 cm. from the middle of the scalp and 16 cm. backwards along the nasion-inion line. This unhealed patch was surrounded on three sides by a horse-shoe shaped incision, which had united firmly. Within lay an irregularly quadrilateral area, where the bone had been removed; this was covered by normal scalp except over the site of the original wound.

When this was plotted on the surface of the brain, it was found to occupy the first temporal gyrus and the Sylvian fissure exactly as in No. 13 (Fig. 8). But the trephined area was more extensive, especially in front and above, and there can be no doubt that it extended forwards to the lower portion of the central fissure.

At first he was too ill for complete examination, but his speech was the most extraordinary jargon. There could be little doubt that he knew what he wanted to say, although the words poured out in phrases which had no grammatical structure and were in most cases incomprehensible. In many instances the words themselves were well formed, but they had no meaning as they were uttered; occasionally, however, sufficient words were correctly placed to make his meaning clear. He could not repeat a sentence said to him and, when he attempted to read, uttered pure jargon.

He was unable to find names for common objects of daily use and yet his correct choice to printed commands showed that he was familiar with their usual nomenclature.

Comprehension of spoken words was obviously defective and he was liable to be puzzled by any but the simplest oral commands. Time after time, in general conversation, he failed to understand what was said and to carry on a subject started by himself. Spontaneous thought was rapid and correct and his intelligence of an extremely high order, but his power of symbolic formulation and expression was hampered by the defects of his internal speech.

He undoubtedly comprehended what he read in the newspaper and demonstrated to us the movements at the Front on large-scale military maps. He understood French and amused himself with a work on Napoleon's Russian campaign. But any attempt to reproduce aloud what he had read resulted in incomprehensible jargon. Asked to read aloud the commands of the hand, eye and ear tests, he could not do so, although the movements were executed perfectly and without hesitation.

Single words were, for the most part, so much more easily written than spoken, that he carried about paper and a pencil to help him out of his conversational difficulties. When at a loss, he would write something sufficient to convey his meaning to his puzzled auditor. But he was unable to read what he had written and this, together with his difficulty in forming phrases and sentences, made it impossible to compose a letter or coherent account of something he wished to convey. He could copy perfectly, but wrote badly to dictation, because of the rapidity with which he forgot the phrase that had been said to him.

He could play the piano, read the notes correctly and evidently recognised the constitution of a chord and the changes of key.

These characteristic defects of speech were associated with extensive signs of cerebral injury. He developed seizures in which he ceased to talk and the right arm fell powerless on to the bed. He was never convulsed and did not appear to become unconscious in all these attacks, although he was ultimately found dead in his bath; but he was unable to speak and found he was powerless to think. These attacks were preceded by a "hot" or "tingling" feeling down the right arm and leg, accompanied by a taste and smell and a peculiar state of mind, which he could not describe in comprehensible terms.

Even when I saw him first, he did not suffer from headache and vomiting. The optic discs were normal and there was no hemianopsia. Movements of the lower part of the right half of the face were defective and the tongue deviated to this side. The deep reflexes on the right half of the body were brisker than those on the left and the plantar gave an upward response; the superficial reflexes from the right half of the abdomen were greatly diminished compared with those of the left. These abnormal signs passed away entirely in about a year from the time he was wounded.

In spite of the difficulty he found in executing movements to command, I was able to show, even in the early stages, that there was no absolute paralysis of the right upper or lower extremity; isolated movements of the fingers were possible, but there was extreme inco-ordination of both arm and leg. Subsequent examination confirmed the original supposition, that his loss of power was mainly afferent in origin.

In consequence of a lesion, which fell mainly over the middle of the first temporal gyrus, this patient suffered from profound syntactical defects of symbolic formulation and expression. His speech, both external and internal, was jargon and he could not write coherently. But the injury produced more severe general effects than those of No. 13. For he not only suffered from seizures, with a characteristic aura of smell and taste accompanied by a dreamy mental state, but also showed in the earlier stages profound incoordination and signs of afferent disturbance in the right arm and leg.

(c) *Nominal Defects*

No. 7[1] was wounded by a fragment of a high explosive shell, which produced a compound depressed fracture of the skull in the left parietal region, with laceration of the dura mater and protrusion of brain substance. He came under my care, nearly six weeks later, with a granulating stellate wound, which destroyed all the structures down to the brain. In front it was 7 cm., behind 9 cm. from the middle of the scalp and it extended between two points 19·5 cm. and 27 cm. on the nasion-inion line. An X-ray photograph showed an area of removal of bone in the anterior parietal region, measuring 4 cm. by 2 cm. at its broadest part, with a fissured fracture running directly forwards. The wound healed finally eight weeks after it was inflicted.

While this injury was plotted on the surface of the brain (Figs. 10 and 11) it was found to occupy an area shaped like an arrow-head, pointing upwards and forwards within the limits of the angular gyrus (area angularis of Brodmann).

On admission to the London Hospital, nearly six weeks after he was wounded, he was so grossly aphasic that no coherent information could be obtained from him. The words he uttered were comprehensible, but he could not find means to express himself in speech or writing. On pp. 282–285 I have summarised his condition at various periods after he was wounded. Throughout, the character of his disabilities remained the same, although he rapidly regained sufficient facility in utterance for daily intercourse; even five years and nine months after the injury his speech was demonstrably abnormal and he was still an excellent example of nominal aphasia.

Fortunately in this case there were no signs pointing to gross injury of the deeper structures of the brain. He suffered from no convulsions or seizures. Vision was in every way normal. Movements of the face and tongue were unaffected and he showed no changes either in motion or sensation. The reflexes, including the abdominals and plantars, were equal on the two sides.

[1] Reported in full, Vol. II, p. 89 et seq.

This man formed a superb example of the condition I have called nominal aphasia, in which the principal defect consisted in want of power to name objects and to recognise exactly the meaning of words presented orally or in print. The lesion lay over the angular gyrus and was comparatively superficial.

No. 2[1] (Figs. 10 and 11) was of much less value for purposes of anatomical localisation. The lesion was extensive and deep, at any rate in

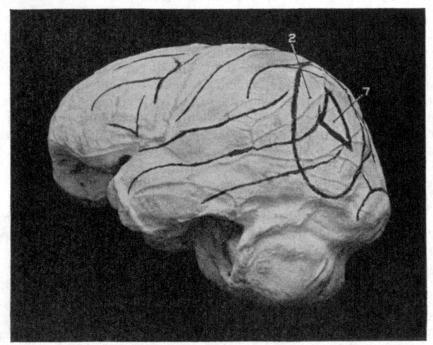

Fig. 10. To show the site of the injury to the brain in No. 2 and No. 7, cases of Nominal Aphasia.

the centre; but the clinical observations were of unusual completeness and interest owing to the great intelligence of the patient, and to my repeated opportunities for examining him over a period of more than four years.

This young Staff Officer received a compound fracture of the skull in the left parieto-occipital region from the kick of a horse. Fragments of depressed bone were removed by operation, carried out within a few hours of the accident, and the brain below the injury was found to

[1] Reported in full, Vol. II, p. 14 et seq.

be reduced to pulp for a depth of about three inches (about 7 cm.). Right hemianopsia and "some degree of aphasia" were present from the first, but motion and sensation were never affected.

When he first came under my care some six months afterwards, the wound was firmly healed, and lay within a depressed oval area, where the skull had been removed. At a subsequent operation we were

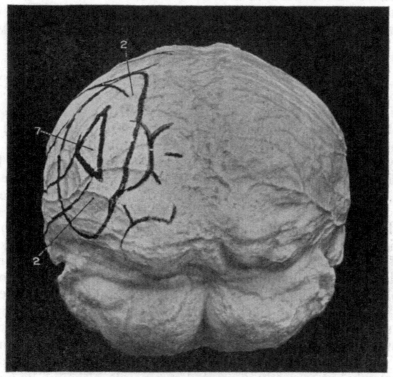

Fig. 11. To show the site of the injury to the brain, seen from behind, in No. 2 and No. 7, cases of Nominal Aphasia.

able to measure the exact limits of this opening; its largest diameter, pointing upwards and a little forwards, was 10 cm., whilst horizontally it measured 5·5 cm. at its broadest part. Looked at from behind, its superior border was opposite a point 23 cm. along the nasion-inion and 3·5 cm. to the left of the middle of the scalp; below it reached a point 33 cm. along the nasion-inion line and 3·5 cm. to the left.

During the operation to repair this opening, Mr Trotter cut a piece of rubber of the exact size and shape to act as a guide. This was subsequently of great help in plotting out the site and extent of the injury, for we were able to fix this oval patch on to the skull of the cadaver and drill through to the brain to mark its boundaries. (Figs. 10 and 11.)

In this way we found that the area of loss of bone occupied the angular, superior parietal and parieto-occipital gyri; its anterior border extended as far forward as the middle of the supra-marginal. But we must bear in mind that this gives the extreme limits of the injury, within which the destruction of brain tissue occupied an unknown but smaller extent.

This patient suffered from profound loss of power to name common objects or colours, and to use nominal expressions in ordinary conversation. Most of the words at his disposal were well pronounced and intonation was normal, but, when he had difficulty in finding a name, he would try various combinations of sound more or less related to the word he was seeking. He was able to give long explanations of his inability to find the right names, and could use appropriate metaphorical expressions to designate colours that he could not name. If he failed to find a word, he could repeat it accurately after it had been said to him.

He showed obvious difficulty in grasping the exact meaning of what was said, especially such words as "up" and "down," "back" and "front," "to" and "past" the hour, when contrasted with one another. He could choose familiar objects slowly but correctly to oral commands; with colours, he hesitated greatly and made several mistakes. He could not set the hands of the clock or carry out the complex hand, eye and ear tests to orders given by word of mouth.

He was unable to read a newspaper to himself or to comprehend exactly the meaning of a printed paragraph. Common objects were chosen slowly but correctly to printed commands, although he hesitated greatly with colours. If the order to set the clock was given in printed words, it was badly executed; but he had no difficulty when they were replaced by numbers. The hand, eye and ear tests were performed extremely badly if he read the words silently; when, however, he read them aloud the orders were executed without fail.

He wrote his signature, but could not add his address, and was incapable of writing a letter or giving a written account of what he had heard, seen or read. Later, he regained this power somewhat, although his spelling was so incredibly bad that many of the words were scarcely recognisable. Writing to dictation was faulty, and he copied printed letters accurately in capitals, but could not transcribe them with certainty into ordinary handwriting.

He could count aloud, but wrote the names of the numbers extremely badly. He was unable to carry out even simple arithmetical operations and had difficulty in expressing the relative value of two coins, although he was evidently conscious of their fundamental relation.

He could make an excellent drawing from a model and reproduce it later from memory; but his drawing of an elephant to command was absurd, though, when trying to explain the difficulties of transport in Mesopotamia, he produced spontaneously a spirited sketch of a camel.

He was unable to draw a ground-plan, in spite of the fact that he possessed strong visual images and orientation was not fundamentally affected.

He suffered from no fits or seizures at any time. There was complete right hemianopsia to movement, form and colour, which remained unaltered throughout; apart from this, vision was normal. Otherwise there were no abnormal signs of any kind in the central nervous system.

This is a splendid example of what I have called "nominal" aphasia in a man of unusual intelligence and education. The power of naming and appreciating verbal meaning was defective, although he retained the capacity to formulate the end and aim of a symbolic act. We do not know exactly the situation of the brain lesion, but it must have lain within limits which comprised mainly the angular, superior parietal and parieto-occipital gyri. It thus includes the whole of the more localised lesion found in No. 7.

(d) *Semantic Defects*

No. 10[1] was wounded accidentally over a small area in the left parietal region by the premature explosion of a hand-grenade. At the operation next day the dura mater was found to have been perforated in two places and two small fragments of bone were removed from the brain.

When he came under my care, thirty-four days later, the wound had healed completely. Bone had been removed over an oval area 2·5 cm. by 1·25 cm., extending between two points 15·5 cm. and 18 cm. along the nasion-inion line at a distance of 8 cm. from the middle of the scalp.

On plotting the site of this lesion, it was found to occupy the anterior portion of the supra-marginal gyrus, bounded in front by the

---

[1] Reported in full, Vol. II, p. 151 et seq.

post-central fissure (Figs. 12 and 13). It was of small size (less than 2·5 cm. by 1·25 cm.) and did not extend deeply into the substance of the brain; this was confirmed at an exploratory operation carried out whilst he was under my care.

This patient was a splendid example of what I have called semantic defects of speech. He could name objects or colours shown to him and had no difficulty in finding or articulating words to express his ordinary

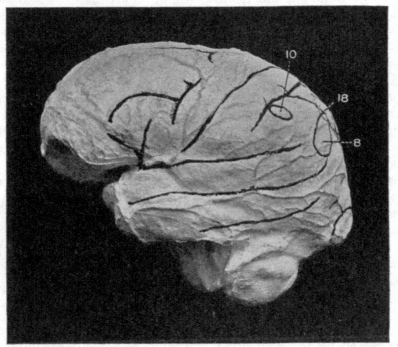

Fig. 12. To show the site of the injury to the brain in No. 8, No. 10 and No. 18, cases of Semantic Aphasia.

needs; his phrases were perfectly formed and spaced. But in general conversation he paused like a man confused, who had lost the thread of what he wanted to say. Words and phrases said to him were repeated correctly, provided they did not contain a number of possible alternatives.

He chose an object or colour named by me, but had obvious difficulty in setting the clock or carrying out the hand, eye and ear tests to oral commands. He was easily puzzled and became confused as to the aim of the task set him.

He understood the significance of printed words and short sentences provided they did not contain a command. But he gave a poor account of the general meaning of a series of short paragraphs he had read silently to himself; his narration tailed away aimlessly, as if he had forgotten the goal for which he was making.

He read aloud simple sentences without mistakes, but tended to doubt the accuracy of the words he had uttered correctly.

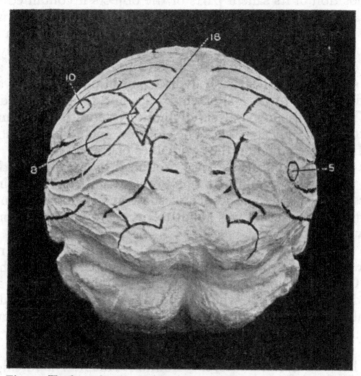

Fig. 13. To show the site of the injury to the brain, seen from behind, in No. 8, No. 10 and No. 18 to the left and No. 5 to the right of the middle line. All these patients suffered from Semantic Aphasia.

His handwriting was profoundly altered; he wrote with extreme rapidity, as if afraid of forgetting what he wanted to transfer to paper, and he tended to employ the same symbol for d, f, o, r, t, and v. Apart from the bad writing and the use of this peculiar letter, he copied correctly; he showed the same defects to dictation and, in addition, he repeatedly forgot what he had been told to write.

Although he counted excellently, he was unable to carry out the simplest arithmetical operation; and this was the more remarkable as he had been an accountant, accustomed to handle complex masses of figures. He was confused by the relative value of coins and had much difficulty in ordinary life with change and the price of his purchases.

He could not draw from the model or from memory, and was completely unable to delineate an elephant to command. He failed entirely to draw a ground-plan of a familiar room and was unable to express the relative position of its salient parts or the objects it contained.

Orientation was gravely affected; he was liable to lose his way in the street or hospital, and had difficulty even in finding his own room.

He could play no games and "puzzles" worried him greatly.

These defects of symbolic formulation and expression were associated with no other signs of structural disorganisation. Vision was perfect and the fields were of normal extent. Face and tongue moved well and equally. There was no paralysis of motion; sensation was unaffected, even to the most delicate tests. The reflexes, including the abdominals and plantars, were equal on the two halves of the body.

In this case the sole disturbance produced by a lesion in the supra-marginal gyrus was inability to comprehend and to maintain in consciousness the general significance of some symbolic representation, or the intention of an act he was about to perform, either to command or on his own initiative.

No. 5[1] (Figs. 13 and 14) was the only left-handed man in my series, and the wound, due to a rifle bullet, was situated in the right parietal region. On admission to the Base Hospital, this was a minute punctured opening, from which exuded cerebro-spinal fluid mingled with small quantities of disintegrated brain matter. The bullet had bored a circular hole in the skull, perforated the dura mater, and was extracted from a point in the brain about 4 to 5 cm. in depth.

When he was admitted to the London Hospital a fortnight later, the wound of entry was healed and covered by a minute scab, situated 20·5 cm. backwards along the nasion-inion line and 11 cm. from the middle of the scalp. The semicircular surgical incision had healed by first intention.

On plotting the position at which the bullet had entered the brain, it was found to lie over the inferior and posterior portion of the supra-marginal gyrus (Figs. 13 and 14). The removal of the bullet, lying some 5 cm. deep in the brain, undoubtedly produced more destruction of substance than in the case of No. 10.

Here again the most striking feature was his inability to formulate,

[1] Reported in full, Vol. II, p. 64 et seq.

to recognise and to retain in his mind the exact general intention of some action requiring symbolic representation.

Articulation was perfect, words were produced without difficulty and the rhythm of the phrase was unaffected. His sole defect was shown in a tendency to forget the exact general intention of what he wanted to express; sentences died away without reaching their formal conclusion. He could name common objects or colours correctly, and

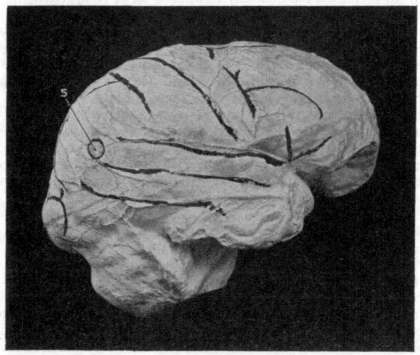

Fig. 14. To show the site of the injury to the brain in No. 5, a left-handed man suffering from Semantic Aphasia.

repeat single words or even sentences, provided they did not comprise many independent statements. The first few phrases of a long paragraph might be repeated correctly, but as the test proceeded he would lose touch and complain that he could not remember what I had said.

On superficial examination he seemed to understand what was said to him and chose all the common objects accurately to oral command; with colours he was not so exact. But he made gross mistakes, in setting the clock and in carrying out the hand, eye and ear tests to orders given by word of mouth. His greatest disability appeared when he was asked to render the general sense of some story I had told him; after the first few phrases, he broke off, saying, "I don't know what it is."

He chose common objects with ease to printed commands and made no gross errors in the selection of colours. The hands of the clock were ultimately set correctly and the hand, eye and ear tests perfectly executed. His difficulty lay not so much in understanding the meaning of a word or phrase read silently to himself as in comprehending their general significance.

He wrote his name and address rapidly and with ease. But the names of common objects or of colours were badly written, although the nomenclature was correct, and he made many mistakes when writing down the time from a clock shown to him. He was unable to round off and bring to a logical conclusion a letter which began intelligibly.

He would copy with ease and certainty, but, when writing from dictation, he tended to shorten the sentence, to omit some part of its content and to substitute words which differed from those said by me.

He counted perfectly up to the seventies or eighties, and then became slower and less accurate. Simple arithmetical exercises were imperfectly carried out and he seemed unable to correct his mistakes.

He drew the rough outline of a jug placed before him and reproduced it almost exactly from memory; but he absolutely failed to draw an elephant to command.

Orientation was defective and he was unable to construct a ground-plan of the ward in which he occupied a bed, although he gave undoubted evidence of the possession of visual images.

These defects in symbolic formulation and expression were unaccompanied by any other signs of gross destruction in the nervous system. Vision was normal and the field of full extent. Movements of the face and tongue were unaffected. There was no paralysis of motion or sensation and the reflexes, including the abdominals and plantars, were equal on the two halves of the body.

In this case profound semantic defects in a left-handed man were associated with a small cortical and sub-cortical lesion situated in the lower and posterior portion of the right supra-marginal gyrus.

No. 8[1] (Figs. 12 and 13) was another excellent example of the same defects of speech. The lesion was, however, more severe and of considerably greater extent than that in either of the two preceding cases; but it is of interest from the point of view of localisation, because the

[1] Reported in full, Vol. II, p. 108 et seq.

superficial area, occupied by the wound of entry, served to unite that of the last patient (No. 5) with that of No. 18, lying over the superior parietal lobule.

No. 8 was struck by a fragment of shell casing in the left parietal region; this traversed the brain almost directly from side to side, and was removed through a small trephine opening over the right supra-marginal region.

When he first came under my care a month later, there was a small pouting wound on the left side, which lay in the centre of a trephined area measuring 4 by 2·75 cm. This healed in a fortnight. It extended between two points 26 to 29 cm. along the nasion-inion; above it was 2·5 cm. and below 8 cm. from the middle line of the scalp, seen from behind. The opening on the right side, from which the missile had been removed by operation, had healed completely on admission.

When the extent of the trephined area, over the wound of entry, was plotted on the surface of the brain, it was found to occupy the supra-marginal gyrus and part of the superior parietal lobule (Figs. 12 and 13). The lowest point just touched the site of the lesion in No. 5, and from this the long axis of the oval extended upwards and a little backwards to just beyond the interparietal fissure.

This patient was a splendid example of semantic aphasia, and his condition at various periods has already been summarised on pp. 286–288.

In this case there were other signs of gross injury to the brain, apart from these semantic defects. Four months after he was wounded he developed epileptiform attacks, in which he became unconscious, and was slightly convulsed. Under the influence of worry, confusion and noise, these became somewhat frequent; but with treatment and a quiet life in the country they have been greatly reduced in number.

The most striking physical abnormality consisted of defective vision over the right half of the field. His visual acuity was perfect with either eye, but he tended to miss letters towards the right of any line he was reading, unless his attention was concentrated directly upon them. Over the right half of the field a moving object could be appreciated up to the periphery, but a stationary white square was frequently unrecognised. Moreover, if two discs were exposed simultaneously, one to the left and the other to the right of the visual field, he never failed to appreciate the former, though he was frequently uncertain to the right. This condition has remained unchanged to the present time.

On admission, the optic discs were blurred at the edges, showing traces of previous swelling, which had subsided. The pupils reacted well, even when the light was thrown on the affected half of the visual field. Face and tongue moved normally. The reflexes, including the abdominals and plantars, were equally brisk on the two sides. Careful examination failed to discover any affection of motion or sensation.

There were no abnormal signs of any kind on the left side of the body, corresponding to the opening in the right half of the skull through which the foreign body had been extracted.

This young and highly intelligent officer suffered not only from semantic defects of speech, but also from loss of vision of a high cerebral type over the right half of the field. The wound of entry, which was responsible for these signs and symptoms, lay mainly over the supra-marginal gyrus, but extended on to a portion of the superior parietal lobule. It was probably the sub-cortical passage of the bullet that was responsible for the presence of the partial hemianopsia.

In the next patient, No. 18[1] (Figs. 12 and 13), the lesion lay somewhat higher than in any other case of this group, occupying mainly the superior parietal lobule; but there was definite evidence of considerable sub-cortical destruction. The semantic defects were less profound, although he showed a complete hemianopsia, and sensibility was slightly disturbed in the right hand.

He was wounded by shrapnel, rapidly became unconscious, and woke to find himself in a Base Hospital. When admitted under my care exactly a month later, no operation had been performed, and the wound consisted of a long granulating area, which, at the site of its maximum breadth, covered a small stellate fracture of the skull. In the centre of this portion opened a small sinus, leading into the substance of the brain.

This orifice was allowed to close; but suppuration continued in deeper parts. Finally, we explored the track and several fragments of bone, lying about 1·5 cm. from the surface, were removed from the sub-cortical tissues. The wound then became reduced to a minute sinus, extending for 8 cm. downwards, forwards and inwards; this healed completely, seven weeks after the operation, and exactly eight months from the date of the injury.

The position of this opening in the bone could be determined with greater precision in 1921, when he again came under my care; I shall therefore depend on these measurements for localising the site of the lesion. The wound was then a firm, deeply depressed scar covering a roughly quadrilateral area, where the bone had been destroyed. This measured 2 cm. in either direction, and the superior border reached to

---

[1] Reported in full, Vol. II, p. 259 et seq.

1·25 from the middle line of the scalp; it extended between two points 22·5 cm. and 24·5 cm. along the nasion-inion line.

If this area was plotted on the surface of the brain, it was found to lie over the superior parietal lobule; but, when interpreting the signs and symptoms presented by this patient, we must not forget the definite evidence of sub-cortical destruction of tissue (Figs. 12 and 13).

No abnormality could be noticed in the course of ordinary conversation beyond a certain hesitancy and diffidence in expression. Intonation, the distribution of the pauses, and the syntax of each phrase were perfect; and yet there was a tendency for his talk to die out before it had reached its full logical conclusion. He named correctly and repeated everything he heard with ease. He understood what was said to him and could carry out simple orders, although the more complex oral commands of the hand, eye and ear tests confused and puzzled him. He read silently or aloud, and understood the meaning, if it was simple and not complex. He wrote his name and address correctly, but, when he attempted to write down the gist of what he had been told or had read to himself, he was liable to make curious errors. He wrote with great rapidity, as if afraid of forgetting what he wanted to express. These defects were particularly evident when, after reading a printed paragraph silently, he was told to narrate or to write down what he had gathered from it. He even found difficulty in writing the alphabet, though he could say it correctly. Simple arithmetical exercises were badly performed; in fact, he started in each instance from left to right. It was not the detailed significance of numbers that was at fault, but rather the general conception of the acts of addition and subtraction. Once this had been corrected in his mind the same problems were easily solved. Orientation was not so grossly affected as in some of the other patients of this group; but the plan he drew of the room, in which we had so often worked, was defective, although he could indicate orally the relative position of its salient points. He had great difficulty in formulating the general intention of some act he was about to perform spontaneously or to order; he could not even lay the table with certainty. But he was able to copy simple actions with ease, provided they did not demand recognition of several alternatives. Oral, pictorial, and printed commands suffered to an almost equal extent. He understood straightforward pictures; but those which demanded coherent composition or the simultaneous comprehension of a printed legend, usually failed to convey to him their full meaning. He could play no games with pleasure and disliked puzzles, which confused him.

The other signs and symptoms, pointing to gross destruction in the central nervous system, remained the same throughout the history of the case. He suffered from no fits or seizure of any kind after the wound had finally healed. In 1921, he showed a complete right hemianopsia; he was blind to colour, form and movement over this half of the field, and the pupil did not contract to light, thrown on to the nasal side of the right and the temporal portion of the left retina. Face and tongue moved equally on the two sides. Individual movements of the digits could be carried out perfectly with the eyes open; but, when they were closed, the fingers of the right hand performed these finer movements more clumsily and less perfectly than the left. Moreover the digits on the right side were slightly atonic. These defects were obviously afferent in origin and, on closer examination, the power of recognising posture and passive movement was found to be somewhat diminished. The compass-test, localisation, tactile sensibility and discrimination of shape, weight and texture were unaffected. All the reflexes, including the plantars and abdominals, were normal and equal on the two sides.

This perfect example of semantic defects of symbolic formulation and expression was due to injury of the superior parietal lobule, combined with sub-cortical destruction. Bone fragments driven into the tissues of the brain had led to suppuration, and it is impossible to determine to what extent this sub-cortical lesion played a part in the speech affection; but it was evidently responsible for the gross hemianopsia and probably also for the changes in sensibility.

§ 3. THE RELATION OF THE FORM ASSUMED BY THE APHASIA TO THE SITE AND NATURE OF THE LESION

In each example dealt with in the previous section I have attempted to map out on the surface of the brain the approximate limits of the injury. Since the impact of the blow came from without, the cortex was affected in every case; but in addition all showed more or less evidence of sub-cortical destruction. In some instances this was severe and of considerable depth; in others the amount of deep structural change must have been comparatively slight.

But, if my contention is correct that such lesions produce their effect by interrupting a highly complicated form of behaviour, the additional presence of sub-cortical changes is not of fundamental importance with regard to the nature of the manifestations, although it has a profound effect on their severity and duration. Were aphasia due to destruction or ablation of specific centres for speech, strict limitation of the lesion to the cortex would be a necessary preliminary to any attempt at anatomical localisation of function. But such conditions have rarely if ever been fulfilled even in the most satisfactory cases where a careful microscopical examination has been carried out. Destruction was sometimes confined to sub-cortical tissues; but, if it affected the cortex, the deeper structures were almost always more or less involved.

These changes interfere with the orderly march of a highly integrated series of voluntary and automatic processes, which require perfect action of cortical and sub-cortical mechanisms. Now, in all my aphasic patients with gun-shot wounds of the skull the injury of necessity affected the surface of the brain, to whatever depth it may have penetrated. It is impossible, therefore, from such material to deduce any specific difference between the results produced by a cortical or sub-cortical lesion. We can, however, conclude that the deeper it extended the more severe and lasting was the disorder of speech.

Bearing these facts in mind, can we draw any conclusions from such cases with regard to the relation between the site of the lesion and the nature of the aphasic manifestations? The number of my patients in whom the injury was sufficiently limited to be of any localising value is lamentably small; but in all of them the clinical signs and symptoms were worked out with unusual care and they have been under observation for long periods, extending in some instances over many years. This material, though of great scientific value for determining the forms assumed by disorders of speech, is in no sense ideal for anatomical localisation. But, with many reservations, I think it is capable of leading us to certain tentative conclusions.

Thus, in all three cases of uncomplicated verbal aphasia, the lesion lay mainly within or beneath the central convolutions. No. 6 was an ideal example; for his wound consisted of a longitudinal incision, 5 cm. in length, which penetrated to the brain and lay over the lower portion of the precentral gyrus. The only abnormal sign, apart from his affection of speech, was transient weakness of the right half of the face and tongue. Motion, sensibility, and the reflexes were entirely unaffected.

No. 20, in whom an extracerebral tumour pressed upon the lower part of the precentral gyrus, is also of interest in this connection. The operation for its removal was followed not only by severe verbal aphasia, but also by motor hemiplegia unaccompanied by any form of sensory disorder. The abnormal physical signs cleared up rapidly and even the affection of speech diminished to a profound degree, although to the end it maintained its specific verbal character.

No. 17 was of much less importance from an anatomical point of view; for, although the superficial extent of the wound fell over the lower portion of the pre- and post-central gyri, the gravest lesion was an abscess in the substance of the brain beneath them. This was responsible for the gross hemiplegia, both motor and sensory, on the right half of the body. But, in spite of the extent of these destructive changes, the aphasia assumed a purely verbal form and passed away almost completely.

So far we are justified in stating that a lesion situated within the lower portion of the central convolutions, or the structures beneath them, is liable to evoke what I have called verbal defects of symbolic formulation and expression. These parts are not centres for any constituent element of speech; but injury in this region produces defects in the use of language, which tend to assume this specific form.

When we turn to the three traumatic cases of syntactical aphasia, we are led to an equally definite conclusion. Pick[1] has always contended that a disorder of speech, consisting of true jargon, or as he calls it "agrammatism," is associated with lesions of the temporal lobe. With this conclusion I am in entire agreement; all my three patients, who suffered in this way, had lesions of this portion of the brain.

In No. 15, the bullet entered close to the root of the nose and passed backwards through the left temporal lobe to make its exit just above the left ear. The left eye was destroyed, but the field of vision in that which remained showed the upper quadrantic blindness described by Cushing[2] as characteristic for lesions within the substance of the temporal lobe. There was slight paresis of the right half of the face and tongue with an upward plantar response and loss of abdominal reflexes on the same side; but there was no paralysis of the limbs, motor or sensory, at any time. Subsequently the patient developed characteristic seizures, preceded by an abnormal "smell" and associated with a "dreamy state," each of which was followed by some increase in the degree of syntactical aphasia.

In No. 13, the original wound seems to have consisted of two separate perforations of the skull, which led down to independent suppurating foci. Of these, the uppermost lay in the neighbourhood of the central fissure, whilst the lower one fell over the first temporal gyrus and inferior lip of the Sylvian fissure. The nature of the clinical

[1] See Part I, pp. 126, 127.   [2] [33].

manifestations seemed to indicate that the latter injury was mainly responsible for the affection of speech. But in addition there was slight paresis of the right half of the face and tongue, which rapidly passed away, associated with some weakness and high-grade changes in the postural sensibility of the right hand. The reflexes and visual fields were entirely unaffected.

The lesion in No. 14 fell exactly over the same area on the surface of the brain as that of the lower wound in the previous case. It occupied the first temporal gyrus and fissure of Sylvius, but evidently extended more deeply into the sub-cortical tissues; for it was associated on the right half of the body with a gross sensory hemiplegia, absent abdominal reflexes and an upward plantar response. At first speech was extensively affected, but finally the aphasia assumed a purely syntactical form. This patient also suffered from seizures associated with a "dreamy state" and an unpleasant taste or smell, so characteristic of lesions of the temporal lobe.

Thus the temporal lobe was the one constant site of the injury in all these cases of pronounced syntactical aphasia (Nos. 15, 13 and 14) and two of them were accompanied by other characteristic signs and symptoms of a lesion in this situation.

So far, the anatomical conclusions to which I have arrived do not diverge materially from those of other observers. Granting that my views of the nature of the clinical manifestations differ fundamentally from those usually held, it is obvious that what I have called "verbal defects" of symbolic formulation and expression comprise the more specific examples of "motor" aphasia. These morbid states are notoriously evoked more readily when the lesion falls mainly on the lower half of the central convolutions and the parts which lie immediately beneath them. My three cases bear out this conclusion.

Moreover, true jargon has long been associated with disease of the temporal lobe, and this form of defect of speech is comprised amongst the manifestations of syntactical aphasia. This localisation is supported by my three examples of gun-shot injury, where the loss of symbolic formulation and expression assumed this form.

But, when we consider the effect of lesions situated behind the post-central fissure, the material at my disposal is unsuitable for strict anatomical localisation. The injuries were too diffuse and the limits of the various structural areas on the surface of the brain are less easy to define. Clinically, however, there can be little doubt that unilateral lesions situated between the post-central fissure and the occipital lobule, including the supra-marginal and angular gyri, are liable to evoke two diverse forms of disorder in the use of language. One group of defects, which I have called "nominal," is shown by difficulty in recognising the meaning of such symbols as words or figures and by inability to find appropriate names for objects. The other, or semantic form of aphasia, appears as a more general lack of logical sequence in word or deed, accompanied by defective appreciation of the ultimate significance of statements communicated orally, in print, or by means of pictures.

If we first consider the cases which belonged clinically to this semantic group, No. 10 is the most satisfactory from an anatomical point of view. A hand-grenade, exploding prematurely, had produced a small fracture of the skull over the left parietal region. Fragments of bone pierced the dura and produced an injury of the supra-marginal gyrus, which did not extend deeply into the brain. The clinical manifestations formed a perfect example of semantic aphasia, uncomplicated by any other signs or symptoms of injury to the central nervous system.

No. 5 was the only example amongst my collection of war injuries where a right-sided lesion in a left-handed man was associated with disorders of speech. A rifle bullet had entered the brain in the neighbourhood of the contingent parts of the supra-marginal and angular gyri; it was removed from a depth of about 4 to 5 cm., and the wound healed in a fortnight. Clinically this patient was a perfect instance of semantic aphasia, unaccompanied by any other signs or symptoms of injury to the central nervous system.

No. 8 was an equally characteristic example, accompanied by partial hemianopsia. The missile had traversed the brain almost directly from side to side, but I could find no abnormal signs corresponding to the injury of the right hemisphere. The wound of entry, which was responsible for all the morbid manifestations, both of speech and vision, lay over the supra-marginal gyrus and part of the superior parietal lobule.

In No. 18, the fourth example of this clinical group, there was definite evidence of sub-cortical suppuration. The orifice of the small but deep wound had been allowed to close prematurely and, at a subsequent operation, we removed several fragments of bone lying about 1·5 cm. from the surface of the brain. The external injury lay over the superior parietal lobule. Although the semantic defects were less severe than in the other cases, he showed in addition gross hemianopsia and slight sensory changes in the right hand.

Thus in all four instances where the disturbance of speech assumed a semantic form the main lesion lay behind the post-central fissure, in the neighbourhood of the supra-marginal gyrus and the superior parietal lobule.

Nominal aphasia forms one of the most distinctive abnormalities of speech. But in two only of my patients was the condition due to injury of the skull and in one of these the area of destruction was too wide to be of any value from the point of view of anatomical localisation.

In No. 7, the wound was an arrow-shaped fracture, about 4 cm. by 2 cm., which lay over the angular gyrus. Beyond the nominal aphasia, he showed no signs or symptoms pointing to injury of the central nervous system.

No. 2 was clinically one of the most perfect examples of this group, and I have watched his progress for nearly five years. But the injury was a wide-spread fracture of the skull, which covered an area corresponding to the angular gyrus, superior parietal lobule and arcus parieto-occipitalis; its anterior border extended as far forwards as the middle of the supra-marginal gyrus. We must, however, bear in mind that this gives the extreme limits of the injury within which the destruction of brain tissue occupied an unknown but smaller extent. The lesion extended sufficiently deeply to produce a complete right hemianopsia; but there were no further abnormal signs or symptoms.

No definite anatomical conclusions of differential value can be deduced from these examples of semantic and nominal aphasia. Both forms of defective use of language can be evoked most readily by injuries which fall over an area lying between the post-central and interparietal fissures, that is, over the supra-marginal and angular gyri and the parts beneath them. But it would seem as if a lesion producing nominal aphasia tended to lie somewhat farther back than one which was associated with semantic disorders of symbolic formulation and expression.

CHAPTER III

GENERAL CONCLUSIONS AND SUMMARY

§ 1. GENERAL CONCLUSIONS

THE use of language in its various forms is acquired during the life of the individual, and finally comprises a number of habitual actions, mental and physical, which can be modified at will. An act of speech is a march of events, where one changing condition passes insensibly into another. When speech is defective, this easy motion or transition is impeded; one state cannot flow into another because of some mechanical imperfection in the process. The power of finding words, the rhythmic modulation and balance of a phrase, the appreciation of meaning and intention, verbal or general, are thrown into disorder.

The processes which underlie an act of speech run through the nervous system like a prairie fire from bush to bush; remove all inflammable material at any one point and the fire stops. So, when a break occurs in the functional chain, orderly speech becomes impossible, because the basic physiological processes which subserve it have been disturbed. The site of such a breach of continuity is not a "centre for speech," but solely a place where it can be interrupted or changed.

But the term has been habitually employed in a more inclusive and different sense. Cortical "centres" for motion, sensation or speech are supposed to be areas on the surface of the brain within which certain forms of neural activity are originated. A function is "localised" in a more or less restricted group of cells, and ablation or injury in this region destroys the power to generate the "energy" requisite for some particular form of behaviour. This view is a heritage from the doctrine of "faculties," reinforced by the results obtained on experimental stimulation of the cortex.

Most so-called "centres" in the nervous system are strictly speaking nodal foci, where central neural activities undergo integration and other changes in relation to one another. Like the points on the railway, they determine the subsequent course of events. This may happen automatically or voluntarily, just as the passage of a train may set the track for its successor, or the mechanism may be manipulated at the will of the man in the signal box in response to information received from without. Such a "centre" also forms a shunting station where one group of impulses is guided in one direction, whilst another passes on into some fresh combination.

Whenever a primitive function is rendered more perfect and is given a wider range of purposive adaptation, the structures which are primarily responsible for its existence become linked up with those on a higher anatomical plane of the nervous system. But many of the more mechanical processes and the actual force expended may still be furnished by the lower functional levels. No fresh "energy" is generated by this higher integration, but the response gains in freedom; it can be more closely regulated according to the needs of the moment and brought into harmony with the reaction of the organism as a whole. This is the purpose of that series of complex integrative changes which start with the birth of afferent impressions at the periphery and continue until their ultimate consequences act on the final efferent path.

Speech, reading and writing are acquired at a period when the central nervous system is structurally complete. They require the perfect interaction of widely different forms of behaviour, both psychical and somatic, combined at the moment to a single end. There is nothing exclusive about acts of symbolic formulation and expression; they employ highly integrated functional arrangements, developed originally for other simpler purposes. These in turn depend on the integrity of a series of arcs or circuits, subserving processes on the most diverse physiological levels, the highest of which are to be found in the cortex.

Even motor reactions, aroused by electrical stimulation, consist of a march of events with a definite temporal relation; for the response obtained at any one moment depends on what has happened before. Motor "centres," even in the cortex, cannot be the sole and primary foci from which movements are initiated and determined; they form rather the means by which we are enabled to interfere with otherwise automatic acts, modifying them in accordance with our voluntary requirements. Their function is that of a switch, facilitating, diverting, or even reversing the habitual course of events. Injury or destruction interrupts these processes for a time; but readjustment occurs if the lesion has not been too extensive or profound. Although the "centre" has been completely removed, the movement can be performed, perhaps a little more slowly and uncertainly, but otherwise with no noticeable defect.

The structural mechanism required for the normal use of language not only comprises parts of the cortex exercising functions of various levels in the neural hierarchy, but also requires the synergic activity of centres on a deeper anatomical plane. A lesion at some appropriate place on the surface of the brain can interrupt speech for a time. Sooner or later the flow is re-established; but, the deeper and more acute the injury, the greater will be the severity and duration of the disturbance. The reaction tends to assume a stereotyped form; it is evoked slowly and after an undue expenditure of effort. The deeper the destruction of tissue, the greater is the resistance interposed between the initiation and completion of the processes required for some particular act of speech.

The power to express ourselves in spoken words is acquired by voluntary effort, but ultimately becomes almost automatic. In the same way, when learning to play the piano, the fingers are at first laid laboriously on each key, and a complicated apparatus is thrown into action, which sounds the note. Soon, with practice, the fingers move automatically and consciousness is occupied in reading the musical symbols on the printed page. Finally, with increased facility, even this becomes almost automatic; the expert musician scarcely sees the page, for the nature of the musical phrase suggests to him the sequence of the accompanying harmonies.

Any high-grade aptitude, such as the use of language, acquired by conscious effort, is carried out with practice more and more unwittingly and the functional adaptations on which it relies become gradually engulfed in the automatic activities of the central nervous system. As this habituation proceeds, the particular mode of behaviour in question depends to an increasing extent on the orderly sequence of a series of predetermined reactions. Gross organic injury does not remove the structural basis of a "faculty" or the repository of "images," but disturbs the march of events necessary for the perfect accomplishment of some acquired act; this can be re-learnt, even after ablation of the whole of its "cortical centre."

The form and extent of the disorder of function depend on the stage in the life of the individual at which this mode of behaviour was developed; more recent aptitudes suffer in excess of those acquired earlier in ontological history. Each human being learns to speak and to understand what is said to him during his earliest years; the arts of reading and writing, on the other hand, become possible only after he can already express himself fluently in words, and the vast mass of mankind remain permanently illiterate. Anything which disturbs the free use of language will therefore tend to affect the power of reading and writing to a profound degree. Articulated speech, the oldest acquisition racially and individually, exhibits the most specific and particular changes, whilst the recently developed powers of reading and writing are more massively and indifferently affected. The condition of articulated speech and the power of comprehending spoken words are therefore the best indication of the form assumed by an aphasia, and the names I have selected have been chosen to characterise this aspect of the disorder.

These diverse defects of speech do not reveal the elements out of which the use of language is built up; on the contrary, they show the way in which a highly complicated series of acts can be disturbed by lesions of certain parts of the brain. It is the custom to assume that, when some particular form of behaviour is thrown into disorder, the manifestations reveal the functions which combined for its development, exactly as a chemical salt can be analysed into an acid and a base. But in most instances this is not true, as far as the negative phenomena are concerned; they are morbid variants of the disturbed form of behaviour.

Although the negative effects of a lesion are expressed in terms of the affected process, the positive manifestations may reveal activities which under normal conditions are controlled or suppressed. A glass fire-screen allows the light to pass, but shuts off most of the heat. Should it be broken, the fragments do not reveal the elements out of which it was made, though it may be possible empirically to determine that one came from the upper, another from the lower corner. On the other hand, removal of the obstructing pane of glass now permits the heat of the fire to radiate freely into the room. The various forms of aphasia, being for the most part negative effects of the lesion, show how the use of language can be broken up rather than the elements out of which it is composed.

The more definitely the injury destroys the lower portion of the pre- and post-central convolutions and the parts which lie beneath them, the more likely are the defects to assume a "verbal" form. A lesion in the neighbourhood of the upper convolutions of the temporal lobe tends to produce "syntactical" disorders of speech. Destruction round about the region of the supra-marginal gyrus causes lack of appreciation of general symbolic significance and intention, defects which I have called "semantic." A lesion situated somewhat more posteriorly in the neighbourhood of the angular gyrus seems to disturb the power to discover, to understand, and to employ names and other "nominal" expressions.

No one part of this wide area on the surface of the brain is associated exclusively with the processes of speech; activities of a lower order can be disturbed coincidently with the use of language. Thus, a lesion of the precentral convolution on the left side not only produces verbal aphasia, but is accompanied in the acuter stages by defective movements of the face and tongue. But these various disorders belong to different levels of functional integration and the term "motor" cannot be transferred from the defective movements to the lack of ability to employ verbal symbols. Moreover, the two disorders of function obey Jackson's law, in that motion returns to the face and tongue before the more highly integrated and recently acquired power to employ words in speech.

§2. SUMMARY

1. There are no "centres" for speaking, reading, writing or other forms of behaviour comprised in the normal use of language.

On the other hand, there are areas of the brain within which structural injury can produce disorders of symbolic formulation and expression. This is manifested in diminished capacity to employ words and figures in certain ways and under certain definite conditions.

2. Disorders of speech and similar high-grade defects of function are produced by injury to a single hemisphere, which in strongly right-handed persons is usually the left. At this level the problem of localisation consists in determining the exact nature of the disturbance in the use of language associated with lesions in different parts of the brain.

3. The form assumed by an aphasia may differ with the site of the lesion. The structural injury interrupts in various ways the sequence of complex processes necessary for ordinary speech, and so produces diverse clinical manifestations.

4. If the lesion falls over the lower portion of the central convolutions and the parts beneath them, the patient has difficulty in finding verbal forms in which to express his thoughts. Injury to the temporal lobe, on the other hand, leads to disordered rhythm and want of grammatical structure; speech tends to become true jargon. A lesion lying between the post-central fissure and the occipital lobule disturbs the appreciation of meaning, either verbal or general. Should the destruction occupy the neighbourhood of the angular gyrus, it is mainly the nominal value of words which suffers. If on the other hand it lies in the region of the supra-marginal gyrus, the patient finds difficulty in recognising the ultimate significance of logical conceptions evolved by himself, or placed before him orally, in print or in pictures.

5. Cortical and sub-cortical mechanisms participate in every act of language. The deeper a lesion extends from the surface into the substance of the brain, the more definite and permanent will be the disorders of speech. But there is no absolute qualitative difference or other criterion by which the results of cortical injury can be distinguished from those due to destruction of deeper parts of the brain.

PART IV

CHAPTER I

VIGILANCE

THE neurologist grows so familiar with the various forms of loss of function, produced by an organic lesion of the central nervous system, that he is liable to consider them all in anatomical or regional terms. Motor paralysis, defective sensibility, or disorders of speech seem to him to be equally explicable, provided he can discover the exact limits of the destruction of tissue to which they are due. He is liable to forget that, between these structural defects and the affection of sensibility or of speech, lie intermediate vital processes of profound importance. These have a determinant action on the form assumed by the manifestations. The effect of the structural changes does not depend only on their extent and severity; the mode and rapidity of onset and the general condition of the nervous system at the time are of even greater importance in determining the nature of the loss of function.

Now there is little difficulty in correlating a motor paralysis with destruction of cells and fibres in the spinal cord or even in the brain; we know that, so long as they live, they govern the function of muscular movement. Even loss of sensation seems easily explicable; for the neurologist is liable to consider mainly the destination of afferent impulses and to ignore the fact that sensation is a process of mental activity. So many of the duties exercised by afferent impulses are concerned with control and guidance of motion or other acts, which are performed outside consciousness, that the essentially psychical nature of sensation is neglected or forgotten. To many "afferent" and "sensory" are equivalent terms.

But when we consider disorders of speech, the mental aspect of the loss of function cannot be ignored. There are consequently three factors which equally demand recognition. First, the extent and nature of the anatomical destruction; secondly, the physiological disturbance it evokes, and lastly, the nature of the psychical manifestations we speak of as aphasia.

It is the second term of this chain that is habitually slurred over. The loss of tissue can be determined by anatomical examination and the clinical manifestations are patent to anyone who will take the trouble to observe them; but no intervening link is discoverable between them. Few to-day go the length of those stiff-necked anatomists who assert that single words are located in single cells or cell complexes; or that each psychical group of functions possesses an independent anatomical substratum, formed of certain cortical centres in combination with appropriate association paths. Yet, few have attempted to consider the steps by which a structural change evokes a physiological disorder which in turn is manifested as some defect of a specific psychical process.

We are accustomed to associate a violent injury to the head with loss of consciousness and other symptoms of concussion; empirically we are equally familiar with that curious unwitting state, which precedes the patient's complete recovery, during which he is liable to act apparently reasonably, but in a purely automatic manner. But we make no attempt to explain how a local lesion of the brain can abolish certain specific mental activities, leaving other independent functions of the mind intact. In reality, all these phenomena are aspects of the same problem, though familiarity with the facts has staled the wonder they ought to excite within us. For in the phenomena of aphasia, we are face to face with the relation of body and mind in a form capable of experimental examination, and we are compelled to ask ourselves how a diminution in physiological activity can be associated with specific psychical defects.

§ 1. WHAT IS MEANT BY "VIGILANCE"

But before we can attempt to answer this question it is necessary to take into consideration certain facts in the physiology of the central nervous system.

When the spinal cord is divided, or so grossly injured in man that conduction is destroyed, the lower extremities lie flaccid and atonic on the bed in any position into which they may be placed. The urine is retained, the patient has no power of evacuating the bowels, and at first the skin is dry. All deep reflexes are abolished, and scratching the sole of the foot may either produce no movement of the toes, or one that is feebly downwards.

Should the injury be acute and the patient young and otherwise healthy, particularly if he remains free from cystitis, bed-sores or fever, the deep reflexes reappear as the period of spinal shock passes away. First the ankle-jerk, and then the knee-jerk can be obtained; gradually the plantar reflex begins to assume a form characterised by an upward movement of the great toe. The field from which it can be evoked enlarges and finally, in successful cases, the spinal cord becomes so excitable that stimulation anywhere below the level of the lesion may be followed by a characteristic upward movement of the toes. But this now forms a small portion only of the reaction to superficial excitation; ankle, knee and hip are flexed and the foot is withdrawn from the stimulus applied to the sole. Not infrequently the abdominal wall is thrown into contraction and every flexor muscle below the lesion may participate in an energetic spasmodic movement. Stimulation of a small area on the foot has evoked a wide-spread response from the whole extent of the spinal cord below the lesion[1].

Still more remarkable evidence of this diffusion of afferent impulses in the isolated cord is given by the behaviour of the bladder and rectum. For a considerable period after the injury, the patient is unable to pass either urine or faeces; but, in favourable cases, this merges into a condition where both bladder and rectum are emptied automatically. At this stage of excitability, evacuation can be facilitated by scratching the sole of the foot or by any manipulation which produces a flexor spasm. At the same time, passing fluid into the bladder or rectum may evoke an upward movement of the great toe, accompanied by other characteristic flexor manifestations of the lower extremity[2].

This condition has been called a "mass-reflex," because any afferent excitation below the level of the lesion is liable to produce motor effects, not only in the parts normally thrown into action by such a stimulus, but also in organs that do not usually lie within the arc of its reflex influence. The bladder can be excited to action by stimulating the sole of the foot, and movements of the toes can be evoked by filling the bladder with fluid.

Once this condition has been established, the mechanism by which it is produced may become astonishingly sensitive, and comparatively slight stimuli applied to any part below the lesion may evoke violent and wide-spread movements. But if the patient develops fever, in consequence of toxic absorption from a bed-sore or septic bladder, his condition may fall back to that found shortly after the injury. The deep reflexes disappear, the field for the plantar response becomes restricted to the sole or lower portion of the leg, and evacuation of bladder and rectum can no longer be facilitated by stimulating the lower extremities or surface of the abdomen. Not only has the excitability of the cord diminished, but the nature of the response to stimulation reverts to its earlier condition. This may also occur after some operative procedure carried out

1 Riddoch, G. [119].
2 Head, H. and Riddoch, G. [67], and [62], p. 467.

within the spinal canal, especially if the dura mater is opened. Even a gastro-intestinal disturbance, unaccompanied by fever, may produce the same signs of lowered activity. If the toxaemia or other abnormal state passes away, the isolated spinal cord gradually regains its power of responding vehemently to afferent stimuli and the mass-reflex may be evoked as vividly as before. But anything which tends to lower the vitality of the isolated spinal cord will diminish these manifestations of high neural potency.

These observations on man are in complete agreement with the animal experiments of Sherrington[1] and his pupils[2]. Suppose, for instance, that the spinal cord of a cat has been transected in the region of the medulla oblongata; twenty minutes later prick the hind paw with a pin and no general reflex results, but the toes make an opening movement. Gradually the response becomes more wide-spread, until the whole of the limb may be thrown into flexion and the opposite one extended by a stimulus of the same nature and intensity. Not only has the motor response become brisker and more extensive, but the skin area from which it can be evoked has greatly increased. Pinching the superficial structures over any part of the limb may now cause flexion, accompanied by extension of the opposite extremity.

The deep reflexes reappear rapidly and the character of the knee-jerk shows that the quadriceps has regained tone to a considerable extent. As the spinal preparation improves in excitability, even the scratch reflex may reappear; it is, however, easily fatigued and the foot is not brought up to touch the spot stimulated on the body.

When the spinal cord has reached this high condition of activity, the administration of chloroform causes rapid regression. Knee-jerk and ankle-jerk disappear and finally the only reflex that can be evoked is a slight movement of the toes, elicited from the pad of the foot only. Pricking any other part of the limb no longer produces any effect.

Let the preparation recover and, as the narcosis passes away, the receptive field enlarges rapidly; full flexion, with contralateral extension, is again evoked by pricking any part of the limb. At the same time knee- and ankle-jerks reappear; at first they consist of a short twitch, but, as

[1] Sherrington, C. S. [121].

[2] For the opportunity of seeing these experiments and of watching the effect of chloroform in the spinal and decerebrate preparation, I am indebted to the kindness of Sir Charles Sherrington. I also wish to express my thanks to Professor Bazett, who was then working in the physiological laboratory at Oxford, for showing me his animals and giving me much information about them (Bazett, H. C. and Penfield, W. G. [9]).

the muscles recover their spinal tone, these reflexes regain their previous character.

It is obvious, therefore, that, even when completely transected, the spinal cord is capable of various degrees of activity, manifested not only in a brisker reaction, but also in different forms of reflex response. A toxaemia, or anything which lowers vitality, tends not only to diminish the response, but to change its nature. This may be temporary and cannot be due to gross structural disorganisation, for it can be produced in a purely transient form by the action of chloroform. Here we are face to face with a profound coming and going of function in the completely isolated spinal cord, associated with certain vital or physiological conditions, which cannot be caused by gross anatomical changes.

This is still better exemplified in the decerebrate preparation[1]. If the head is removed just in front of the anterior colliculi the cat is capable of a large number of discriminative reflexes. Water placed in the pharynx is swallowed in a normal manner, and, when a small quantity of alcohol is added, the tongue makes a wide sweeping movement, curling at the tip as if to lick the lips. On the other hand, oil produces no movement of the pharynx or tongue. Several different reflexes can be evoked from the pinna, each of which is adapted to the nature of the stimulus; if it is pricked it folds down, but touching the hairs within the ear causes a movement, which would be most effective in dislodging a flea. A drop of water placed in the pinna is followed by a rotation of the head, which brings the stimulated ear downwards, followed by a rapid shake admirably adapted to displace the fluid.

Sometimes a preparation of this kind can purr; it will respond vocally in an appropriate manner to the singing of a canary or the bark of a dog, and at the same time the tail makes the movements customary with such states of excitement.

Normally a decerebrate animal is rigid in extension and if balanced can support its own weight; that is to say, it can stand with help. It sits up with head erect, the forepaws stretched out on either side and the hind limbs tucked beneath it. But if it is put aside in a quiet place, and, after an interval, is approached with great care, it may be found lying on its side relaxed, with its limbs flexed as if asleep. Jarring contact, or even a slight noise, provided it is capable of responding to auditory stimuli, will cause it to assume its natural state of rigid extension. It has woke again from the reflex relaxation proper to sleep.

---

[1] Bazett and Penfield [9], p. 214.

Hold up such a preparation so that it stands on its four limbs, or place it in a seated posture on the table and then administer chloroform. It will sink together exactly like a normal animal; the head falls forwards, the legs double up and the tail ceases to curl at the tip. Then the reflexes become diminished and the knee-jerk loses its characteristic decerebrate form; it becomes a simple jerk, like that of a spinal animal, unaccompanied by increase in extensor tone. The pinna reflexes cease to exhibit their diverse and appropriate forms; swallowing is no longer produced by a drop of water in the pharynx and even alcohol evokes no response.

So long as spontaneous respiration continues, the limbs do not become completely flaccid; but if chloroform is pushed until breathing ceases and artificial ventilation becomes necessary, even the knee-jerk may disappear and all postural tone becomes abolished in the hind limbs.

At this stage remove the chloroform, but continue artificial ventilation. As the effects of the anaesthetic wear off, postural tone is restored, spontaneous breathing returns, swallowing is again possible, the pinna reflexes become differentiated according to the form of the stimulus, and the knee-jerks recover their plastic character. Finally, the preparation may return exactly to its original condition. This regression and restoration of function under the influence of chloroform can be watched time after time in the same decerebrate animal, if care is taken not to abolish the heart-beat.

The spinal and decerebrate preparations differ profoundly from one another in their reactions to external stimuli; but, in both alike, the nature of the response varies greatly according to the general state of vitality in the particular part of the central nervous system which has been isolated from higher control. The transected spinal cord of man can live and function on a level characterised by low-grade reactions; but, under favourable conditions, its activity may increase, until there is scarcely a part below the lesion from which a movement of the toes and a flexor spasm cannot be evoked or evacuation of the bladder and rectum facilitated. The vigour of such a response varies from day to day, and is diminished by any state which lowers the general vitality of the isolated spinal cord.

In the same way the spinal cat at first yields reflexes of a low order; but, with the improvement in its condition, the most complicated move ments can be obtained involving mutual inhibition of flexion and extension. The animal may even regain the scratch reflex in an incomplete form. On administering chloroform all these reactions disappear, to be again recovered as the influence of the anaesthetic passes off. In man this degradation can be produced by a temporary toxaemia, and the restoration of the various forms of response can be watched step by step during recovery from its evil effect.

Now, it is scarcely sufficient to say that these phenomena are manifestations of heightened or lowered excitability. If we say that some part of the nervous system is in a state of raised excitability, we mean that it responds in the same manner to a stimulus of diminished strength. The excitability of a tissue is measured by the ease with which it can be provoked to activity by a suitable external stimulus and is therefore inversely proportional to the strength of the excitation needed to produce any recognisable sign of activity, in fact to its threshold value[1]. But, in the phenomena we are discussing, the main factor is not the diminution or increase in the strength of the stimulus which is required to evoke a reaction, but the fundamentally divergent nature of the response according to whether the preparation is in a high or low state of vitality. At one time it is not only more prepared to receive and react to external impressions than at another, but an identical stimulus produces a different result and, during a high state of vitality, tends to evoke more or less high-grade adapted movements.

These reach a marvellous complexity and perfection in the decerebrate animal. Here the nature of the movement of ear or tongue depends on the form and quality of the stimulus rather than on its strength. The response is truly discriminative, but can be abolished by any condition inimical to a high state of neural vitality, such as sepsis, haemorrhage into the wound, or the lighter degrees of chloroform narcosis. Apart, however, from such hostile influences, the decerebrate preparation may occasionally be found with its limbs in a state of flexion, as if asleep; any contact, or in some instances even a noise, will rouse it, and all four extremities at once reassume the characteristic posture of tonic extension. If we were dealing with an intact animal, we should say that these differences were associated with the presence or absence of consciousness.

---

[1] It is sometimes used with a meaning more akin to the German *Leistungsfähigkeit*. It then signifies the responsiveness of the tissue to a given stimulus and would be measured by the strength of the response, e.g. the height of contraction in a muscle evoked by a stimulus above the threshold value. This is misleading. It is true that a tissue which gives a large response can often be activated by a weak stimulus; but there is no invariable correlation between the value of the threshold stimulus and the size of the response. In fact, there are many cases where a raised threshold is associated with a relatively increased reaction; once a stimulus is sufficient to evoke a response the effect produced is both greater in amount and more extensive than under normal conditions.

But such an explanation of the reactions of the spinal or decerebrate preparation is unsatisfactory, and I would suggest that we employ the word "vigilance" for this state of high-grade physiological efficiency. Shortly after division, the spinal cord of man is in a condition of low vigilance. It is still excitable, for scratching the sole of the foot may produce a movement of the toes. Under favourable conditions the vigilance of the cord increases, until at last it is in a state of intense readiness to respond to excitation. In the cat the reaction may now assume a form of a series of complex movements, involving both lower extremities and necessitating coordinated excitation and inhibition. The tone of the flexor muscles has increased profoundly and, even in the extensors, has become sufficient for reappearance of a knee-jerk.

As revealed in the decerebrate preparation of Sherrington and his fellow-workers, vigilance is expressed in heightened extensor postural tone and acutely differentiated responses. This high state of physiological efficiency differs from a pure condition of raised excitability; for although the threshold value of the stimulus is not of necessity lowered, it is associated not only with an increased reaction but with highly adapted responses. These may vary profoundly according to circumstances, which are not inherent in the nature of the stimulus.

§ 2. AUTOMATIC ACTIONS

If we did not know that the whole of the brain had been removed, we should say that the actions of the decerebrate animal were directed by consciousness. It initiates no movement spontaneously, but purposive adaptation is evident in every response. The character of its purring varies with the nature of the auditory stimulus; irritation of the ear excites a variety of highly differentiated movements, each of which is accurately designed to the end in view. Thus, every one of these actions may be purely automatic. Their formal recognition, if present, would be accessory to a mode of behaviour which can be carried into execution without it.

Both the decerebrate preparation and the normal cat react in an equally discriminating manner, when a flea or a drop of water is placed in the ear. The reactive significance of each stimulus is registered, and suitably adapted responses are prepared on a purely physiological level. But, whenever a reaction shows these characteristics, it demands a high state of vigilance in those parts of the nervous system necessary for its performance. The more highly differentiated the act, the greater degree of vigilance does it require and the more easily can it be abolished by toxic influences, such as chloroform, or by other conditions unfavourable to physiological activity. Experimentally we can watch the various responses disappear step by step under the influence of the narcosis.

Many actions acquired during the life of the individual tend to be carried out on the physiological level. A child has to be taught not to wet the bed at night, and this control of a spinal reflex becomes so completely automatic, that it is maintained even in the deepest sleep. But anything which lowers the vigilance of the central nervous system, such as dyspnoea or a debilitating illness, is liable to disturb this control and the bed is again wetted at night.

The same law is illustrated in many aptitudes, such as flying, shooting and out-door games, which are acquired and maintained by conscious effort. They never reach a high degree of perfection until the necessary movements are carried out unwittingly. The counter-stroke of an expert lawn-tennis player is determined at the moment when the ball leaves the opponent's racquet, whilst the tyro waits until it has bounded on his side of the net; a good shot watches the bird and pays no attention to his gun. Moreover, anything which at the moment concentrates the mind on the various stages of a mechanical action, diminishes the likelihood that it will be carried out successfully. The performer must concentrate on the goal or intention of his desires, and trust to habitual skill for its mechanical execution. But all these aptitudes are profoundly influenced by conditions of general health or by anything which lowers physiological vitality. A common cold, a gastro-intestinal attack or even mental worry may materially diminish any form of mechanical skill.

Every automatic act demands retentiveness and can be disturbed by vital states, which have nothing to do with consciousness. What wonder that the complex powers demanded by speech, reading and writing, can be affected by a lesion, which diminishes neural vitality. Vigilance is lowered and the specific mental aptitudes die out as an electric lamp is extinguished, when the voltage falls below the necessary level. The centres involved in those automatic processes, which form an essential part of the conscious act, may continue to live on at a lower vital level, as when under the influence of chloroform; they do not cease entirely to function, but the vigilance necessary for the performance of their high-grade activities has been abolished by the fall of neural potency.

§ 3. SENSATION AND ITS SUBSERVIENT PHYSIOLOGICAL DISPOSITIONS

The changes produced by a cerebral lesion in all forms of sensation yield striking proof of the wide range of physiological processes underlying the more limited field of specific consciousness. Thus, before the afferent processes caused by the movement of a joint can evoke a perception, they must be integrated and brought into relation with physiological dispositions, which are the result of antecedent changes in posture. Complete recognition of spacial relationships occurs with the appreciation of serial changes in certain directions. On a taximeter the measured distance we have travelled is presented to us already translated into shillings and pence; so the final product of spacial changes rises into consciousness as a measured postural appreciation.

For this standard against which all subsequent changes in posture are measured before they appear in consciousness we have proposed the word "schema[1]." By means of perpetual alterations in position we are always building up unwittingly a model of ourselves, which is constantly changing. Every new posture or movement is registered on this plastic schema and the activity of the cortex brings into relation with it each fresh group of afferent impulses, evoked by a change in the position of the body. The psychical act of postural recognition follows, as soon as this relation is completed on levels that are not associated with consciousness[2].

The only constant and continuous record of our movements in space exists in the condition of these schemata. For innumerable changes in posture occur which are not represented in consciousness, and, were it not for these physiological dispositions we have called schemata, the inception of a voluntary movement would often find the part to be moved in an unsuitable attitude. Unless postural impulses continuously modified these unconscious activities in consonance with every change in bodily attitude, we might will a movement that was impossible owing to the situation of the limb. This is evident in every case of ataxy.

In order that any part of the body may be able to spring off, like a runner, at the word of command, its postural tone must be normal. Should it be posed atonically the voluntary act has to gather in slack

[1] Head, H. [62], pp. 605, 722. Head, H. and Holmes, Gordon [66], p. 186.
[2] It must not be forgotten that the theory of schemata involves two conceptions, the schema building and the schema built. The first is an activity corresponding to all those processes discussed in this work, the second is a state which results from the activity.

before the limb can begin to move. Normal posture and normal tone are coincident terms.

Any lesion, which disturbs postural schemata, will interfere with static tone. For in order that any part of the body at rest may retain a normal posture, afferent impulses must exert a constant constructive influence on postural schemata. The physiological state brought about by this stream of afferent impressions not only checks and controls voluntary movement, but insures that the static tone of the part shall be adapted to maintain its position. Consciousness is in no way necessary for such coordination; in fact, tonic innervation, though dependent on afferent impulses, is determined and regulated entirely on the physiological level. Any lesion, which destroys postural schemata, may diminish static tone, if the other conditions are suitable. It will only affect sensation when the want of these spacial dispositions disturbs the activity of some centre habitually associated with conscious processes. For instance, if the vigilance of the so-called "sensory" cortex is lowered, either temporarily or in consequence of organic destruction, not only will postural sensibility be disturbed in the appropriate parts of the body, but their static tone will be diminished. This is not due to the loss of postural sensations, but to the destruction of those physiological processes on which they are based. For static tone is automatic and depends on a constant stream of influence exerted by the action of ever-varying postural schemata.

When the highest centres, though themselves intact, no longer receive normal afferent impulses, the affected part of the body seems "numb" and the patient complains of "loss of feeling." But, if the schemata are destroyed or eliminated by a lowering of physiological activity, the limb or some portion of it disappears from consciousness.

The following case is an instructive illustration of these principles. A patient of mine had received a gun-shot injury, which had disorganised the elbow-joint and completely destroyed the ulnar nerve. For five months we hoped to be able to save the limb, but were at last compelled to amputate through the lower third of the arm. From the time he was wounded, there were the usual changes, both motor and sensory, associated with complete ulnar paralysis; but the little finger alone was devoid of all forms of sensibility, superficial and deep. So long as he retained his limb, this finger seemed to him a dead object attached to the hand. But the phantom hand, which appeared after amputation, had four digits only. During the five months of total insensibility, the schemata associated with the little finger, no longer reinforced from the periphery, had gradually died away and, when the actual hand was removed, this digit was absent from consciousness. A portion of the body, cut off from the central nervous system, but attached to structures endowed with sensibility and movement, may continue to exist as a "dead" part of ourselves; it occupies a certain place in our spacial activities[1]. But, as soon as the structures on which it is based are removed, it disappears from consciousness, whilst the normal parts of the amputated limb are represented in phantom form.

§4. THE CONTINUITY OF CONSCIOUSNESS

In all discussions on the relation of body and mind stress is laid on the continuity of consciousness. But this continuity is produced by habitually ignoring the gaps. However long the period of dreamless sleep or chloroform narcosis, the processes of the mind seem to have been uninterrupted. A sufferer from minor epilepsy may become completely unconscious and yet remain ignorant that he has had an attack; the stream of mental processes seems to him as unbroken as that of the astonished spectators. But during this period of unconsciousness he can carry out the most elaborate acts, guided and governed by what appear to be reasonable though extraordinary motives.

The mind, acting as a whole, not only ignores these gaps in general consciousness, but habitually neglects many possible experiences even on some specific level, such as that of sensation. The normal individual does not recognise that he is colour-blind over a considerable area of his retina. Close one eye, so as to exclude the compensating effect of binocular visions, and the world around seems unchanged. If, whilst we fix an object in front, someone then brings a red or green square of suitable size from behind forwards, it appears first of all to be either dark or light grey, although otherwise clearly visible. It will have lost its colour; but so little are the peripheral parts of the visual field concerned with this aspect of sensation, that we fail to notice its absence. In the same way we ignore the blind spot, even in uniocular vision.

Still more remarkable are the conditions found with an homonymous hemianopsia of cerebral origin. The patient knows nothing of any defect in his visual field. A man, who has lost an eye or suffers from destruction of the optic nerve, recognises that he is partly blind; but one who is deprived of sight over one-half of the field from cerebral causes is

[1] A dental plate may become so much part of ourselves that we project our sensations to the end of the artificial teeth. But the discomfort produced by a minute crumb or pip between the jaw and the plate converts it into a foreign body lying in the mouth.

ignorant of any abnormality in his vision. He wonders that he so frequently collides with objects on one side rather than on the other and
cannot understand why they seem to disappear prematurely in this
direction.

Such abolition of a specific form of psychical activity, without leaving
a trace on consciousness as a whole, may occur as a temporary phenomenon. After injury to the brain a slight Jacksonian seizure, a severe
bout of headache, or even fatigue and worry may be accompanied by
profound loss of somatic sensibility. But this disturbance of function
appears in consciousness as absence of the hand or some part of the limb.
It does not seem "numb" or devoid of sensation; it simply ceases to
exist. With recovery from this temporary condition of lowered vigilance
in the nervous centres the lost part returns to consciousness and the
patient may then recognise that its sensibility is abnormal, complaining
that "it feels wrong."

§5. PURPOSIVE ADAPTATION

Purposive adaptation is sometimes said to be a distinctive mark of
mental activity. But if we analyse this mode of behaviour, its essential
elements are found to a varying degree in reactions, whether conscious
or not, from all parts of the central nervous system.

It depends fundamentally on three factors. The character of the
response must vary with specific differences in the quality of the stimulus
and not only with its relative amount. Secondly, the form assumed by
the reaction is determined more or less by the sequence of events and
is not dependent solely on the excitation of the moment. Lastly, the
spacial elements, present in afferent impulses, lead not only to coordination of muscular movement, but to projection of qualitative differences
on to those external objects which evoked them.

Once a stimulus applied to a peripheral nerve is effective, the result
is the same in kind, varying in amount only. But, in the spinal cord,
diverse forms of stimulation tend to produce specific and individual
reactions; these may be mutually antagonistic and, should they clash,
are not summed, but one or other may be inhibited. As we ascend the
nervous system this mode of adaptation becomes developed to an even
finer degree; the decerebrate preparation, for example, exhibits purposive
responses of a very high order in harmony with differences in the nature
of the stimulus. For a flea in the ear has a different significance from a
drop of water, and behaviour varies accordingly. Thus, even in these
lowly circumstances, certain characters of an external event are accepted

whilst others are ignored and the object acquires a "meaning" for the
reacting organism. Differential selection occurs from amongst the massive presentations and this determines the form assumed by the response.

The second factor, which plays a part in purposive adaptation, even
on the physiological level, is the influence exerted by past events on the
reaction of the moment. The central nervous system does not function
on the principle of an automatic machine, where a coin thrust into one
slot produces chocolates, into another a box of matches or some other
article. What we obtain, when we throw a stimulus into some part of
the central nervous system, depends to a great extent on what has
happened before. A neural response of this order is a march of events
and not a series of disconnected episodes; the past is active in the present,
and within it lies implicit the form of future reactions. Here we find the
germ of the conscious processes of memory and intention.

The third element, which renders possible purposive adaptation on
a physiological level, is comprised under the term "projection." Afferent
impulses fall into two groups; if consciousness is present, one set arouses
qualitative sensations and effective states, whilst others are concerned
with finer discrimination or with diverse forms of spacial recognition.
The latter coordinate the motor side of the response and render it in this
way effective; under their guidance the scratch reflex is exactly adapted
to remove the source of irritation in the flank. These spacial afferent
elements also enable the body to behave as an object amongst objects
in the world around, even in the absence of consciousness.

But, without the phenomena of simultaneous and successive contrast,
these three factors, the power of endowing an event with reactive
significance, physiological memory and projected characters, would be
insufficient to account for the diversity of response yielded by the central
nervous system. For, provided the stimulus remained unchanged both
in strength and quality, an apparatus, working on purely mechanical
principles, would continue to turn out identical products. This is
notoriously not the case, even with the isolated spinal cord. A physically
constant stimulus produces a steadily decreasing neural effect, and no
two successive excitations, however similar, are followed by the same
result. Contrast, simultaneous or successive, is one of the fundamental
characteristics of vital processes in the central nervous system.

If we remain for a sufficient length of time in a room illuminated
by red light, it will ultimately seem to be colourless. Adaptation has
occurred, and the constant physical stimulus no longer produces its usual
effect. But, when we emerge, everything seems to be tinged with green,

an indication of the extent to which the neutral point has become displaced by physiological contrast during the action of the red light on the retina.

A constant physical stimulus cannot excite a constant vital effect within the central nervous system. At first, it is true, facilitation may occur; the reaction is obtained with greater ease and the field from which it is evoked is increased in extent. But soon the phenomena of reversal and deviation appear. The same stimulus, applied under apparently the same conditions, leads to an opposite result and may even inhibit the original reaction. Or some new feature appears, as when stimulation of a point on the cortex, previously associated with contraction of the face, suddenly yields movements of the elbow[1].

Such diverse and varying modes of response allow of close purposive adaptation, even on a physiological level; but they demand a high degree of vigilance in the structures responsible for the particular reaction. What wonder that a structural lesion of the brain, which affects speech, can disturb appreciation of the logical significance of internal or external events and destroy that habit-memory requisite for the perfect performance of symbolic formulation and expression.

§6. PSYCHICAL AND SOMATIC BEHAVIOUR DEPENDENT ON THE STATE OF VIGILANCE OF THE NERVOUS SYSTEM

Any one of the specific mental processes, which enter into the general stream of consciousness, may be eliminated without materially disturbing its other components. Provided the manifestations of the lesion are purely negative, any aspect of sensation, perception, images, various forms of symbolic formulation, and even elementary states of ideation may be lost independently of one another. Sensation can be gravely affected, but images remain intact; the visual images of a patient, who has long suffered from hemianopsia, do not differ from those of a normal man. Certain aspects of speech may be disturbed without any loss of general intelligence, except in so far as these particular acts are necessary for formal thinking. A lesion of the left pre-frontal region of the brain may affect the elementary processes underlying ideation, in such a way that it becomes possible to formulate and to act upon two fundamentally incompatible statements. One of my patients, who had received a small wound in the left frontal region, which injured the brain, appeared to be in every way normal. In daily intercourse he behaved rationally and

---

[1] Leyton, A. S. F. and Sherrington, C. S. [85], and several papers by Graham Brown in the same Journal [28 and 29].

showed executive ability in the work of the ward; but he wrote a long letter, asking detailed questions about the family, to his mother, although he recognised that she had been dead for three years. He thought that there were two towns of Boulogne, one of which, on the homeward journey from the Front, lay near Newcastle; the other one, in France, was reached "after you had crossed the sea." He had lost that fundamental sense of reality which would render two statements of this kind incompatible to the normal person. This lack of mental cohesion lies at the basis of Korsakow's psychosis, so commonly the result of toxic agents, such as alcohol.

These various mental activities, sensation, perception, imagery, symbolic formulation and ideation may be affected independently by an organic lesion, because the physiological processes, which subserve them, are bound up with the vitality of different parts of the brain, any one of which can be destroyed without of necessity affecting the others. Each such local disturbance is associated with some specific psychical loss of function. But the activity of the mind as a whole is uninterrupted; removal of one aptitude does not cause collapse of the whole structure like a house of cards. The field of consciousness remains continuous as before; it closes over the gap as the sea leaves no trace of a rock that has crumbled away.

Perhaps these conceptions will be rendered clearer by the following simile. Intelligence of the movements of a hostile army can be gained from the air by the use of observation balloons, aeroplanes and dirigibles. Suppose that each form of aircraft depended for its existence on a separate aerodrome; any one class of machine could be eliminated independently, either by destroying its base or by reducing the number of skilled observers, pilots and mechanics below the level of efficiency. Now the sum of knowledge gained by observation from the air depends, not only on the messages communicated to the ground, but also on information signalled from one air-craft to another. Total disappearance of any one form of machine would diminish the sum of aerial knowledge without of necessity causing a break in continuity; but, on the other hand, the absence of this specific source of information could be recorded from the air as an observational fact.

As we pass in review, from below upwards, the various functions which depend for their existence on the integrity of the central nervous system, sensation is the first to reveal the workings of consciousness; it forms the lowest mental level. But the afferent impulses, on which it depends, have already reached a stage of profound integration and, in the absence of the higher centres, are capable of initiating and controlling elaborate and purposive responses. Moreover, the anatomical centres, which govern sensation, are also responsible for a vast number of purely non-conscious and automatic functions. The same afferent impulses subserve sensation, maintain postural tone, and coordinate muscular movement.

Let us examine more closely the automatic activities of the central nervous system, to discover what relation they bear to those normally associated with some form of consciousness. I leave out of account altogether those mental states, termed sub-conscious, which have once formed part of the life of the mind and, although at the moment repressed or outside the focus of attention, may under favourable conditions exert some direct psychical influence. I am concerned solely with those processes which can manifest themselves when the highest cerebral centres are out of action.

Many of these responses, as I have already indicated, show a high degree of purposive adaptation. The various integrative processes which have occurred insure reaction of the body as a whole; a reflex in a decerebrate cat may extend from its ears to the tip of the tail. This direction of behaviour towards a definite end is brought about by three factors.

Firstly, the central nervous system exercises selection amongst the diverse and massive physical influences acting on the organism from without; some of these are effective in arousing a neural reply, others pass unnoticed. Each adequate stimulus is followed by an appropriate response, which becomes increasingly specific with each rise in functional level. But if any two are applied together, the reaction which follows does not of necessity express their algebraic summation; more often one is favoured at the expense of the other. Qualitative selection has occurred in the absence of consciousness, and external objects have acquired a reactive significance.

Secondly, the response at any one moment is not an isolated phenomenon, but forms part of a march of events in which the past exerts a profound determining influence; at the same time the future is implicit in the present. This insures that the activities of the central nervous system shall possess duration, the basis of physiological memory.

Lastly, the spacial elements in afferent impulses endow even non-conscious functions with projection. The responses of a decerebrate animal are directed, not only to a certain end, but also to a definite place. Its behaviour is governed both by relations of space and time.

Sensation, by endowing us with awareness of these reactions, contains the elements of consciousness. As we ascend further step by step in the nervous system, each specific nodal point of vital activity is associated with some more highly developed psychical aptitude and the mental functions increase in complexity with each rise in physiological level.

But, so long as we confine our attention to those specific aspects of psychical defect, which follow lesions of the higher anatomical centres, we find no function that cannot be discovered in primitive form amongst the reactions of the isolated nervous system. Selective responses give meaning and purpose to external and internal events. Memory and intention are developed out of that march or sequence of occurrences which constitutes duration. A succession of momentary happenings would have no continuity; a series of perishing "nows" would be useless, even at the lowest level of neural activity. Finally, the power of spacial projection enables us to endow external objects in the world around with those qualitative attributes which are developed out of selective responses to physical stimulation.

Consciousness stands in the same relation to the vigilance of the higher centres as adapted and purposive reflexes to that of those of lower rank in the neural hierarchy. When vigilance is high, mind and body are poised in readiness to respond to any event external or internal. But if it is lowered by injury, want of nutrition, chloroform or any other toxic influence, these high-grade functions may suffer in general or in part, whether they are associated with consciousness or not.

There is no absolute criterion by which an external observer can distinguish conscious from unconscious behaviour. A man may respond, in an apparently normal manner by act or cry to a painful stimulus, when insensible from chloroform, and can babble intelligibly during delirium or sleep.

Mind and body habitually respond together to external or internal events. The aim of the evolutionary development of the central nervous system is to integrate its diverse and contradictory reactions, so as to produce a coherent result, adapted to the welfare of the organism as a whole. This unification is the product of its vital activity from the lowest spinal to the highest cerebral centres. There is no more difficulty in understanding how an act of consciousness can affect a physiological process, than to comprehend how one reflex can control and modify another of a lower order.

Consider, for example, the conditions which govern micturition. When the fluid in the bladder reaches a certain variable amount, the muscular wall contracts, the sphincter relaxes and the contents are expelled. After transection of the spinal cord, this whole process may occur automatically. Should the cord reach a high state of vigilance, the act can be greatly facilitated by scratching the sole of the foot or other parts of the body below the lesion, and the bladder is emptied at a smaller volume. But, as soon as the controlling influence of the mid-brain can be exerted upon the spinal centres, this facilitation ceases; the stimulus to be effective must be applied within the limited field of the bladder itself.

Psychical conditions have a profound effect upon this reflex. It may become urgent and uncontrollable under the influence of fear; animals evacuate the bladder preparatory to flight, and the language of schoolboys has preserved this association between states of emotion and the passage of urine. On the contrary, it can be checked by an idea; all desire to micturate dies away with the knowledge that place and time are unsuitable for the performance of the act.

Here mind and body are intimately associated in facilitation and control of one of the lowest reflex actions of the spinal cord. We can recognise by introspection that, at any one moment, consciousness played a part or was absent from the sequence of events; but, whatever the level, conscious or automatic, on which this control is exercised, it would have been impossible without a high degree of vigilance. Lowered vitality in the spinal, or mid-brain, or cerebral centres governing micturition will be associated with some variety of incontinence or retention of urine. The common factor in psychical and physiological processes is vigilance; to express this relation and avoid the words "conscious" and "unconscious," we might speak of "psychical" and "somatic" reactions.

This is even more evident, when we consider the manifestations of a high intellectual aptitude, such as speech. It is acquired during the lifetime of the individual, not as an isolated faculty, but as a sequence of psychical and physiological processes. It is a mode of behaviour in which mind and body are inseparable. The one essential and obligatory condition is a state of vigilance in the cerebral centres that participate in the act.

Perfect symbolic formulation and expression demands the capacity to manipulate freely and at will images, meanings, intentions, feelings and ideas, for a specific purpose. In aphasia and kindred disorders of speech all these psychical functions are more or less affected, in so far as they participate in this mode of behaviour; apart from it, they may remain entirely undisturbed. A specific form of psychical activity and its subservient physiological processes have been thrown into disorder, but general consciousness and the mind as a whole remain intact.

CEREBRAL LOCALISATION

WE have already seen that the usual conceptions of localisation of function are not only unsupported by experiment, but are entirely inadequate to explain the phenomena of aphasia and kindred disorders of speech. The so-called "centres" in the cortex are not conglomerations of cells and fibres where some particular and more or less exclusive function is initiated, to be abolished by their removal. They are points where the progress of some mode of action can be reinforced, deviated or inhibited; in fact they are foci of integration.

A destructive lesion of one of these "centres" throws some highly organised function into disorder. Vigilance is lowered at that point and the tissues of the brain can no longer carry on those high-grade physiological processes necessary for the consecutive development of some particular somatic or psychical activity. This is hindered or blocked and a new adjustment occurs, which results in what we call the abnormal response.

So far as the loss of function or negative manifestations are concerned this response does not reveal the elements out of which the original form of behaviour was composed. Like all such pathological reactions it is a new condition, the consequence of a fresh readjustment of the organism as a whole to the factors at work at the particular functional level disturbed by the local lesion.

Should inhibition or control of some lower neural activity form one of the normal results of integration in the higher "centre," the abnormal response may comprise positive manifestations due to release of this function. This phenomenon, so common amongst the physiological and pathological activities of the central nervous system, plays comparatively little part in the disorders of speech produced by organic lesions of the brain, which are to a preponderant degree manifestations of functional loss.

According to the older view of cerebral localisation, various functions generated in different areas of the cortex are brought together like fragments of a mosaic to produce some higher form of activity. Should this be disorganised by a lesion of the brain, it was assumed that the elementary processes out of which it was composed must be revealed in their primary character. Thus the phenomena of aphasia were supposed to discover the motor, auditory and visual elements of normal speech.

I have shown that such a conception is completely untenable and is not justified by the facts either of experiment or of clinical observation. No function is "localised" strictly in any part of the cortex and no form of activity, somatic or psychical, is built up into a mosaic of elementary processes which become evident when it is disturbed by a lesion of the brain.

On the other hand, local destruction of tissue prevents the normal fulfilment of some form of behaviour and the reaction which follows expresses the response of the organism as a whole under these changed conditions. Moreover, the abnormal manifestations can be described only in terms of the act which has been disturbed, and do not reveal the supposed elements out of which it has been synthesised.

In the light of such conceptions the term "cerebral localisation" must be employed in a strictly limited sense. Firstly, it signifies determination of the site of the lesion associated with disturbance of some function, such as the use of language; secondly, it implies discovery of the exact nature of the functional disorders which follow injuries to different parts of the brain.

§1. SUGGESTED EXPLANATION OF THE SITE OF THE LESION IN THE VARIOUS FORMS OF APHASIA

That lesions situated in different localities of one hemisphere can produce specific changes in the power to employ language is one of the most remarkable facts which emerge from the study of aphasia. The material at my disposal is in no way sufficient to determine this relation with precision. Moreover, in all attempts to correlate the site of structural changes with defects of function it must never be forgotten that the severity and acuteness of the lesion exert an overwhelming effect on the manifestations.

But in spite of these deficiencies, I think we are justified in drawing the following conclusions from the cases cited in this work. The more definitely the injury destroys the lower portion of the pre- and post-central convolutions and the parts beneath them, the greater the probability that the defects of speech will assume a "verbal" form. A lesion in the neighbourhood of the upper convolutions of the temporal lobe

tends to produce "syntactical" disorders. Destruction round about
the region of the supra-marginal gyrus causes those defects in the use
of language which I have called "semantic"; whilst a lesion centred
around the angular gyrus, in a somewhat more posterior position,
seems to disturb the power to evoke and to understand names or other
"nominal" expressions.

Thus, lesions in certain parts of the left hemisphere tend to be associated with more or less specific disorders of symbolic formulation and
expression. It is impossible to deduce the various forms assumed by
an aphasia from any logical or a priori analysis of the structure and use
of language; but I think some light can be thrown on the peculiar relation between the nature of the defects of speech and the site of the
injury by considering the physiological functions exercised by cerebral
structures in the vicinity of these foci.

Verbal aphasia is more particularly associated with injury to the foot
of the precentral and neighbouring gyri and the parts beneath them.
A lesion within this area, either in the right or the left hemisphere, is
liable to produce some loss of power in the opposite half of the tongue
and lips, which interferes with perfect articulation. With the gradual
acquisition of capacity to use words, this mechanism on the left side
becomes associated with the more definitely verbal aspect of the new
function; yet a disorder of speech which follows destruction in this
region is not "motor," "effector" or "expressive," nor is it purely
articulatory, even in the slighter cases of aphasia. The act as a whole is
disturbed, but the greatest incidence of this loss of function affects the
formative aspect of words and phrases rather than the power to appreciate their significance.

Syntactical aphasia is associated with lesions in and around the upper
temporal gyri and the parts beneath them. This is the neighbourhood
of the so-called "auditory centre." But the defects of speech which are
the subject of this investigation are in no way due to auditory imperception or to a disturbance of auditory images; they are principally
shown by defects of rhythm and inability to form coherent phrases.
Hearing and the interpretation of sounds may remain intact; thus,
No. 14, when playing the piano clumsily, was able to recognise and
correct the wrong notes he struck. Moreover, all the patients of this
group understood and executed oral commands. They showed, it is
true, some difficulty in appreciating what was said to them in conversation; but this was due to want of power to reproduce exactly the phrases
they had heard, rather than to lack of auditory perception.

There is no difficulty in thinking logically without syntax. If I say to myself "Cat...grass...window...mat...fire," I recognise that the cat, walking on the grass, sprang in at the window and lay down on the mat by the fire. Should this "agrammatical" formula be reinforced by visual images of the cat in the act of carrying out these movements, no more is wanted to insure full registration of the facts. But it would be difficult or impossible in many cases to convey to another person the full meaning of a series of nouns or nominal expressions without combining them by means of syntax. A phrase is not solely the conjunction of distinct words; it is thought expressed with a view to appreciation by an auditor[1]. This need not always be another individual; for in silent or internal speech we are often our own listeners. Speech is a mental process which we may or may not exteriorise. "We speak," as Jackson says, "not only to tell other people what we think, but to tell ourselves what we think." As our own auditors we demand a certain normal rhythm together with the power to formulate and emit words arranged syntactically, duly stressed and accentuated. Much silent thought is incoherent, jerky and linked together by non-logical processes. But on certain occasions, especially when writing spontaneously, internal speech is elaborated by means of syntax into strictly coherent phrases.

All speech contains elements that subserve the rhythmic purposes of the phrase, rather than its actual meaning. Syntactical defects increase the difficulty of producing a progressive flow of articulated sounds. Like a running jumper, who is unsuccessful in taking off, the aphasic of this group cannot correct himself; he may go back to his starting-point and try again, but finally gives up in confusion. He usually dashes on hoping that his jargon will be understood; he cannot go slowly and does not as a rule deliberately return to a word wrongly pronounced in the hope of correcting his faulty articulation.

In the course of the development of speech the parts around the upper temporal gyri on the left side become necessary for rhythmic phrasing and a lesion in this portion of the brain tends to disturb more particularly perfect execution of this aspect of speech. The morbid manifestations are not due to primary lack of perception of the meaning of sounds, but to disorders of rhythm, stress, syntax and those factors in speech which are so necessary to weld isolated words into a coherent expression of the speaker's ideas, or to convey them to the comprehension of an auditor.

---

[1] Cf. Gardiner, A. H. "The definition of the word and the sentence." [54.]

It is worthy of note that the temporal lobe is one of the last portions of the brain to reach full development in the history of man. Speech was originally evolved out of cries of fear, joy, or anger intended to express the feelings of the speaker. Powers of oratory were acquired when it became necessary to persuade other members of the tribe of the utility and rectitude of these emotions.

A lesion situated in the left hemisphere between the post-central fissure and the occipital lobule tends to affect more particularly the meaning and categorical use of language. One of the main differences according to Elliot Smith between the brain of man and that of the gorilla lies in the enormous development of this region, particularly the supra-marginal and angular gyri.

When the lesion lies in the neighbourhood of the angular gyrus and the parts beneath it, the defects of speech are liable to assume a nominal form. The patient is unable to name objects, or to choose them with certainty to oral and to printed commands.

If I am asked to name an object placed before me, I recognise that it possesses certain characteristic qualities and attempt to find the verbal symbol which expresses them adequately. Now, in daily life the recognition of these qualities is mainly dependent on sight; detailed meaning, form, colour, place and relation to other objects are largely based on visual impressions. Touch, and to an even less degree smell and taste, play little part in determining the name of an object; for these senses require contact, whereas vision gives information concerning objects at a distance.

The angular gyrus, where a lesion produces more particularly loss of power to evoke appropriate names, is situated just in front of the area striata, where destruction of tissue produces definite localisable disturbance within the visual field. I wish, however, carefully to exclude the idea that perfect vision is necessary for the integrity of symbolic formulation and expression, or that nominal aphasia is directly associated with defects in the visual field. I suggest only that, during acquisition of the power to speak and understand spoken words, certain anatomical structures became necessary for the due performance of these acts. Such topographical associations came about because particular parts of the brain were already required for some lower function, which played a part in the evolution of one of the many aspects of the use of language.

It is less easy to explain the association between semantic aphasia and lesions in the vicinity of the supra-marginal gyrus; for capacity to understand the deeper significance of words and the wider meaning of a whole sentence seems to be dependent on the integrity of this region in the left half of the brain. Injury to this portion of the right hemisphere may be associated with local disorders of somatic sensibility, consisting mainly of inability to recognise differences in the physical qualities and relations of external objects, such as their form, weight, size, texture, together with want of power to appreciate differences in degree of tactile and thermal stimuli.

With the acquisition of speech this area on the left side of the brain became associated with the complete categorical comprehension of relations. Man was not only able to differentiate objects by means of names, but to understand the remote meaning of a logical series of verbal, pictorial or other symbols. Thus, the activities of this region became of profound importance for comprehending and recording the march of events; this resulted in the realisation of space and time as a guide to the aim and intention of action.

Semantic defects consist more particularly in want of recognition of the ultimate meaning of a logical and consecutive statement together with incapacity to keep in mind the intention of the act originated spontaneously or to command. These disorders are manifested in want of orientation and power to comprehend the aim and purpose of speech, thought and action. Can it be that ability to carry out these processes was acquired as a higher development of interest in recognition of mutual relations, qualitative, spacial and temporal, between objects in the external world?

All such attempts to explain how a lesion in a certain part of the brain came to be associated with defects of symbolic formulation and expression are purely hypothetical suggestions and do not form an inherent part of my general thesis. Moreover, these disorders of speech are not necessarily accompanied by any other loss of function. Verbal aphasia may exist without paralysis of the lips and tongue; syntactical defects do not require auditory imperception; nominal aphasia is not of necessity associated with loss of vision, nor the semantic form with disorders of somatic sensibility. Nor is it possible by analysis of the phenomena of aphasia to discover any elements which can be attributed to disorders of motion, sensation, hearing or vision.

§ 2. THE NATURE OF THE DISORDERS OF SPEECH PRODUCED BY A LOCAL LESION OF THE BRAIN

"Symbolic formulation and expression" is a purely descriptive term for the various forms of behaviour which are found by experimental observation to be affected in conjunction with disorders of speech. It is in no sense a definition; because some form of psychical activity cannot be logically included under this term there is no reason why it should not suffer in fact, and conversely there are many symbolic processes which escape. Moreover, the use of a symbol in one way can be disturbed, although it may be employed with ease in some other manner.

I am not attempting to set up a new human "faculty," an elementary class of conscious processes, or even a primary and coherent group of psychical aptitudes. I use the term "symbolic formulation and expression" as a convenient designation for the various actions, which are manifestly disturbed as the result of certain organic lesions. In the same way "verbal," "syntactical," "nominal" and "semantic" are employed to indicate the diverse forms that may be assumed by the defective use of language in consequence of destruction of different portions of the brain.

Although I do not believe that disorders of speech reveal the elements out of which it is composed, I have habitually employed the term "integration" in the following sense. I do not intend to imply that a series of factors are summed algebraically. At each physiological level the organism reacts anew to its environmental conditions, and the character of the response depends not only on the reactive significance of the impulse but on the state of the receptive centre. This is best seen by tracing the fate of sensory impressions from the periphery to the highest functional levels. A multitude of impulses pass into the spinal cord by way of the posterior roots, grouped to a great extent according to whether they originate in superficial or deep structures. These reach their first synaptic junction somewhere between the cells of the posterior horn and those of the posterior column nuclei. Here occurs the first functional integration; the organism reacts to form a fresh pattern of afferent impulses and in this form they are transmitted to the receptive nuclei of the optic thalamus. From this point they pass to act upon the cortex and the essential centres of the thalamus itself. Each of these organs responds in an appropriate manner to produce what we call a normal sensation. But, should some morbid condition exist on either side of this mechanical system, remarkable reactions appear unlike any manifestations which can otherwise occur.

So, when speech is affected, the various processes which commonly act in harmony are disturbed. Each response is a fresh reaction to abnormal conditions; it is a morbid phenomenon due to an attempt of the organism to adapt itself to a new situation created by the defects of function which result from the lesion. No two cases are exactly alike; for the manifestations depend not only on the site and severity of the destruction of tissue, but on the mental characteristics and aptitudes of the patient.

In every instance the names chosen for these specific defects are intended solely to indicate their most salient features. It is a mistake to suppose that, even with the most definite varieties of aphasia, every test yields a distinctive result. One task may suffer diversely with each form of disordered speech, whilst another is affected more or less uniformly throughout. Thus, the abnormal behaviour of patients belonging to the various classes of aphasia is characterised in part only by mutually distinctive responses.

It is of fundamental importance that these names should be understood and employed in an indicative sense only. They are useful labels and not exclusive definitions. Having determined empirically what functions are affected, we can then speak of them as disorders of symbolic formulation and expression. Closer examination may show that still further differentiation is possible. Certain tasks, necessitating articulated speech or the understanding of spoken words, are found on examination to be disturbed in a peculiar manner and to each such class of disorder we are justified in applying a distinctive designation.

But each variety of aphasia comprises defects in excess of those which can be deduced from its name. Verbal and syntactical aphasia consist of more than a disturbance of articulated words and phrases, whilst the nominal and semantic forms interfere with wider aptitudes than the appreciation of verbal or general meaning. The power of setting the hands of a clock to command, of imitating movements made by the observer, of drawing to order or constructing a ground-plan, orientation, and many other actions may suffer in association with more directly linguistic tasks.

Moreover, the loss of power is relative and not absolute. A man who is unable to read or to write under certain conditions can do so if the task is presented to him in some other way. For example, it may be impossible to read aloud or to write to dictation the simple words of the man, cat and dog tests; yet the patient can both find the correct names and transfer them to paper in response to pictures. Visual images may still be available for use in spontaneous thought, although they cannot be employed to command in a normal manner for recalling and registering relations.

This strictly observational method and purely indicative nomenclature makes it possible to correlate the defective psychical aptitudes with the degree of loss of function and so with the extent and situation of the organic lesion. This is entirely impossible if the names given to any specific variety of aphasia are supposed to correspond to some pre-existing psychical category, or if the clinical manifestations are thought to reveal the elements out of which speech is composed. For instance, alexia and agraphia are nothing more than expressions for inability to read and write. Reading and writing signify solely that a human being is behaving in a certain manner connected with the use of language; they are useful descriptive terms corresponding in conceptual rank with the words walking and eating. They cannot be employed as categories of physiological activity; still less can want of capacity to read or to write be associated specifically with destruction in some limited area of the brain.

Such terms as "aphasia," "amnesia," "apraxia" and "agnosia" are even more abstract and still further removed from the actual phenomena. Yet, at one time or another, attempts have been made to correlate each of the morbid conditions designated by these terms with the topography of brain lesions. But aphasia, or inability to speak, does not correspond to any self-contained disorder that can be discovered by examination. Amnesia signifies no more and no less than loss of memory, and there is no memory apart from things remembered; "general memory" is a misnomer. Apraxia is employed to designate a form of behaviour in which the patient cannot perform at will certain high-grade actions prompted from without or in his own initiative; but these form a widely heterogeneous group belonging to various psychical categories. Finally, agnosia comprises conditions so different as visual, auditory or tactile imperception and defects of language characterised by loss of appreciation of symbolic meaning.

So long as we clearly recognise that these words are purely abstract terms corresponding to no constituent groups of phenomena, psychical, physiological or anatomical, they may be employed as summary indications of different varieties of abnormal behaviour. But they can never be correlated in a distinctive manner with the site of any anatomical lesion.

Thus, throughout my work I have used the words aphasia and amnesia solely as shortened indicative expressions to avoid detailed description. But I have avoided the terms agnosia and apraxia in connection with the high-grade disorders of speech which form the basis of this research. As I have already shown, both imperception and that loss of power to execute certain acts at will, known as apraxia, can interfere materially with the use of language; but the defects so produced are of a different order from those with which I am concerned. Moreover, nothing could be more deceptive than attempts to explain the phenomena of aphasia and amnesia in terms of verbal apraxia and agnosia. All such expressions must be employed solely as descriptive of certain forms of abnormal behaviour. Used in any other sense they belong to that deceptive class of clinical terms which, although they explain nothing, produce a fictitious feeling that an absolute classification of the phenomena has been attained.

The progress of medical knowledge has been profoundly hampered by failure to bear these principles in mind. Time, place, quantity and intensity have been inextricably confused in so-called "diagnosis." Disease is an event which manifests itself in certain ways, and our business as practical physicians is to select from the morbid phenomena those which we consider to be important as a guide to our subsequent conduct. Since no two examples can ever be identical, we choose out certain features as significant and, collating them with our previous experience of similar or diverse signs in other cases, we conclude that the patient is suffering from a certain disease. But this entity, which we have erected by conceptual abstraction from the events that are happening before us, has no existence apart from our own intellectual activities and those of persons whom we can persuade to think like ourselves. No disease can be defined exactly; its boundaries are always hazy, and the more closely we limit its characters the less does the final result correspond to actual experience.

All names of diseases and formal collections of signs and symptoms are counters which help us to represent to ourselves what is happening to the patient. This power of intellectualising the observed facts and erecting conceptual categories is a useful aid to action; but these so-called "diagnoses" have no absolute value. Names, such as "angina pectoris" or "epilepsy," cannot be translated into equivalent anatomical terms. Directly we behave as if they possessed any validity other than descriptive, we are liable to fall into the fallacious mode of reasoning which has been so prevalent in the study of aphasia and kindred disorders of speech.

The power to employ language is acquired by every individual in the course of his life-time and is improved and widened by practice and conscious effort. At first it consists solely of capacity to speak and to comprehend spoken words; the majority of human beings progress no further in the art of using these vocal symbols. But civilised man invented writing to perpetuate his utterances and to transmit them to his fellows distant from him in space and time. In order to understand these arbitrary signs and to interpret their significance into action, he learnt to read. Out of simple acts of enumeration sprang arithmetic and higher mathematics, the purest form of symbolic thinking. Pictorial representation, a lowly form of intellectual statement, became refined until it became possible to construct more or less elaborate diagrams, such as a ground-plan.

Education steadily improves the power of employing these procedures for intellectual operations of ever increasing complexity. But essentially they are all developments of simple acts of speaking and comprehension of spoken words. It is here that we must look for the evident diversity in the manifestations caused by organic lesions of the brain.

On the other hand, less primitive, more recently acquired and highly abstract forms of symbolic formulation and expression are liable to be disturbed in a more massive way. Should the patient fail to solve a problem in arithmetic, there may be nothing in the actual record to betray the nature of his defects of speech; yet, from his difficulties in speaking or in understanding what is said to him, it is at once evident to what class his disorder belongs.

Acts such as writing stand in an intermediate position. When the written material is examined from the point of view of formulated thought and expression of meaning, it is liable to show distinct abnormalities corresponding to the various forms of aphasia. But its more structural characters, the formation of letters and spelling of words, tend to suffer in a less specific manner.

The effects produced by an organic lesion of the brain on the more primitive acts of language fall naturally into disorders of verbal formulation and defective recognition of meaning. But it would be a fundamental fallacy to divide aphasia into two exclusive groups according to these categories, as erroneous as the analogous classifications into aphasia and amnesia, or apraxia and agnosia.

So long as the disturbance of function is of slight degree, or the task set extremely easy, the defects of speech may appear to consist almost entirely of want of power on the one hand to formulate, or on the other to understand, spoken words. But, even in such cases during the severer stages of the malady, both aspects of speech are definitely affected. A verbal aphasic is misled by the wrong words he has enunciated, either aloud or to himself, and it is difficult to avoid the intellectual consequences of such false formulation. In the same way, syntactical defects prevent accurate silent reproduction of phrases heard by the patient and so reduce his power of comprehending exactly what has been said to him.

Conversely, want of appreciation of meaning spoils verbal formulation. The nominal aphasic cannot find the right word, whilst the semantic is unable to complete his sentences or to bring thoughts and actions to a logical conclusion.

In every instance we are dealing with an abnormal reaction evoked by morbid physical conditions; one form of intellectual behaviour cannot be abstracted from the other and treated as if they were separable and completely dissociated activities of the mind.

Speech, examined introspectively, appears to be a progressive act, which may be analysed into events appearing at separate moments of time. As a gun is aimed, the trigger pulled and the cartridge explodes, so it would seem as if we first think of what we want to say, then select the terms in which to express it and finally embody them in words and phrases.

But this is certainly a misleading and fallacious method of stating what actually occurs. An act of speech comes into being and dies away again as an alteration in the balance of psycho-physical processes; a state, never strictly definable, merges into another inseparable from it in time. When this transition is interrupted and the evolution of a perfect response is prevented by physical causes, fresh integration becomes necessary and new phenomena appear. These in no way represent temporal elements in a series of normal events. Unimpeded symbolic formulation and expression cannot be analysed into a sequence of semantic, nominal, syntactical and verbal processes which normally follow one another in time. Each specific disorder of speech is an abnormal reaction, manifested in some particular way throughout the whole duration of those acts, which take on a fresh form in consonance with the physical disability. Had these reactions corresponded to the constituent parts of an orderly sequence in normal speech, disturbance at some definite point of time would have prevented the development of all those processes which followed later in the series. This is certainly not the case; these disorders of speech do not reveal the normal order of psychical events. They disturb in certain ways the progressive development of language processes as a whole, and so produce the different varieties of aphasia.

Habitual acts, which have become almost automatic, may be prevented altogether if a task is presented in some unfamiliar manner. Thus, a man who can write his name and address correctly is unable to do so if he is asked to put down those of his mother with whom he lives; the unusual beginning has increased the difficulty and made it impossible to write the words that would otherwise have come easily to him.

Moreover, it is often easier for the aphasic to arrive at a result by following a sequence than by direct recognition of a single word or unit. Individual symbols, such as the days of the week, the months, the letters of the alphabet and numbers can be more readily comprehended and manipulated as part of a series than when they stand alone.

Such a method of using progression is a reversion to an earlier type of response, and is employed when the more highly developed method breaks down. It then becomes easier to arrive at a correct answer by saying over the series until the required word or number is reached than to recognise it without this procedure. Some normal persons, especially when adding up low numbers, count to themselves, a relic of the finger counting habitual in childhood.

That form of behaviour which we call the use of language has a history, and many of the phenomena of disordered speech resemble the stages by which the complete act was developed in each individual. The patient describes an object or mentions its use instead of giving it a name; he spells the words he is reading instead of recognising them directly; he counts on his fingers when he should add or subtract. In fact he falls back in many ways to more infantile modes of response.

But the mechanism underlying symbolic formulation and expression is not a palimpsest from which, when the more recent writing is removed, an earlier text is revealed in a primitive form. The aphasic may return to the less exacting methods of solving a problem which resemble those adopted in childhood; but his mind differs fundamentally from that of a child. In the earlier days, when he was acquiring the use of language, he gradually refined and extended his verbal aptitudes and power of employing symbols of all kinds. When these are disturbed in conse-quence of physiological defects, he falls back on methods of arriving at the desired result corresponding to the steps by which he acquired the art of using language. Thus, he describes a colour by comparing it to a concrete object, although he cannot give its name; blue is like the sky, red is blood and green resembles grass. Apart, however, from this adoption of a form of response more prevalent in childhood, the phenomena of disordered speech do not strictly correspond to stages of its historical development.

Nor do they represent complementary portions of the psychical process itself. Normal acts of speech cannot be analysed into verbal, syntactical, nominal or semantic elements. I have chosen these terms solely to indicate that amongst a group of morbid phenomena the most distinctive loss of linguistic capacity fell mainly on some one of these grammatical features. Each specific form of aphasia is accompanied by disorders of function too extensive to correspond with any constituent element of speech, and the various abnormal manifestations cannot be combined like the pieces of a puzzle to compose a coherent whole. Each group of morbid reactions far exceeds the due proportion of an integral part of the total psychical process.

Every disorder of speech is manifested in psychical terms; but in no instance can the nature and extent of the disturbance be deduced from a priori consideration of the normal use of language. Each particular variety of aphasia represents the response of the organism under the changed conditions produced by physiological defects, and we cannot discover the form it assumes from logical conceptions with regard to the processes of the mind. The morbid phenomena must be determined solely from observation of the actual facts. However unlikely the conclusions may appear at first sight, they must be judged by experimental evidence only. Moreover, it is well to remember that if any two hypotheses equally explain a set of observed facts, there is no inherent reason why the simpler one should lie nearer to the truth. Biological processes do not of necessity conform to the logical demands of the human intellect.

A disturbance of speech represents physiological defects manifested in terms of a psychical act. Let us imagine that, whilst my attention is fixed on the eyepiece of a polariscope, the constituents of the solution under examination are changed without my knowledge in such a way that the rotation they produce shifts from left to right. I am at once aware that the polarity has been reversed and make the necessary adjustments which can be read off on the scale. The alteration in chemical constitution of the fluid becomes evident to me in terms of polarised light. So the physiological changes responsible for disorders of speech can be recognised solely by psychological tests.

Thus the various forms assumed by an aphasia do not correspond to any elementary categories of the act of speech. Although expressed in terms of the defective use of language, they cannot be deduced logically and must be discovered by observation. As the result of defective physiological activity a certain form of behaviour is thrown into disorder; the consequences appear as a morbid psychical reaction, which does not reveal or correspond to any normal group of mental processes.

There is no point to point correspondence between physiological processes and the constituent elements of an act of speech. At one time it was supposed that a certain part of the brain A exercised a certain function A^1 which was directly associated with a psychical process A^2. Destruction of A was followed by manifestations corresponding to loss of A^2. But I have been able to show that this is not the case. An aptitude such as the use of language is gradually acquired during the life of each individual and a high level of physiological activity is required for the performance of these complex acts; should vigilance be diminished from any cause they will fade out and cease to be possible. Simpler, lower-grade activities can still be exercised, and other psychical reactions do not suffer apart from those which stand in direct relation with highly purposive physiological processes normally exercised by the injured structures.

A local lesion produces a limited loss of physiological capacity determined by the site and severity of the injury. This in turn interferes with the efficient performance of those psychical acts which can only be exercised and developed at a high level of vigilance. But the loss of function is determined by a failure of physiological potency, although it is expressed and can alone be recorded in psychical terms.

CHAPTER III

LANGUAGE AND THINKING

THIS is too vast a subject to be dealt with adequately in a single chapter and demands a whole treatise to itself. But I cannot close these theoretical considerations without calling attention to certain questions concerning the mechanism of thought and language which have been elucidated by my observations. I must leave a complete exposition of the problem to others, who may perhaps be able to weave my results into the texture of a more general statement of the facts[1].

Acts of free associative thinking normally comprise a multitude of psychical procedures, both simultaneous and successive, bound together by the most diverse links to form a more or less coherent sequence. Examination of a silent train of thought shows that it depends on fragments of logical reasoning, frequently broken by the upward rush of apparently inconsequent ideas or the intervention of some emotional reaction. To such processes may be added verbal associations, suggestions due to place and time, and images of all kinds. For example, in a strong visualiser like myself the progression of thought is constantly illustrated, illuminated or confused by innumerable more or less appropriate mind-pictures. What is called "thinking" ranges from the fantasy of the day-dream to the formal and logical though silent exposition of an orderly course of reasoning.

Acts of free associative thinking cannot be expressed completely in words; the whole process is inherently illogical, intuitive and punctuated by irrelevancies. As soon as we attempt to express our thoughts even to ourselves, we re-arrange them and drastically prune away redundant and incoherent features. For the purposes of articulated speech or writing this process is carried out still more ruthlessly, and we strive to cast our thoughts into a form that is not only comprehensible to ourselves but to our hearers; the results of unrestricted thinking are refined and ordered in accordance with logical canons.

But in order that these formal products of thought can be expressed in articulated speech or writing they must be clothed in suitable words

[1] I should like to call attention to the valuable and interesting treatment of these problems in the light of modern research by Henri Delacroix in *Le Langage et la Pensée* [40].

and phrases. This facility can be gained only by repeated exercise like any other form of mechanical skill. We learn to speak by constant practice exactly as a lawn-tennis player acquires the power of executing a difficult stroke or a skater some new figure. At one stage the child probably possesses more words than ideas and exercises the art of speaking in and out of season as a golfer practises the use of his clubs. A word or a phrase once acquired is repeated over and over again, often on inappropriate occasions. Moreover, having learnt a number of appellations for the ordinary living creatures that he meets, such as "bow-wow," "moo-cow," "dicky," he is obliged to replace them by "dog," "cow," and "bird," and to adopt other structural forms of adult speech. Spoken language has to be acquired as an habitual act in order that organised thought can be expressed with ease and freedom.

On the other hand, the power of reducing the products of thinking to a logical and grammatical form, in which alone they are capable of verbal expression, is acquired to a considerable degree by formal consideration and study. It is not sufficient to gain a glibness of utterance; we must be aware of differences of meaning and the intellectual value of composition. Thus we study French grammar in order to learn how to communicate our ideas in that language; but we practise speaking French to acquire facility in the foreign tongue.

These two aspects of language, the formulation of thought and its skilful expression, although they may be separable by introspection, are not dissociated as the result of organic lesions of the brain. The superb logician may have difficulty in expounding his ideas and we are familiar with the practised speaker whose words are jejune of thought. But in aphasia both sides are affected, although one may suffer more severely than the other, and I have therefore spoken of these defects in the use of language as disorders of symbolic formulation and expression.

Even in the slighter forms of verbal and syntactical aphasia, where the loss of function appears to be confined to want of skill in manipulating words and phrases, formal thinking is hindered by defective internal verbalisation. The patient may be confused by his own jargon or other defects of speech. If, for instance, when drawing an elephant, he says "horns" instead of tusks, he is liable to represent them on the forehead of the figure and not as emerging from the mouth. In the same way the meaning of a command may be misunderstood because he cannot formulate to himself exactly what he has heard or read.

Conversely, power to discover the correct form of words is profoundly diminished by defective appreciation of meaning. The nominal aphasic, in doubt as to a name, says "mat, mats, match," or speaks of "berloo" and "or-ridge" instead of blue and orange, and he recasts his sentences many times before he can bring them to a satisfactory conclusion. Semantic defects do not as a rule disturb the structure of words, but diminish the power of rounding off a series of phrases to culminate in a distinctly expressed conclusion. The process of thinking is vague and incomplete; speaking is therefore hesitating and inconclusive.

When we consider that the use of language in all its forms is a development of the capacity to speak and to understand spoken words, this intimate and indissoluble unity of meaning and expression is easily comprehensible. Facility in formulation and utterance have been acquired simultaneously and have grown up step by step together. Any other additional processes which are affected suffer because they have become linked up with or are a higher development of speech. In so far as they enter into this connection they are liable to be disturbed in aphasia; but except for their participation in the use of language, they may remain intact.

All substitute signs may properly be treated as language, but some only function as expressions of thought. There are certain acts of speech which have little or nothing to do with thinking, and neither state a proposition nor culminate in action. These remain unaffected in aphasia and kindred disorders. They comprise meaningless words and phrases, emotional ejaculations, such as "Oh! dear me," together with oaths and other familiar expletives. I once had a patient under my care who could utter "yes" but not "no"; for all forms of negation or disapproval he employed the word "damn."

Even in current speech there are many words which, though used idiomatically, have little distinctive meaning in themselves. Many ready-made expressions or clichés are employed habitually in order to start and maintain the progressive flow of speech. These are linguistic tricks, which enable the speaker to utter the essential contents of his mind, and many of them give emotional tone to an otherwise colourless phrase. I once took down the following sentence from the lips of an irate colleague: "[I'll tell you what it is,] he [jolly well] wants [to get] a [common or garden] secretary to make him answer his letters." All the words in brackets are logically unnecessary, but they helped him to express both his opinion and his irritation.

Slang closely approaches this order of verbal utterances. Many educated aphasics, when in difficulty, fall back on this more descriptive and ready-made method of expression. Captain C. (No. 2) characterised a suggestion of which he approved as "a good egg" and, whenever he wished to tell me that a task required much effort, he said he had "to put heavy guns on to it." As his powers of speech improved, he gradually purged his language of slang and talked more in accordance with his abilities and education.

We perpetually enlarge our powers of employing language, not only by learning to formulate our ideas as a coherent sequence, but by practising the art of expressing them freely in articulated words and phrases. During this process the earlier requirements, those most intimately associated with speaking and the comprehension of spoken words, become increasingly habitual; the response becomes more or less stereotyped. A complete mastery of language demands rapid formulation and conscious manipulation of more or less automatic modes of expression. When these forms of behaviour are thrown into disorder, the defects of speech tend to assume diverse forms according to the site and severity of the cerebral lesion. Each variety of aphasia disturbs the power of manipulating and comprehending words and phrases in a different manner. On the other hand, more recently acquired aptitudes, demanding a higher degree of conscious formulation and expression, tend to suffer in a more massive and less specific way.

There are two groups of linguistic processes which tend to become increasingly automatic and can be initiated with comparatively little conscious effort. The one consists of ejaculations and phrases devoid of logical meaning, which serve to betray emotion or to form the preliminary to significant verbalisation. These escape altogether in aphasia, for they have little to do with systematic thinking. On the other hand, there are many acts of speaking and understanding spoken words, which, although they have become by practice almost habitual, remain endowed with significance. However great the facility of diction or of comprehension these processes were developed out of formal thinking and still serve to secure that end. They consequently suffer severely in disorders of symbolic formulation and expression. The hands of a skilful pianist move automatically over the keys to express the harmonic development of the music and he is scarcely conscious of the individual notes on the paper. But his movements and sensations are endowed with intense reactive significance. So the educated and practised speaker concentrates his attention on the subject of his exposition and trusts to acquired automatisms for its expression. Even when listening to others, we fix our mind on the sense and rarely attend to the words in which it is embodied. Such modes of behaviour as speaking and the comprehension of spoken words, charged as they are with meaning, suffer severely in the various forms of aphasia, whilst emotional expressions and meaning-less phrases are not materially affected.

§ 1. ACTS OF DIRECT REFERENCE

When we are faced with a problem demanding an active response, we mobilise all the powers we possess for its solution. Thought pre-supposes the existence of language, but exceeds it widely in range, and there are many forms of behaviour, the result of thinking, which do not require the intervention of a symbol. Percepts and emotions alone may determine the form of the response. We often act without thinking of ourselves as acting, or formulating beforehand the exact nature of the reply to the conditions of the moment. Many actions in a game such as lawn-tennis or in piloting an aeroplane belong to this order. Some fresh situation is dealt with successfully with extreme rapidity; the manipulator is conscious only of the result and he may be unable to recall the movements he has actually performed.

The tests which I have employed in this research comprise a certain number of intellectual operations, based on correspondences of a sensory order or on similarity and difference of perceptions. Such acts are not directly disturbed in aphasia and kindred disorders of speech. All those on the contrary which imply more complex adaptation, the recog-nition of signs, logical symbols or diagrams, suffer more or less severely.

Acts of direct reference do not form a sign-situation and are not affected even in severe examples of disorders of speech, provided the patient can be made to understand exactly what he is expected to do. He can choose a familiar object or a colour from amongst those before him, which exactly corresponds to the one he was shown. Here the act of matching depends on reaction to similarity in successive visual impressions[1].

But suppose some article such as a knife, or even a geometrical figure, is placed in his hand out of sight, the patient has no difficulty in selecting its duplicate, provided no words are employed. Moreover, if he has been given a pyramid cut out of a block of wood, he can match it with any pyramidal object, however greatly the two may differ in relative size and structure. He deduces from the multifarious sensations yielded by his hand certain characteristics, which are also possessed by the object

---

[1] Gelb and Goldstein [57] have shown however that the same patient may fail to sort the various shades of the Holmgren wools correctly. (Vide Part I, p. 132.)

within sight, and ignores the many differences. In both percepts he reacts to a common quality, the pyramidal factor, although the one is the result of tactile the other of visual impressions.

So long as the act to be performed is one of direct matching it can usually be executed in spite of the defective use of language. But as soon as a symbol intervenes between the initiation and performance of any task, the patient is liable to fail to carry it out correctly. Suppose, for instance, he has succeeded in matching a single object shown to him with the one on the table which resembles it. If he is then given two objects at a time, he may fail to select the two corresponding duplicates, because he attempts to register what he has seen in words and to make his choice accordingly. A symbolic formula has been interjected and the act is no longer one of direct matching.

To place the hands of a clock into the exact position of those on one set by the observer is in most cases an act of pure imitation. But should the patient have any difficulty in appreciating the relative significance of the two hands, even this simple task may be badly executed. He confuses the hour and minute hands, or fails to comprehend exactly what he is expected to do.

Certain forms of behaviour, which at first sight appear to be purely imitative, in reality require the intervention of some verbal symbol or formula. If I am seated face to face with a patient and touch an eye or an ear with one or other hand, he may fail to imitate my movements because he cannot bear in mind that our actions are apparently reversed. To carry out this test successfully he is compelled to formulate to himself that my right hand is opposite to his left and that the same is true for eye or ear. In some instances he attempts to express this fact silently in words by saying to himself, "It is the opposite," or even, "His right is my left."

But as soon as I stand behind him and my movements are reflected in a mirror, all necessity for such formulation disappears; the act becomes in most instances one of pure imitation. Many patients express this by saying, "It is easy because I don't have to think." When, however, the disorder assumes a semantic form the essential nature and intention of the movements to be performed become a matter of doubt; the patient grows confused in his attempts to reason out what he is required to do and fails to execute even this simple act of imitation. Any task that leads to "thinking," or the intervention of certain symbols, tends to be badly performed. Thus, even if the patient imitates with ease and certainty my movements reflected in a mirror, he cannot write them down, not because he is unable to form the necessary words in writing, but because a verbal formula intervenes between this mode of expression and what he sees.

To copy capital letters line by line is an act of imitative drawing; it can be executed by a child before he has learnt to write. But to translate them into their small cursive equivalents demands symbolic formulation and is difficult or impossible in many cases of aphasia. This does not depend on any peculiar inherent difficulty in cursive script; for if the letters to be copied are set out in this form, they can be reproduced correctly by the same patient who was unable to translate capitals into common handwriting. All transliteration demands the intervention of a certain degree of logical thinking however slight, and consequently tends to suffer in many cases of aphasia.

In most instances the patient can draw from a simple model and can even reproduce his drawing from memory. Should he fail, however, to appreciate the intention or aim of the action he is expected to perform, he may be unable even to draw from a model; yet he can produce a fair representation of some object that has risen to his mind as a spontaneous image or idea. It is not the mechanical act of drawing which is affected, even in semantic aphasia, but the power to formulate a conception of how to undertake the solution of the problem.

There are certain other acts, which can be performed correctly in spite of these disorders by a process of direct reference, but not by a formal statement of symbolic relations. A patient who cannot state how many sixpences make up half-a-crown, when they are placed before him, can pile up a heap of coins of the exact value of either piece of money. He may be unable to state the price he pays for his tobacco; yet he knows that, when he asks for two ounces and tenders two shillings, he receives threepence in change. Capt. C. (No. 2) was fully aware that his railway journey cost him five shillings minus twopence halfpenny and this sum he expected to receive together with his ticket. Such patients can register an event and act upon it, although they cannot state a formal relation either to themselves or others.

During the period when No. 2 was unable to tell the time from a clock face shown to him, he was punctual for his engagements. Moreover, if the hands pointed to half-past one, he said, "That's when we have dinner," which was correct. He still possessed some appreciation of the passage of time by means of which he regulated his actions, although he could not state the hour formally either aloud or to himself.

In the same way, in spite of the confusion between right and left, he was conscious that the traffic of the streets kept to the left in England, but not in other countries, and could indicate this fact to me by suitable gestures.

Thus, amongst the multifarious processes comprised in unrestricted thinking, some can still lead to the desired result in spite of the existence of aphasia and kindred disorders of speech. These are brought to a successful conclusion mainly by direct reference; but the same tasks may be rendered impossible if an act of symbolic formulation or expression is interposed between their initiation and completion.

§ 2. IMAGES AND THINKING

Images play a double part in unrestrained thinking and may or may not suffer according to the manner in which they are employed. We know very little of the behaviour of auditory images in aphasia; but the direct reproduction of melody and the recognition of time and tune are not affected, apart from the difficulty of forming the words of a song, or reading the notes of the music. Careful interrogation failed to reveal in any of my cases that the patient was in the habit before his injury of hearing the words of his internal speech without moving his vocal organs; nor could I obtain satisfactory evidence of direct auditory reproduction of phrases previously heard or arising spontaneously to the mind.

But I have been able to gather a good deal of information concerning visual imagery from the highly intelligent and educated patients with whom I have been brought into contact. In persons with a strong visual memory all the processes of thinking are accompanied by and at times essentially composed of more or less vivid and detailed imagery. If I think of a horse, it is not the word in any form which springs into my mind, but a picture of a horse. This image assumes a familiar general character, which usually represents a horse to me; it is in reality a nominal symbol or visual noun. If it has been aroused by something I have heard or read, the figure is suitably varied in colour, form or posture in accordance with the descriptive details, and in this way reproduces adjectival meaning. Such images stand in place of words and as such tend to be affected in aphasia.

On the other hand, during spontaneous thinking visual images may appear in a sequence suggested by association, or corresponding to the order in which the objects were originally perceived. Such images form perceptual data, which may remain unaffected in disorders of speech. For instance, No. 10 was able to recall spontaneously the shape and colour of his hives and to see the bees arriving at the entrance laden with yellow pollen.

But visual images are fragmentary and uncertain; each one of them may be vivid and full of detail, but the connecting links with those which accompany or follow it are too weak to lead unaided to a definite intellectual conclusion. Yet they may amply suffice for purely descriptive purposes.

Thus, when No. 2 attempted to give an account of a famous prize fight, he failed grossly so long as he relied on recalling what he had read. But my question "Can you see it?" evoked so lively a series of visual images that he was able to describe many more details correctly; finally, springing out of bed, he assumed the exact attitude of the triumphant Carpentier gazing down on his vanquished opponent.

Even a vivid and accurate series of visual images is insufficient alone for constructive and logical thought. In many cases of aphasia they can be employed for direct reference, but the links between them are too tenuous to insure reproduction of a sequence of events without some kind of verbal formulation. Visual images form isolated points in the complicated mechanism of thought, unless they are connected by symbolic processes adequate to express the relational aspects of constructive thinking. Such links are of the nature of the general or universal, and therefore suffer in aphasia and kindred disorders of speech. When No. 2 was asked to describe how he would walk from the hospital to the War Office, he said he could see the big stores, Westminster Abbey and other buildings he would meet on his way. Each appeared as an isolated event; he could not connect them together and pass with ease from one to the other, in consequence of his want of names. He explained that it was "all in bits," and that he had to "jump from one thing to the other" because he "had no names." For, normally, as each image arises it is fixed by its name or some other appropriate formula, and the final conclusion is recorded as a conceptual statement. Images are less easily manipulated than words; they appear and disappear without being strictly connected in logical sequence. Without some verbal form of symbolic substitution it is impossible to express their essential likeness and difference or their significant relations in time and space.

However vivid and detailed these visual images may be, they are elusive and fleeting; the patient complains, "They seem to go faint and I can't get them when I want to." Once aroused, they recur insistently in no obvious connection with the train of thought, or they disappear before the task is completed. One image not infrequently ousts its predecessor, instead of being added to it. Suppose, for instance, the words "The dog and the cat" are presented orally or in print, the patient may obtain a clear picture of the dog, which is obliterated by the subsequent appearance of the visual image of the cat; the two are not present in consciousness together, but the second displaces the first. Conversely, the word dog may evoke an image so vivid and dominant that the word cat produces no effect. These abnormalities and the want of control over imagery lead to uncertainty in choice, even when two percepts are employed in acts of direct relation.

Such images cannot be freely evoked at will. The greater the effort expended by the patient, the more difficult it is to "get into touch" with those he requires even for non-verbal processes of thinking. Still less can they be recalled with certainty in response to external commands given in the form of spoken or written words, phrases, or a consecutive narration. This inability of a word to evoke an image in persons with a strong visual memory is one of the most obvious signs that it has lost more or less of its meaning as a verbal symbol.

In spite of these defects, visual images can frequently be translated into some form of expression, such as drawing, provided the image and its representation stand in direct relation to one another and no verbal or logical formula intervenes. Thus, No. 2 drew an excellent picture of a camel, when he was attempting to describe the means of transport in the East; yet he was totally unable to draw an elephant to command. No. 23 produced spontaneously a detailed drawing of the house in which he lived, indicating by dark shading the window which had been blocked up and no longer admitted the light.

But images of objects that can be drawn in elevation cannot be transferred to a ground-plan. This demands a higher degree of symbolic representation. The patient may recognise the position relatively to himself of the salient features in some familiar room; he asserts that he sees them clearly. Yet he cannot indicate them on a ground-plan; he tends to represent the various pieces of furniture more or less in elevation, a method which approximates more closely to the form assumed by his visual images. All such acts of translation suffer in accordance with the degree of difficulty of the symbolic formulation demanded.

Under normal conditions, a visual image may be so vivid that it replaces the name we are seeking. I can see a mental picture of an acquaintance with such clearness that I am unable to recall his name. So closely does this visual symbol satisfy the internal situation that I cannot discover its verbal equivalent for the purposes of external expression. Again, an image may produce a false or misleading association; for instance, if I am thinking of Capt. C. and, instead of visualising him as a whole, see mainly the huge opening in his skull, I go off at a tangent and cannot concentrate on his general behaviour and mode of speech. Finally, an image may produce an affective state which interrupts a train of logical thought; grief at the loss of a dead friend may inhibit my comprehension of the meaning of a passage in a book which recalls him to my mind. All these processes, recognisable in normal persons with strong visual imagery, operate even more powerfully in many aphasics.

Thus, visual images suffer or escape in aphasia according to the part they play in the processes of language and thinking. They can frequently be evoked spontaneously and used for direct reference; but they are employed with difficulty as symbols or substitution signs. Moreover, the closer the disorder approaches want of power to appreciate either the detailed significance or the general meaning of a situation, the less easily can a visual image be summoned at will or to command.

§ 3. THE USE OF SYMBOLS IN THINKING

When man learnt to speak and to understand spoken words, he acquired the power of registering relations. Action was no longer determined by perception or unformulated emotional responses. He not only drew near to a fire to experience its heat, but was able to state, either for his own information or that of his fellows, that "a fire makes me warm." The use of symbols materially shortened the processes and extended his powers of thinking.

Now we have already seen that, although all substitute signs may rightly be treated as language, some only function as expressions of thought. True symbolic reference postulates subsequent behaviour, or the assumption of an attitude, in consequence of the intervention of a symbol, and it is this aspect of thinking which suffers most profoundly in these disorders of speech. The greater the difficulty of the task from this point of view, the more likely is it to be affected. Under normal conditions statement of a problem in symbolic terms increases the ease and certainty of its solution, whilst in aphasia exactly the opposite is true. Even acts which can be performed spontaneously may be imitated with difficulty if they necessitate the use of a symbol. Thus the patient is unable to repeat to command a word or phrase he can utter unprompted, and, although he can copy my movements reflected in a mirror, he may be unable to do so when we sit face to face; for in this case some kind of linguistic formula is required between perception of my actions and their exact imitation.

In the same way, when an aphasic is shown a common object, he can pick out its duplicate from amongst those on the table by relating the two similar perceptions. But, if two familiar objects are presented to him at the same time and he then attempts to choose those which correspond to them, he is liable to fail because he attempts to register what he has seen in some form of words. When, for instance, a normal person is shown a knife and a key, he tends to record the fact by saying the names to himself in order to reinforce his memory, whilst he searches for the two objects amongst those on the table. It is here that the aphasic tends to fail; for he cannot find or retain the suitable words he requires for this dual operation.

The first method by which the use of symbols aids thinking and facilitates action is by obviating the necessity of trying several alternatives. It is no longer necessary to adopt the lengthy process of trial and error. Given a bottle and a number of corks, we may try them one by one until we find that which fits the opening. Or, if we have become expert by practice, we reject the majority of them as too large or too small, setting aside a few for systematic trial. But if we know the diameter of the neck of the bottle and each cork is marked with a number on the same scale of measurement, all necessity for trial is avoided and we at once select the cork which satisfies the situation.

In the same way, if I am told to take the second turning to the right, I am precluded from choosing any one on my left hand and also the first on the right. But many aphasics, unable to comprehend or retain the exact terms of a command, fall back on the method of trial and error. Having taken a false turning, they look around to discover that the objects actually in sight do not correspond with those they expected. They then cast back and explore other ways until, catching sight of some familiar landmark, they walk on confidently towards their goal.

This return to a more primitive method is particularly evident during the tests with the alphabet. Given the twenty-six letters on separate blocks, the normal man looks them over and selects without trial the one which is required to make a direct sequence; A leads to the choice of B, B to C, and so on. Having placed a letter, for example M, in position, he formulates some symbol, verbal or visual, for N and fixes his attention on finding it; or his procedure may be even more direct. But the aphasic tries the most unlikely combinations one after the other until he discovers the particular letter which fits the sequence.

Symbolic formulation also assures and amplifies the processes of thinking by enabling us to record the likeness or dissimilarity of two percepts and all forms of identity or difference. When we are shown a pyramid, we recognise at once that it resembles an object of similar shape on the table and that it differs fundamentally from a cone. Most aphasics can carry out this test correctly because it is based on direct perceptual relations; no verbal symbol is required. But if, when shown a pyramid, the patient attempts in vain to name it before making his choice, he may subsequently be unable to select the object of the same shape from amongst those placed before him. Direct perception of the likeness of the two figures has now been complicated by failure to record their similarity by means of a name. On the other hand, in normal persons the power of recording likeness and difference by means of a symbol enormously extends the power of conceptual thinking and underlies all scientific classification.

Words and other symbols knit together and give permanence to non-verbal processes of thought, which would otherwise be fleeting. This is particularly evident in the case of visual images. Should an aphasic possess this kind of memory in a strongly developed form, images may still arise spontaneously and play a considerable part in his mental processes. But he cannot evoke them at will or to command; nor can he unite them to a coherent logical sequence without the help of verbal symbols. They are episodic, fleeting and transient; they arise and perish without leaving behind them any permanent or certain addition to thought. Without names we cannot record their relation in time or space, nor their essential likeness or difference.

Logical thinking holds in check and diminishes affective and intuitive responses. An animal, or even man under certain conditions, tends to react directly to the perceptual or emotional aspects of a situation; but symbolic formulation enables us to subject it to analysis and to regulate our behaviour accordingly. We thereby gain the power of breaking up a situation for the purpose of selective action; but many aphasics are compelled by reason of their disability to fall back on more primitive methods of solving a problem.

When an article of familiar use is presented to our senses, we formulate certain of the more characteristic impressions which it makes upon us and designate them " qualities." These aspects of the event we attribute to something outside ourselves, which we call the " object"; we speak of them as the " elements " out of which the " object " is composed, whereas they are in reality the formulated results of selection from the total reaction to a situation.

The form assumed by this selection depends on the use we are about to make of our knowledge. Choice is regulated in each instance by our attitude of mind. When we "recognise an object," the use to which we intend to put it determines the name it receives. A treasury note is paper currency, a sovereign, twenty shillings, four and a half dollars, an interesting sociological document, or a printed slip of peculiar colour and design, according to the manner in which it is employed. The inexhaustibleness of Nature is due to the fact that we can never come to the end of such possibilities of selection; however rigorous and exacting the analysis, there is always something over, when we have completed a categorical examination.

Such systematic analysis would be impossible without symbolic formulation, of which the commonest manifestation is the power of naming. Now a name is a descriptive label employed to designate some aspect of an event, selected for special attention with a view to subsequent behaviour. We speak of a name as concrete, when it covers a small group of "objects," whilst a more abstract designation is applicable to a wider range of events. Thus the word "knife" is more concrete than the word "red." For the former can be applied to a small group of things only, which have many characters in common, whilst the latter expresses a "quality" to be discovered in articles of profoundly different use, shape and texture. A concrete name or description is attached strongly to the thing it designates, whilst an abstract term is more mobile and of wider application.

Thus to find a name for a colour is a categorical act of higher intellectual order and is liable to suffer more severely than the power of naming articles of familiar use, especially if the defects of speech assume a nominal form. But with verbal aphasia, this is not the case; for here the main difficulty is to discover the correct verbal form, and in this respect all names, abstract or concrete, are equally words.

When abstraction is carried still further and the task set to the patient demands expression of the formal relations between two or more abstract terms, he is still more likely to fail to execute it correctly. Should capacity to carry out the required operation be a comparatively recent acquisition, the loss of response is liable to assume an extreme form; this is particularly the case with tests based on arithmetic or a knowledge of foreign languages.

On the other hand, when an aphasic cannot employ more abstract terms, he can often use descriptive phrases, similes and metaphorical expressions in an appropriate manner. They are less definite and are more closely allied to the use and manipulation of the object; they place before the hearer a wide range of points of attachment, whilst an abstract term tends to hit or miss the mark.

It is common knowledge that such descriptive designations are frequently employed by aphasics; unable to discover the name of an object, they fall back on the easier method of describing its use or composition. Given a pair of scissors they either perform the act of cutting or reply, "Something to cut with"; they may even approach more closely to a name with the words, "The tweezers you cut with," or, like one of Jackson's patients, call a kitten, "A little fur-child."

Similarly both No. 2 and No. 22 were unable to name colours correctly; but the former succeeded in designating them by using similes such as "What you do for the dead" to indicate black, and the latter, who was a house painter, described to me exactly how he would compose each colour from the materials used in his trade.

We are accustomed to think of an object as possessing "qualities," such as colour, which can be considered apart from the remaining impressions it makes upon us. My observations seem to show that, in these disorders of speech, capacity to formulate the relations of objects to one another in space may be affected in association with want of power to select any one of them in response to a command given orally or in print.

When the patient is shown a familiar object or colour and is asked to indicate the one he has seen, he not only makes a correct choice, but rapidly learns the order in which the duplicates lie on the table before him. If the screen, which hides them from his sight, is not removed with sufficient rapidity, he may place his finger exactly over the position of the one he is seeking to indicate. So long as the act consists of matching one percept with another he has no difficulty in moving at once to the right spot. But as soon as the selection depends on the name presented to him orally or in print, his finger wanders up and down the set of objects or colours on the table until he finds the one he wants.

This relative position in a series is as much part of the characteristic features of an object as its shape or colour. So long as an aphasic is not required to formulate these characters and makes his choice directly as an act of matching, he behaves as if he knew its position. But whenever he has difficulty in recognising the meaning of a verbal symbol, he loses the power to formulate the relative position of the object to which it corresponds. He is not only uncertain about such qualities as its shape and colour, but also with regard to its spacial relationships.

These relational factors are a part of perceptual data and, as far as symbolic formulation and expression are concerned, behave like other characters of this order. So long as the act to be performed can be carried out by matching two percepts, the response is prompt and accurate. But, whenever it requires the intervention of some symbolic formula, the patient may be unable to execute the task correctly and with ease.

Right and left, up and down and similar designations for relative positions in space are the formal expression of direct perceptions. With nominal aphasia power to appreciate their exact meaning and to apply them correctly suffers in the same way as other names, such as those for form or colour. This difficulty in expressing spacial relations leads to some confusion in action; but the patient is not fundamentally disorientated. He still possesses a general conception of right and left and can communicate it by gestures, although he cannot employ the appropriate terms. He may be unable to remember whether he should take a turning to the right or to the left; yet, if he chooses the wrong one, he stops and turns back, because he does not perceive the landmarks he expected. He possesses a sense of direction and can guide himself by recognising the familiar objects on his course. But he lacks the power of employing spacial nomenclature both for his own use and that of others.

On the other hand, the patient with semantic aphasia has lost the power of appreciating or formulating general space data. He cannot think out a route beforehand and does not guide himself by recognisable landmarks. He forgets in which direction he was walking, becoming helplessly confused should he take a wrong turning. He may even lose himself in the hospital, unable to find his room, or the bed he occupies in the general ward. His disorientation is general and comprises more than loss of power to formulate detailed spacial relations and to express them in symbolic terms.

With the progress of mental development and education we gain increasing capacity to generalise with the help of abstract terms or symbols. This reaches its highest development in certain mathematical procedures. But as soon as symbolic formulation and expression are affected, the patient reverts to more primitive methods of solving the problem. In many instances he succeeds in bringing out a correct answer, but the means he employs are clumsy, uncertain and difficult. For example, instead of adding 6 and 3 he counts on his fingers, "Six, seven, eight, nine"; or told to multiply 5 by 3, he replies, "Five and five is ten and five is fifteen." When a penny and a shilling are laid before him and he is asked how many of the former go into the latter, he answers, "Eleven"; he states the number it would be necessary to add instead of the multiple.

Again, when reading we snatch the sense of phrases or even long sentences without actually formulating the words of which they are composed. The aphasic is compelled to adopt a more childish method, deciphering each word as an isolated task and spelling out the more difficult ones letter by letter. This mode of reading is less likely to convey a complete impression of the meaning than a more rapid generalisation. Even a normal reader, compelled, when correcting proof for the press, to pay attention to the structure of the words, fails to appreciate their full significance.

The primitive methods adopted by the patient may be insufficient to furnish an answer in the form demanded, although the essential fact can be expressed in some less abstract manner. He may be unable to state the relation of two pieces of money and yet he can pile up a number of coins exactly equal to either of them in value. He remembers the situation of the salient objects in some familiar room with regard to the position he usually occupied in it, but cannot formulate their relation to one another. The first act is less categorical and therefore easier, whilst the latter requires a higher degree of symbolic aptitude.

Symbolic formulation enables us not only to analyse a situation, but to combine a series of diverse events into a coherent and logical conception. When we look at a picture, we receive and register a general idea of its meaning; should it contain many details, we consider them one by one and reinforce or correct the first impression. It may be that a printed legend is necessary for complete comprehension of the picture; if so we combine what we gather from the words with the pictorial details into a general formula for the benefit of ourselves or others. Should the picture convey a command, the full significance of its various parts must be appreciated as a whole before the order can be executed.

It is this power of synthesising detail so as to produce a general conception of its meaning for the purposes of thought or action that is so gravely affected in cases of semantic aphasia. An intelligent man, who has constructed the pieces of a cupboard or the sides of a wooden bee-hive, cannot fix them together. Miss S. built up a model out of blocks on a scale of an inch to the foot, but had no conception of its general dimensions. These patients cannot lay the table for a meal and are puzzled how to fit the various utensils into a general scheme. They cannot play billiards, because they are unable to foresee the effect of striking the ball on one side or the other and the results that will follow a rebound from the cushion. They have lost the power of exhibiting that "togetherness of things" which is their general significance.

It is not necessary that this should be expressed in actual verbal symbols. My observations seem to show that an organic lesion can disturb the power of formulating without words the general aim or intention of an act to be performed in response to spontaneous suggestion or to command.

The existence of pre-linguistic formulation has been hotly disputed and affirmed. Pick[1] attempted to divide the processes of speech into a sequence consisting of intuitive thought, the proposition, the grammatical schema and the explicit verbal statement. Van Woerkom[2] has also erected four stages: massive conception of the idea, a psychical process of analysis and synthesis in time and space, schematic conception of the phrase without verbal symbols, and the choice of words[3].

Such detailed analysis seems to me to fail because an act of speech does not come into being and run its course in this diagrammatic manner. The processes which occur between the genesis of an idea and its expression in words, or conversely between verbal recognition and consequent assumption of a mental attitude, comprise a total alteration in psychical conditions. These changes are not composed of stages strictly and uniformly sequent in time; they consist of a state of mind which develops out of one set of dispositions and merges inseparably into another.

But pathologically the total act can be disturbed in such a way that non-linguistic formulation is more particularly affected. The patient has plenty of words and names, but he cannot summon up and manipulate with ease those general symbolic conceptions which are necessary for all consecutive action or logical thought. Such defects form the principal manifestations of semantic aphasia which is more particularly distinguished by inability to appreciate or formulate the total meaning of a situation.

Even in normal persons words, phrases and other symbolic modes of expression assume a form determined by the attitude of the speaker to his hearer and to the matter in hand. This becomes particularly evident in aphasia. The ease or difficulty with which a desired meaning can be conveyed has a profound effect on the means employed for its expression; the patient adopts that style of utterance which enables him to transmit to his auditor at any rate something of what he wants to say. Thus, a verbal aphasic employs single words or short syncopated phrases with a simple grammatical structure, helped out by gestures; a man with

---

[1] See Part I, p. 125.   [2] [133], p. 730.
[3] Cf. Delacroix, H. [40], pp. 398–403.

nominal defects perpetually attempts to clarify his meaning by uttering one more or less appropriate name after the other and by the use of descriptive or metaphorical appellations. The syntactical aphasic, on the other hand, rushes on in the hope that his volubility may convey something to his hearer.

Both the power and mode of expression are profoundly affected by the relation of the patient to his auditor. One person can help an aphasic, whilst another produces an inhibitory effect, even on his capacity to think. We all adopt a different method of expressing ourselves to an adult or a child, and we watch the effect of our words, prepared to repeat them in some other form, if they do not lead to the desired response. So the intelligent aphasic adapts his defective speech to the necessities of the moment, although his power to execute such variations is greatly diminished. I was able to carry on lengthy conversations with one of my patients, aided by maps, pictures and his use of a pencil, although his wife reduced him to incomprehensible jargon and insisted that he was out of his mind. Sometimes the patient does not trouble to correct his faults and confesses, "I just let myself go and hope it will be understood"; if he finds that this is the case, his pleasure greatly increases his power of subsequent expression. On the other hand, disappointment or anger may profoundly affect both the character and ease of utterance. If he is encouraged to write freely and carelessly and is then allowed to correct and copy his manuscript, he may be able to produce a coherent and intelligible document; yet, when he pays meticulous attention to the structure of each word, he cannot produce a single perfect sentence and gives up the attempt in disgust.

Conversely, when an aphasic attempts to understand what he has heard or read, his powers of comprehension depend not only on the inherent difficulty of the task, but also on his intellectual attitude as a whole. Much that is said by an educated person is incomprehensible to one on a lower grade of education; he accepts just enough to enable him to execute a given command, hoping that what he has understood may be sufficiently accurate for practical purposes. Now an aphasic of high intelligence may be reduced to this level; recognising his defects, he jumps to a conclusion without the usual logical steps. He no longer possesses the normal means of certain comprehension and his responses are sometimes right and at others wrong. Moreover, he is compelled to adopt childish methods of arriving at an answer, such as spelling out the words letter by letter as he reads, or counting on his fingers during the solution of arithmetical problems.

Nothing is more puzzling to the intelligent aphasic than the diffuse and tentative modes of expression so common in ordinary conversation. On the other hand, a short well-turned phrase frequently conveys its meaning at once in spite of its apparent complexity. Thus No. 2 explained that he understood "clever people," because they expressed what they wanted to say in a few words, whereas he was puzzled by the diffuseness of others.

The attitude of the patient towards the nature of the task in hand is of fundamental importance for the formulation and comprehension of symbolic signs. Interest in the subject has a profound effect on the ease and rapidity both of expression and understanding. Miss S.[1] laid particular emphasis on the importance of arousing this attitude of mind towards the task in hand. She confessed, "Just as one word...turned me off the whole thing, so one word or sentence bearing upon something of interest will jog my attention in the same way and cause me to read a passage or a page over and over again, until I get its full meaning. But this has to be done, and, if the interest is not there to 'jog,' the effort is not made because one is unconscious that an effort is needed."

Thus the employment of substitute signs facilitates and secures consecutive thinking; in fact logical thought would be impossible without them. The statement of a problem in symbolic terms increases the ease and certainty of its solution. For their use gives permanence to perceptual and other non-verbal methods of thinking, records similarity and difference of all kinds and avoids the cumbrous procedure of trial and error. It enables us to subject a situation to analysis or to synthesise details into a coherent whole and so permits of the widest categorical distinctions and generalisations.

When the power of symbolic formulation and expression is disturbed, all these activities suffer more or less severely. The patient is compelled to revert to more primitive methods of thinking, not only because they are the way by which he acquired his power of using language, but because under pathological conditions they are easier of fulfilment and present a simpler intellectual task.

[1] No. 25, p. 387.

CHAPTER IV

CONCLUSIONS AND SUMMARY

§ 1. GENERAL CONCLUSIONS

BEHIND every conscious act lie many integrations most of which take place on a purely physiological level. Consider for instance the various changes to which afferent impulses are subjected before they can form the underlying basis of a sensory experience. If I take into my hand a glass containing hot water, I receive the impression of its size, shape, weight, temperature, roughness and smoothness; I may also know that it causes me pleasure or discomfort according to the heat of the water it contains. Recognition of each of these qualities has behind it many different impulses, which have been modified and regrouped between their peripheral origin and central termination. The nature of the actual afferent impressions produced by a glass of water cannot be deduced from any a priori considerations. All we can discover by introspection are certain sensory or perceptual qualities; we must for ever remain ignorant of the non-mental factors apart from which they would not be recognised. But by observing the result produced on sensation by interference with the normal integrative processes at various known points in the nervous system, we discover that many impulses are intercepted, and others are profoundly modified, before they reach the highest receptive centres. By analysis of disorders of sensibility due to lesions at different levels of the nervous system it is alone possible to unravel that vast mass of dispositions which lie normally outside the field of consciousness.

These abnormal phenomena reveal the various integrations required to evoke sensation, which is essentially a conscious process. But there are many physiological reactions, which, though not themselves directly associated with consciousness, normally influence the operations of the mind. To this order belong postural schemata, the neural dispositions forming the underlying data on which all power of recognising the position of the limbs in space is based. So long as these physiological reactions are performing their normal function in the integrated complex of sensation, they cannot be discovered introspectively or by any other method; but a disturbance of these processes is manifested in a definite set of symptoms and signs.

Another example of the influence of somatic processes on the operations of the mind is the effect produced by cerebellar incoordination on the judgment of weight. A lesion of the cerebellum may produce profound want of control and incoordination of movements on one half of the body, unaccompanied by any disturbance of sensibility or loss of recognition of posture. If both hands are fully supported and the patient is asked to compare two weights placed one on each palm, his answers correspond to those of a normal person; for his power of estimating relative pressure is intact. But, when told to "weigh" the two objects by raising and lowering his hands in the usual manner, he tends to think that the weight on the affected side is heavier. As soon, however, as both weights are placed one after the other on the affected palm, he can again judge their relation correctly, even though he lifts them; for he is now testing both objects by means of the same defective mechanism. Here imperfect muscular coordination, unaccompanied by loss of sensibility, is liable to disturb the accuracy of a high-grade mental response.

Moreover, the field of consciousness is always liable to be invaded by the consequences of some new physiological integration or abnormal sensation. When a single cold-spot in the skin is stimulated with a sufficiently small metal rod at a temperature of 45° C., a sensation of cold is evoked. But if the surface covered by the stimulating object is large enough to include both heat-spots and cold-spots, the response is the normal one of heat. "Paradox cold," never spontaneously experienced by normal human beings, can be evoked in any one of us by suitable experimental means.

A man may pass through his whole life-time without calling into action that vast mechanism capable of evoking the referred pains of visceral disease. Multitudes of afferent impulses, arising in the viscera, are inhibited or pass unheeded and never give rise to sensation. Yet, when they once succeed in arousing consciousness, the mind is dominated by the abnormal responses and the whole personality of the patient may be profoundly changed.

In every reaction there are two factors, the nature of the impulses generated by the stimulus and the functional state of the reacting organism. Either of these may vary independently of the other. A series of identical stimuli may be followed by inconstant results, for some change in the condition of the integrating centre can fundamentally alter the nature of the response. Thus factors, usually operating on an unconscious level, may become conscious, whilst impulses, normally associated with the activities of the mind, cease to manifest themselves in psychical terms. The state of consciousness is profoundly susceptible to the influence of reactions, which at any one moment may or may not be manifested as a psychical response.

Conscious acts employ every psycho-neural process, even those of the lowest functional levels, capable of evoking the desired adaptation. Faced with a new situation, the organism puts out all its powers, conscious, sub-conscious and purely physiological, in order to produce an adequate response directed towards its welfare as a whole. In many voluntary acts every process, with the exception of the primary initiation, occurs on non-mental levels. The part then played by consciousness may be compared to the turning of a switch, which throws into action mechanical processes, thus generating an electric current that causes the lamps to glow.

Thus every aspect of mental activity is based on a multitude of conscious and unconscious processes, which, as the result of a series of integrations, culminate in a unitary response adapted to the total situation. This is manifested as some form of behaviour in which it is impossible to define the exact part played by psychical or somatic activities. But all these reactions, from the highest to the lowest, are intimately dependent on a state of vigilance in various parts of the nervous system. Any condition, organic or functional, which lowers neural potency in an appropriate portion of the brain or spinal cord, may abolish altogether some specific form of response without of necessity affecting any other function not directly dependent upon it. Thus, a cortical lesion can disturb sensibility in certain directions and make it difficult to appreciate the spacial and other relations of external stimuli; but this in no way affects other unrelated conscious responses. It does not even diminish the capacity to recognise purely qualitative differences of sensation. Even when a lesion of the brain has destroyed the power of symbolic formulation and expression, the patient can still think, except in so far as the affected form of behaviour is necessary for thinking. The mind as a whole is not affected, but specific psychical processes are interrupted or rendered difficult.

On the other hand, if the diminution of vigilance in any particular part of the nervous system is of slighter degree, the loss of function may disturb certain aptitudes and not others of the specific group. Newly acquired facilities and highly complex tasks suffer more than those which are simpler and less exacting. Processes belonging to the same order, which have become with time and practice more automatic and more strictly organised, tend to escape or to be affected in a less massive manner.

These adapted reactions demand as their physiological basis a condition of vigilance in the central nervous system, and any material lowering of this vital state prevents the response from assuming a high-grade functional form. But there is no point to point correspondence between the normal production of a psychical act, such as speaking, reading, or writing, and the independent activity of any particular group of cortical cells. Such "centres" are solely integrating foci; when they are affected certain adapted reactions are interrupted or rendered difficult. As vigilance dies down, various forms of response disappear one by one according to the degree of neural potency necessary for their production; certain special functions become no longer possible, whilst others can be carried out in part only.

Consciousness is a form of integrative vital reaction which enables the organism to adapt itself more perfectly to certain situations, conditioned by its internal state and the impressions produced upon it by external forces. So long as we consider the phenomena as the product of a disintegrated reaction, there can be no separation between mind and body. It matters little whether the lesion disturbs the lowest spinal centres or the highest mental activities, we can only record the results empirically in terms of abnormal behaviour.

At whatever level of integration a function or act is disturbed, two factors may emerge and become apparent in the morbid manifestations. Firstly, the particular group of processes which suffers is destroyed or thrown into disorder apart from all others, and, should it participate in a more complex act, this aspect only of behaviour is affected. The use of language may be grossly defective without of necessity disturbing those intellectual activities which do not depend on symbolic formulation; emotional speech and gesture may remain intact, although the patient cannot express himself otherwise. Such negative manifestations do not represent fractional elements combined synthetically to form the normal act, but are an expression of the manner in which it disintegrates. The reaction at the moment, however insufficient, is a fresh adjustment of the organism to the new conditions. No one group of defects corresponds exactly to an integral portion of the normal mode of behaviour, although such negative phenomena may reveal factors necessary for its complete development.

Secondly, any subservient function or mode of activity, which has been repressed or modified in the course of integration, may reveal itself positively. This is also true of forms of behaviour displaced during the life-history of the individual by those apter for the purpose. As far as motion and sensation are concerned, such positive manifestations reveal crude reactions from lower integrative levels which have escaped from control. But disorders of speech do not exhibit that violent contrast between the normal and abnormal modes of response seen for instance in thalamic or protopathic over-action. Both these morbid phenomena depend upon the release of impulses of a lower functional order and are manifestations of incomplete adjustment of the organism to the impact of physical forces. The cortex exerts a definite controlling effect upon the activity of the thalamus and, when this is diminished, the reaction exhibits abnormal positive characters consisting of over-response to the affective aspects of sensation.

On the other hand, those disorders of speech, which can be strictly classed as aphasic or amnesic, are produced by injury to the cortex or immediately sub-cortical tissues of the left hemisphere. These structures belong to the same developmental level, and, although they all work to one end, no single integrative centre is subservient to another. There is consequently little evidence of that release of function, so common in cases where the normal reaction results from the activity of portions of the nervous system belonging to different hierarchical levels.

But the diverse acts comprised in the use of language are acquired at various periods and to a profoundly different degree during the life of each individual. Some persons develop the power to employ abstract symbols for the most elaborate processes of thought, whilst, on the other hand, the majority of human beings can neither read nor write. Even the art of articulated speech has to be learnt, although the new-born child can express its emotional states by distinctive sounds.

More recently acquired aptitudes are not only the first to be affected, but tend to suffer massively as a whole. Thus, if the patient was master of two languages, he may entirely lose the power of employing the foreign one, whilst his mother tongue shows those specific abnormal characters which signalise some distinctive variety of aphasia. Should the power of solving arithmetical problems be affected, it is usually impossible to determine from the records alone the exact form assumed by the disorder of symbolic formulation and expression; yet this may become evident at once from the condition of articulated speech and comprehension of spoken words. The older and more primitive acts are deeply fixed, more completely organised, and tend to be affected in a specific manner. In consequence, the defects of function assume distinct varieties and the morbid response is the normal act deformed in certain directions.

These disorders of language form an excellent example of the lines on which a mental reaction is organised. The simplest method is the temporal sequence; facts can be remembered and produced in the order of their occurrence. Acts of direct reference, which do not form a sign-situation, belong to this class of response and are not affected even in a severe case of aphasia, provided the patient can be made to understand exactly what he is expected to do. So long as he has to deal with two perceptual patterns, even though they originate from dissimilar senses, such as touch and vision, he can cope with the sign-situation. But he fails to do so if these patterns are employed as general symbols. Temporal organisation is abundantly manifested by the reactions at low psychical levels and much of it may be non-mental and purely physiological.

The image is the product of a higher form of mental activity. It is a piece of experience which is taken out of its setting and employed as a method of defining a situation where some practical difficulty of adjustment has arisen. As a means of thinking, images are apt to fail because they cannot deal fully with the solution of the problem. More-over, used in juxtaposition, even a vivid and accurate series of images is insufficient alone for constructive and logical thought. They represent perceptual data, which may remain unaffected in disorders of speech; but the links between them are too tenuous to lead with certainty to propositional conclusions without the aid of some kind of general, non-perceptual formulation.

All consecutive and logical thinking demands the free use of cate-gorical formulae[1]. Here the reaction is organised by any factors which can lead to a proposition. These formulae express relations that cannot be imaged, and so act as links between the welter of psychological processes which occur during the activity of the mind.

When the power to employ speech in the normal manner is diminished the patient ceases to be able to form a proposition. The use of symbols is affected in so far as they express the relational processes of constructive thinking. The aphasic tends to fall back on images, so long as they do not express a formal relation, and on more primitive methods of temporal association. As Jackson said, "He thinks, but he is lame in thinking."

Even acts demanding definite symbolic formulation differ profoundly in intellectual difficulty. The easiest task is identification of an object, as for instance recognition that a certain coin is a shilling. A more severe task is to explain the object, that is to reduce it to previously recognised data and to state that a shilling contains twelve pence. Finally, to erect and state a law from facts of observation demands a still higher

---

[1] By this term I mean formulae expressive of classes and relations.

capacity for formal thinking. A patient who remembers exactly what he paid for his tobacco cannot say how much it cost an ounce.

Throughout this work I have frequently spoken of some task set to the patient as "easier" or "harder" than another. In some instances this difference exists even for the normal individual; for example, addition is the simplest of all arithmetical operations. But the aphasic, owing to his disability, may find certain tests unusually difficult and adopt a method of solving the problem which is easier for him though not for a normal person. Thus, he counts on his fingers, when adding two or more numbers together, instead of summing them directly; a clumsy method has become easier under pathological conditions. In the same way, he describes an object shown to him and enters into an elaborate statement of its use, instead of naming it categorically. I have therefore employed the terms "easier" and "harder" strictly to characterise the attitude of the subject towards the test he is asked to perform and the method he adopts for its solution. In pathological instances he may thus reproduce some more primitive mode of facing the situation, although this is by no means always the case.

What we call behaviour covers more particularly those activities by which the organism adapts itself to a particular situation and the processes we designate conscious are phases of this total response. All high-grade reactions, both somatic and psychical, possess certain characters in common. Qualitative selection from amongst the impulses generated by the impact of external forces adapts the form of the response not only to the intensity of the stimulus, but also to its specific nature. Duration allows dispositions due to events in the past profoundly to influence the present state of the organism and so renders the reactive process continuous rather than episodic. Lastly, the power of projection enables the individual to adapt the response to the spacial relations of the stimulus and to those of his body as an object in the world around.

Even high-grade reflexes possess reactive significance and all purposive responses enter into and form part of a system adapted to a certain end. When this system is a psychical one, we speak of the acts as conscious; should they consist of words, we say they are endowed with meaning. For to understand a word is to react to it, and such reactions are subject to the same laws as other forms of psycho-physical adaptation.

A conscious act is a vital process directed towards a definite end and the consequences of its disintegration appear as abnormal modes of behaviour. Certain tasks can no longer be performed, whilst others are still possible. The nature of this disorder of function must be determined by direct observation, amplified by the statements of the patient, and described in terms of the affected process. The categories under which these abnormal phenomena are grouped must be dynamic rather than static. When the final response is considered as a form of behaviour there is no necessity to separate mind and body; we can investigate and record on the same principles every morbid reaction from the lowest reflex to the highest form of mental activity. In this way alone is it possible to discover the forms assumed by defects of such high-grade aptitudes as the use of language under the influence of injury or disease. The only link between the facts of anatomical destruction and a disorder of some psychical function lies in a study of morbid behaviour, recorded in categories of the affected process.

On the other hand, the same act can be considered from the point of view of mental content, and we are accustomed to think of it as made up of sensations, perceptions, images, concepts, etc. These are convenient abstract terms for real elements of cognitive material. Such elements are discoverable by introspection, but they do not form the categories into which fall naturally the content of disintegrated mental processes. When, for instance, sensation is disturbed owing to injury to the cortex, total sensibility to pain, heat and cold is not affected, but the patient loses the power of appreciating differences of intensity together with spacial and other relations between stimulating objects. In the same way, with disorders of speech we cannot state that visual images as a whole are or are not disturbed; the defects consist of loss of power to employ them in a certain manner and with a distinct purpose. Even symbols can be used in direct relation, provided they do not require some propositional formulation.

"Sensation," "perception," "images" and "concepts" are abstract terms, the result of introspective analysis of the contents of the mind. They are names for cognitive material rather than for the processes of cognition and may be conveniently employed in the formulation of certain facts. For instance, it is useful to be able to state that visual images are affected, when they form part of a certain situation, but not under other conditions. But all such introspective examination is bounded by the limits of consciousness. It is only by probing and analysing morbid phenomena in terms of function that we can arrive at any conception of the integrative processes and reactions which underlie normal behaviour.

Consciousness not only forms one of the factors in behaviour, initiating, regulating and adapting vital reactions, but it enables us to obtain an inside view of the event. The mind is aware of its own activities and is conscious of itself as an object amongst objects. This power to appreciate the occurrence of a reaction and its functional significance makes a profound difference to the life of the organism. The basis of consciousness is awareness of something and that something implies a process. From such elementary beginnings development occurs by a steady increase of discrimination and categorical distinction.

When the response to a situation is a conscious one, it is not only manifested as a form of external behaviour, but at the same time is known and registered by the reacting organism. This internal response is in itself a form of behaviour which can be observed solely by the individual who responds. Once formulated, however, even in the simplest manner, it may exert an active influence on conduct.

There is no dualism between conscious processes and external behaviour. But, when the mind examines a conscious reaction introspectively, it can take account solely of the phenomena within the field of consciousness at the moment. Everything outside these narrow limits is closed to introspective observation.

The multitude of dispositions, associations and interests which, should the focus of attention change, may profoundly modify consciousness, are for the time hidden from this inside view. They are not subject to introspective exploration, and form those truly non-conscious processes which would remain unrecognised except for their power of modifying behaviour, or their appearance as factors in a morbid reaction.

The field of consciousness, which is alone open to introspection, appears to be continuous and has no gaps. This continuity is not the result of direct synthesis, but is produced by the total exclusion of all phenomena which do not belong to the particular system dominant at the moment.

In this it resembles the field of vision which appears to be uniform in function and continuous. And yet we can discover by examination that the peripheral portions are colour-blind and that the area corresponding to the entry of the optic nerve is insensitive to light. In fact, the field of vision and the field of consciousness are built up on the same principles of ignoring parts devoid of sensation or reactions outside the focus of interest.

When the mind becomes aware of its own experience, one of the simplest consequences is capacity to formulate the qualitative aspect of reactive significance. If my hand comes into contact with an unpleasantly hot body, it is rapidly withdrawn and at the same time I am aware that I am being hurt. Conversely, if the stimulus is pleasantly warm, my hand is attracted and not repulsed. In both cases consciousness records little more than the significant features of the reaction. We register for future reference the character of the response and, by appreciating that one process is pleasant, the other unpleasant, we give a reason to ourselves for our behaviour.

Moreover, even on physiological levels, an adaptive reaction is obviously conditioned and regulated by spacial factors. An animal deprived of its brain attempts to remove an irritating object by well-directed movements of the limbs. Should consciousness be present, we become aware that the source of our discomfort is something external to ourselves. This is little more than recognition of the projected factors of reactive significance.

Thus, the most elementary processes of introspection, based on the physiological characters of the reaction, yield as data the fact that I am being affected by something situated in a certain position outside myself. As soon as we can designate by whatever means the source of this external stimulation, we achieve a simple proposition, such for instance as "Fire hurts me."

We rapidly learn to connect external events not only with ourselves but with one another; for, whenever two items are mentally presented in a unitary response, we may become aware of relations between them. These we express in some form of proposition which in itself forms a reason for conduct.

When we say "Fire burns wood," both nouns are what we call "concrete." But, in such a statement as "Blood is red," the second term is an abstraction. Colour does not exist except as a "quality" reached by conscious analysis of some external event. Such abstract terms play a fundamental part in the normal activities of the mind. Related to one another in the form of general propositions, they enable us to coordinate a multitude of integrated responses with a view to ultimate action.

This employment of substitute signs facilitates and secures consecutive thinking; in fact logical thought would be impossible without them. Their use gives permanence to perceptual and other methods of thinking, records similarity and difference of all kinds, and avoids the cumbrous procedure of trial and error. It enables us to subject a situation to analysis or synthesis and so permits of the widest generalisations.

If the data of psychological activity are subjected to introspective analysis, the content of the mind appears to be built up out of sensations, perceptions, ideas and other similar units. But, when we treat states of consciousness as if they were composed of such elements, we are talking purely symbolically. Sensations and the like are not constituent portions of mental processes, but are the results of abstract introspective analysis. They are names for states of mind and not for conscious processes. Thus, when a conscious mode of behaviour disintegrates, as the result of physiological defects of organic or functional origin, the phenomena cannot be grouped within these abstract categories. They can be expressed solely in terms of the process itself.

Introspective analysis gives us the means for constructing a proposition and recording events, and so shortens the preliminaries to action. In fact, the growth of the mind and consecutive behaviour would be impossible if it were not for the continuous and progressive development of abstract categorisation.

Thus, it is of value to speak of sensations and percepts, although they do not exist as isolated elements of mental activity. In the same way, images are undoubted phenomena of the mind, but do not form unitary responses or categories of conscious activity. These are the terms of the inner conscious life; they do not correspond to factors of the reaction or behaviour of the organism as a whole. The total response, normal or abnormal, at whatever stage of integration, is a unity. It is not built up of sensing, perceiving, imaging or any other abstract mental categories. Developed as a form of behaviour, it can be described in empirical terms only.

Thus, the effects produced on sensibility by a cortical lesion assumes forms which could not have been deduced by a priori consideration of the nature of somatic sensations as they are known introspectively. Similarly, in severe examples of visual or auditory imperception, the disturbance of function far exceeds the limits of isolated appreciation of sights or of sounds; on the other hand, if the disorder is less severe, some percepts are duly recognised, even though the afferent impulses on which they are based originate in the sense affected. This pathological state, an affection of a total psychical reaction, cannot be comprised under the abstract term perception, but must be described empirically as disorder of a particular process of mental activity.

The fact that all conscious responses are recorded introspectively in conceptual terms has a profound effect on the subsequent conduct of the individual. This is in itself a form of inner behaviour and as such can be disturbed by underlying physiological changes; the power of logical analysis and synthesis suffers in the same way as any other reaction.

The mode of behaviour which has formed the subject of this book is concerned with formulation and expression of relations by means of some more or less abstract symbol. Words and phrases are the material factors of a situation to which the organism adapts its response. For to understand a word is to react to it, and to discover an appropriate symbol is a purposive mental action.

The use of language is a peculiarly fruitful field for observing both the result of physiological defects on a high form of conscious behaviour and, at the same time, recording the interaction of categorical abstractions as part of the life of the mind. Thought exceeds the mechanism of speech, but presupposes, at any rate in man, the power of propositional formulation. This in turn requires the use of symbols in some form or another together with the capacity to express their relation.

Thus, introspective experience and the consequent power of analysis and synthesis have a profound effect on the life of the organism as a whole. The products of this activity of the mind may not correspond to the phenomena of functional disintegration; but they are none the less mental facts, because they form the basis or point of origin of subsequent reactions. I cannot therefore accept the position of those who deny the existence of consciousness or state that it makes no difference to the ultimate result attained by the response of the organism. When considering some mental form of behaviour, it would be as absurd to neglect the products of introspection as to attempt to establish the laws of normal speech by investigating a man congenitally deaf and blind.

In conclusion, I have attempted to show that, when some act or process is disturbed in consequence of an organic or functional lesion, the abnormal response is a fresh integration carried out by all available portions of the central nervous system. It is a total reaction to the new situation. The form assumed by these manifestations cannot be foretold by a priori consideration, but must be determined by observation and described in terms of the affected process.

In such reactions conscious processes play their part as a mode of response. Certain aspects are psychical, others somatic, but there is no separation of mind and body. The mind-body problem does not exist so long as we are examining the consequences of functional disintegration.

On the other hand, introspection reveals certain states of mind we call sensations, images, etc. These are categorical abstractions. Although they are not portions of an integrative reaction, they are facts which appear when the mind examines its own activities. Thus, we are justified in stating that under certain conditions sensation is changed in a particular manner or that images can be employed for one purpose but not for another. All such psychological terms are symbols for certain mental abstractions.

The field which is open to introspection is limited to the facts of consciousness. Like the field of vision, it appears to be continuous and gaps are ignored. On the other hand, the consequences of disintegration may reveal a multitude of processes which participate in the response. These do not form part of the continuum of consciousness, and under normal conditions are not susceptible to introspective examination.

§ 2. SUMMARY

1. The central nervous system is capable of reacting as a whole or in part with different degrees of physiological efficiency, which varies with its vital condition. When this is raised, a response to stimulation is not only obtained more easily, but shows signs of belonging to a higher order than when it is low.

2. The extent to which the activities of a particular portion of the central nervous system exhibit at any moment signs of integration and purposive adaptation indicate its vigilance. When vigilance is high, the body is prepared to respond to an effective stimulus with a more appropriate reaction.

3. Vigilance is diminished not only by structural changes in the central nervous system, but also by toxic influences such as chloroform, sepsis, or anything which tends to lower physiological capacity.

4. This is profoundly evident in all automatic actions, even those which have been acquired during the life of the individual. These aptitudes rise and fall according to the vigilance of the parts responsible for their execution.

5. In all specific modes of behaviour, conscious and automatic processes are inextricably mingled. Normal sensation demands not only some conscious response to qualitative and spacial differences, but also accurate registration on a physiological level of the results produced by previous afferent impressions.

For example, the same class of impulses which determines the realisation of spacial relationships is responsible for purely physiological conditions, such as the maintenance of some forms of muscular tone and coordination. Normally, mind and body must be prepared to respond immediately with an appropriate reaction.

HAI   35

6. Purposive adaptation is more or less evident in all responses, somatic or psychical, which occur in a high state of neural vigilance.

Three factors are responsible for this character in the response. Firstly, certain qualities in the stimulating object are ignored, whilst others give rise to reactions; these in turn struggle among themselves for mastery and their final integration gives significance to one aspect of the stimulus rather than another. Secondly, the form assumed by the response at any one moment depends profoundly on dispositions due to past activities, and the future is to a great extent implicit in the present. Thus, the behaviour of the central nervous system, in whole or in part, becomes an orderly march of events and is not a series of isolated episodes. Thirdly, afferent impulses endow the response with spacial relations; the resultant action is coordinated to a definite end in space and time.

7. The same factors in a more developed form can be discovered in all conscious modes of behaviour, which are affected specifically by disorders of the central nervous system. The meaning of a psychical act is formulated on reactive significance; duration forms the basis of memory and intention; whilst the power of projection enables us to attribute to external or internal events those characters we have selected from amongst the impressions they have left upon us.

8. Conscious processes bear the same relation to the life of the higher centres of the nervous system as purposive reflexes to the vitality of those lower in the neural hierarchy. All alike are the expressions of physiological vigilance.

9. Local destruction of the tissues of the brain prevents the normal fulfilment of some specific form of behaviour, and the reaction which follows expresses the response of the organism as a whole to the new situation. No function, somatic or psychical, is a mosaic of elementary processes which become manifest when it is disturbed in consequence of a cerebral lesion. The abnormal phenomena can be described only in terms of the act affected.

10. The names chosen for these defects of speech are employed in an indicative sense only and refer solely to their more salient features. Each variety of aphasia comprises abnormal forms of behaviour in excess of those which can be logically deduced from its name. Moreover, the loss of power is relative and not absolute.

This observational method and purely indicative nomenclature alone makes it possible to correlate defective psychical aptitudes with the degree of loss of physiological function, and so with the situation and extent of an organic lesion.

CH. IV]   CONCLUSIONS AND SUMMARY   547

11. All use of language is essentially a development of simple acts of speaking and comprehension of spoken words; it is here that we discover that diversity of manifestations which enables us to divide aphasia into different classes. On the other hand, less primitive and more highly abstract modes of symbolic formulation and expression tend to be disturbed in a more massive and less distinctive manner.

12. Although the defects produced by an organic lesion of the brain fall naturally into disorders of verbal formulation and defective recognition of meaning, we cannot divide the manifestations of aphasia according to these categories into two mutually exclusive groups. For the use of language as a whole is more or less affected; defects of verbalisation, if sufficiently severe, disturb the full appreciation of meaning, and want of recognition of meaning prevents the normal formation of words and phrases.

13. Unimpeded symbolic formulation and expression cannot be analysed into a sequence of semantic, nominal, syntactical and verbal procedures following one another in time. The disorders of speech to which these names have been applied do not reveal the normal order of psychical events, but disturb the progressive development of language processes as a whole.

14. The form of behaviour we call the use of language has a history, and many of the phenomena of disordered speech resemble steps by which the complete act was acquired in each individual. The patient may revert to a more primitive mode of response. Apart, however, from the tendency to adopt such methods of executing some particular task, the abnormal manifestations do not strictly correspond to any stages in the historical evolution of speech.

15. Every disorder of speech is manifested in psychical terms, but in no instance can the nature of the morbid phenomena be deduced from a priori consideration of the normal use of language. Each particular variety of aphasia represents the response of the organism to a new situation produced by physiological defects, and we cannot discover the form it assumes from any logical conceptions concerning the processes of the mind.

16. The two aspects of language, the formulation of thought and its skilful and exact expression, are not dissociated as the result of disturbances produced by an organic lesion of the brain.

17. Two groups of linguistic processes tend to become increasingly automatic and can be initiated with comparatively little conscious effort.

The one consists of ejaculations, oaths and words or phrases devoid of categorical meaning. These escape altogether in aphasia, for they have little to do with systematic thinking.

On the other hand, many acts of speaking and verbal comprehension have become by practice and habit almost automatic; but however great this facility, the symbolic formulae remain endowed with significance. The whole process was developed out of formal thinking and still serves to secure an end. Such modes of behaviour suffer severely in aphasia and tend to reveal specific defects which differ according to the site of the lesion.

18. Acts of direct reference do not involve a situation in which a general sign is used and are not affected even in severe examples of disorders of speech, provided the patient can be made to understand exactly what he is expected to do. So long as the task to be performed is one of direct matching, it can be executed correctly; but, as soon as a general symbol intervenes between the intention and performance of the action, the patient is liable to fail to carry it out.

19. There are certain acts of thinking which can be brought to a successful termination in spite of these disorders of speech by a process of direct reference, but not by a formal statement of symbolic relations. The patient can register certain facts and act upon them correctly, although he cannot express them as a relation. Thus, he cannot tell the time, but is punctual for his appointments. He is unable to employ or comprehend with certainty the words right and left; yet he recognises that in England the traffic of the streets keeps to the left, whereas abroad it moves on the opposite side of the roadway.

20. Visual images suffer or escape in aphasia according to the part they play in the processes of language and thinking. They may be evoked spontaneously and used for direct reference, but they are employed with difficulty as symbols or substitute signs.

21. The employment of substitute signs facilitates and secures consecutive thinking; in fact logical thought would be impossible without it. The statement of a problem in symbolic terms increases the ease and certainty of its solution. For their use gives permanence to perceptual and other non-verbal methods of thinking, records similarity and difference, and avoids the cumbrous process of trial and error. It enables us to subject a situation to analysis, to synthesise various details to a coherent whole, and so permits of the widest categorical distinctions and generalisations.

When the power of symbolic formulation and expression is disturbed, all these activities suffer more or less severely. The patient is compelled to revert to more primitive methods of thinking, because they are more easily brought to a successful termination and present to him a simpler intellectual task.

22. When some act or process is disturbed in consequence of an organic or functional lesion, the abnormal manifestations are the result of a fresh integration carried out by all available portions of the central nervous system. It is a total reaction of the organism to the new situation, in which conscious processes play their part as a mode of response. Certain aspects are psychical, others are somatic, but there is no separation of mind and body so long as we are examining the consequences of disintegration.

23. On the other hand, introspection reveals certain states of mind which we call sensations, images, etc. These are categorical abstractions; although they are not portions of an integrative reaction, they are facts which appear when the mind examines its own activities. The field open to such introspection is limited to the phenomena of consciousness. But the consequences of disintegration reveal a multitude of processes which participate in the response, although they do not form part of the continuum of consciousness and are not normally open to introspective examination.

END OF VOLUME I

Printed in the United States
by Bookmasters

Printed in the United States
By Bookmasters